Basic CPT/HCPCS Coding

2006 Edition

Gail I. Smith, MA, RHIA, CCS-P

American Health Information
Management Association®

The Web sites listed in this book were current and valid as of the date of publication. However, Web page addresses and the information on them may change or disappear at any time and for any number of reasons. The user is encouraged to perform his or her own general Web searches to locate any site addresses listed here that are no longer valid.

Portions of this volume were originally published in *Clinical Coding Workout 2006,* AHIMA product number AC201506.

ISBN 1-58426-152-8

AHIMA Product Number AC200606

Claire Blondeau, Project Editor
Melanie Endicott, MBA/HCM, RHIA, CCS, Reviewer
Elizabeth Lund, Editorial Assistant
Melissa Ulbricht, Editorial/Production Coordinator
Ann Zeisset, RHIT, CCS, CCS-P, Technical Reviewer
Ken Zielske, Publications Director

American Health Information Management Association
233 North Michigan Avenue, Suite 2150
Chicago, Illinois 60601-5800

www.ahima.org

Contents

About the Author

Gail I. Smith, MA, RHIA, CCS-P, is an associate professor and director of the health information management program at the University of Cincinnati in Cincinnati, Ohio. She has been an HIM professional and educator for more than thirty years. Prior to joining the faculty at the University of Cincinnati, she was director of a health information technology associate degree program and was health information manager in a multihospital healthcare system.

Ms. Smith also is a coding consultant and a frequent presenter at conferences throughout the United States. An active member of the American Health Information Management Association (AHIMA), she has served on the board of directors and several of AHIMA's committees and task forces.

Ms. Smith received a bachelor of science degree in health information management from The Ohio State University in Columbus and a master of arts degree in education from The College of Mt. St. Joseph in Cincinnati.

Preface

This workbook provides basic training and practice in the application of procedural codes from the *Current Procedural Terminology* (CPT) and the Healthcare Procedural Coding System (HCPCS). CPT is published by the American Medical Association (AMA). Updated annually on January 1, CPT is a proprietary terminology created and maintained by the AMA. Its purpose is to provide a uniform language for describing and reporting the professional services provided by physicians. HCPCS is maintained by the Centers for Medicare and Medicaid Services (CMS). Its purpose is to provide a system for reporting the medical services provided to Medicare beneficiaries. HCPCS is made up of two parts: Level I is composed entirely of the current version of CPT; HCPCS Level II provides codes to represent medical services that are not covered by the CPT system, for example, medical supplies and services performed by healthcare professionals who are not physicians.

Like previous editions, the 2006 edition of *Basic CPT/HCPCS Coding* is intended for students who have limited knowledge of, or experience in, CPT/HCPCS coding, and also as a resource and review guide for professionals. The instructional materials in this workbook are not specific to any particular practice setting, and they apply to both hospital-based and office-based coding. The exercises provide hands-on experience in coding some of the more common procedures and services provided by physicians and other healthcare professionals.

Many healthcare facilities and providers develop their own systematic methods for assigning CPT codes to frequently performed diagnostic procedures. For this reason, this workbook provides only minimal practice in assigning CPT/HCPCS codes for diagnostic procedures.

The CPT/HCPCS coding process requires coders to apply analytic skills in combination with a practical knowledge of medical science. To become effective coders, students must be able to apply their knowledge of medical terminology, anatomy and physiology, pathophysiology, pharmacology, and medical–surgical techniques. This workbook assumes that students will already have a basic understanding of these subject areas.

The primary objectives of this workbook include the following:

- To provide a basic introduction to the format of CPT codes as well as CPT coding conventions

- To demonstrate different ways to locate CPT codes through the use of the codebook's index

- To identify ways to ensure accurate code assignment through the application of coding guidelines from the AMA and CMS

- To deliniate the documentation necessary for code assignment

Specifically, chapter 1, Introduction to Clinical Coding, discusses the purpose of CPT/HCPCS codes. It also addresses diagnostic coding and the Medicare requirements for claims submission.

Chapter 2, Application of the CPT System, introduces the CPT coding conventions and explains the application of CPT codes for healthcare reimbursement.

Chapter 3, Modifiers, provides an overview of the purpose and use of CPT and HCPCS Level II modifiers.

Chapter 4, Surgery, reviews the coding guidelines associated with the surgical procedures performed to treat illnesses and injuries of the various anatomical systems. It emphasizes the surgical procedures that are performed most commonly in the ambulatory setting.

Chapter 5, Radiology, discusses the claims process for radiology services performed by physicians and hospital-based outpatient providers. The chapter also discusses the principles of radiology code reporting.

Chapter 6, Pathology and Laboratory Services, addresses the code assignment process for common laboratory tests and procedures performed, supervised, or interpreted by pathologists and other physicians.

Chapter 7, Evaluation and Management Services, provides a concise explanation of the evaluation and management section of CPT. The chapter also provides practice exercises designed to address the complexities of assigning evaluation and management codes.

Chapter 8, Medicine, provides a general overview of the procedures and services described in the medicine chapter of the CPT codebook.

Chapter 9, Anesthesia, introduces the codes used by the physicians who provide or supervise anesthesia services.

Chapter 10, HCPCS Level II, reviews the format and usage of HCPCS National Codes and modifiers.

Chapter 11, Reimbursement in the Ambulatory Setting, explains the claims process for ambulatory services, which is based on correct CPT code assignment. A skills practice at the end of this chapter asks students to review sections of a CMS-1500 form to determine the accuracy of code assignment. This practice reinforces the students' understanding of the CPT/HCPCS coding principles and guidelines discussed in the preceding chapters.

The 2006 edition of *Basic CPT/HCPCS Coding* has been expanded and updated in several ways this year. As in previous editions, review exercises are interspersed in each chapter. Appendix C of *Basic CPT/HCPCS Coding* has been expanded and updated to include new exercises and operative reports. A new appendix D includes keys to these chapter review exercises for student reference. Also included this year is a chapter test at the conclusion of each chapter. Keys to the chapter tests and appendix C exercises and operative reports are available in the supplementary materials for instructors.

This book must be used with the 2006 edition of *Current Procedural Terminology* (CPT 2006) (code changes effective January 1, 2006), published by the AMA. The HCPCS Level II codes included in this publication were current as of October 1, 2005. The most current version of the HCPCS Level II codes can be found under the Utilities/Miscellaneous heading on the CMS Web site: www.cms.gov/providers/pufdownload/.

Students beginning a CPT course of study should have several additional references to help them assign codes. Suggested references and recommended readings that may be helpful to students are listed in appendix A of this workbook.

Chapter 7 of this publication is based on the evaluation and management documentation guidelines developed jointly by the AMA and CMS in 1997. For additional information on these guidelines or to check for additional revisions, students and educators should visit the CMS Web page at www.cms.gov.

The Web sites listed in appendix A and elsewhere in this workbook were current and valid as of November 1, 2005. However, Web addresses and the information on Web sites may change or disappear at any time and for any number of reasons. Students and educators are encouraged to perform their own Web searches to locate the current addresses of any sites that can no longer be found under the addresses provided in this workbook.

AHIMA provides supplementary materials for educators who use this workbook in their classes. Materials include lesson plans, keys to practice exercises in appendix C, PowerPoint slides, and other educational resources. All answer keys are available to instructors in online format from the individual book page in the AHIMA Bookstore (imis.ahima.org/orders), and also are posted on the AHIMA Assembly on Education Community of Practice (AOE CoP) Web site. Instructors who are AHIMA members can sign up for this private community by clicking on the help icon within the CoP home page and requesting additional information on becoming an AOE CoP member. An instructor who is not an AHIMA member or a member who is not an instructor may contact the publisher at publications@ahima.org.

Acknowledgments

AHIMA wishes to acknowledge

Rita A. Scichilone, MHSA, RHIA, CCS, CCS-P, CHC;
the late Rita Finnegan, RHIA, CCS;
and Toula Nicholas, RHIT, CCS, CCS-P,
who served as authors of previous editions of *Basic CPT/HCPCS Coding,*

the members of the AHIMA Professional Practice Resources team
who prepared *Clinical Coding Workout 2006,*
for generously agreeing to republish portions of their work in this book
(June Bronnert, RHIA, CCS;
Melanie Endicott, MBA/HCM, RHIA, CCS;
Susan Hull, MPH, RHIA, CCS, CCS-P;
Rita Scichilone, MHSA, RHIA, CCS, CCS-P;
Mary Stanfill, RHIA, CCS, CCS-P;
and Ann Zeisset, RHIT, CCS, CCS-P),

as well as the many internal and external reviewers who have contributed
throughout the years to this publication.

Chapter 1

Introduction to Clinical Coding

Several medical terminologies and classification systems are used to document and report information related to healthcare services in the United States. The *International Classification of Diseases, Clinical Modification,* currently in its ninth revision (ICD-9-CM), is used to describe and report the illnesses, conditions, and injuries of patients who require medical services. ICD-9-CM is made up of a series of numerical and alphanumerical codes and code descriptions that represent very specific illnesses and injuries.

Similarly, the services provided by physicians and other healthcare professionals are described and reported by using terminologies and classification systems. The *International Classification of Diseases, Clinical Modification,* provides a system for coding medical procedures performed in the inpatient departments of hospitals, but two other systems apply to the services provided by physicians and other medical providers in hospital-based outpatient departments, physicians' offices, and other ambulatory settings: the *Current Procedural Terminology* and the *Healthcare Common Procedure Coding System.*

Current Procedural Terminology

The *Current Procedural Terminology* (CPT), published by the American Medical Association (AMA), provides a system for describing and reporting the professional services furnished to patients by physicians. CPT generally applies to the services provided to patients who are not covered by the federal Medicare program.

CPT was initially developed in 1966 and was designed to meet the reporting and communication needs of physicians. The system was adopted for application to the Medicare reimbursement system in 1983. Since that time, CPT has been widely used as the standard for outpatient and ambulatory care procedural coding and reimbursement.

The information represented by CPT codes is also used for several purposes other than reimbursement, including:

- Trending and planning outpatient and ambulatory services
- Benchmarking activities that compare and contrast the services provided by similar non–acute care programs
- Assessing and improving the quality of patient services

The CPT codebooks include several additional appendixes and an index of procedures. CPT codebooks and codes are updated annually, with additions, revisions, and deletions becoming effective on January 1 of each year. A new edition of the CPT codebook is published annually, and the new edition should be purchased every year to ensure accurate coding. Healthcare providers are expected to begin using the newest edition for encounters on January 1, and there is no longer a grace period during which claims based on out-of-date codes will be accepted.

CPT Category I

The CPT codebook includes a general introduction followed by six main sections that together make up the list of Category I CPT codes:

Evaluation and Management
Anesthesia
Surgery
Radiology
Pathology and Laboratory
Medicine

Specific coding guidelines are provided for each of the main sections.

The Category I codes in each of the main sections are further broken down into subsections and subcategories according to the type of service provided and the body system or disorder involved. For example, code 76645—Ultrasound, breast(s) (unilateral or bilateral), B scan and/or real time with image documentation—appears in the radiology section under the subsection entitled Diagnostic Ultrasound and the subcategory Chest. Similar procedures are grouped to form ranges of codes. For example, the range of codes from 19140 through 19240 represents the various types of mastectomy in the subsection covering the integumentary system in the surgery section. The codes in each of the six main sections (or Category I) of the CPT codebook are composed of five digits and are arranged in numerical order within each section.

CPT Supplementary Codes

CPT also provides three types of supplementary codes: Category II codes, Category III codes, and modifiers. Each of these code sets is listed and explained in a separate section. The Category II and III sections are placed after the medicine codes in the codebook. The list of modifiers and the coding guidelines for modifiers are included in appendix A of CPT 2006.

CPT Category II Codes

Category II provides supplementary tracking codes that are designed for use in performance assessment and quality improvement activities. CPT Category II codes are composed of five characters: four numbers and an alphabetic fifth character, capital letter F. Codes 1000F and 1001F, for example, describe a specific aspect of patient history, specifically, assessments of patient tobacco use. The assignment of Category II CPT codes is optional. Category II supplementary codes are updated twice each year, on January 1 and July 1.

CPT Category III Codes

CPT Category III includes temporary codes that represent emerging medical technologies, services, and procedures that have not yet been approved for general by the FDA and so are not otherwise covered by CPT codes. Level III codes give physicians and other healthcare providers and researchers a system for documenting the use of unconventional methods so that their efficacy and outcomes can be tracked. Like CPT Category II codes, Category III codes are composed of five characters: four numbers and an alphabetic fifth character, capital letter T.

> **Example:** Code 0017T represents a procedure for destroying macular drusen by the application of photocoagulation.

Updated Category III codes are released semiannually via the AMA's CPT Web site. The complete list of temporary codes is published annually in the CPT codebooks.

CPT Modifiers

A third set of supplementary codes known as *modifiers* can be reported along with many of the Category I CPT codes. The two-character modifier codes are appended to Category I five-digit CPT codes to report additional information about any unusual circumstances under which a procedure was performed. The reporting of modifiers is meant to support the medical necessity of procedures that might not otherwise qualify for reimbursement.

> **Example:** Suppose that a surgeon successfully performed a percutaneous translu-
> minal balloon angioplasty to remove a blockage from a patient's renal
> artery, but later that day it became evident that the artery had become
> occluded again. If the surgeon who performed the original procedure
> were not available, another surgeon on call would repeat the procedure to
> remove the blockage. Code 35471 would be reported by the first surgeon
> to identify the original angioplasty, and the second surgeon would report
> 35471–77 to identify the repeat angioplasty.

Most of the two-character modifiers for Category I codes are numerical. (Chapter 3 of this workbook includes a list of the CPT modifiers in CPT 2006.) However, there also are some alphanumeric modifiers to indicate the physical status of patients undergoing anesthesia. These modifiers begin with a capital letter P, as follows:

P1   A normal healthy patient
P2   A patient with mild systemic disease
P3   A patient with severe systemic disease
P4   A patient with severe systemic disease that is a constant threat to life
P5   A moribund patient who is not expected to survive without the operation
P6   A declared brain-dead patient whose organs are being removed for donor purposes

(Chapter 2 of this workbook provides additional guidelines for applying CPT codes, and chapter 3 discusses modifiers in more detail.)

Healthcare Common Procedure Coding System

The Health Care Financing Administration (HCFA) developed the original version of the *HCFA Common Procedure Coding System* (HCPCS) in 1983. HCPCS was designed to represent the physician and nonphysician services provided to Social Security beneficiaries under the federal Medicare program. HCFA's name was changed to the Centers for Medicare and Medicaid Services (CMS) in 2001. The official name of the coding system was also changed, and the system is now called the Healthcare Common Procedure Coding System. CMS is the division of the U.S. Department of Health and Human Services that administers the Medicare program and the federal portion of the Medicaid program.

The purpose of HCPCS as implemented in 1985 was to fulfill the operational needs of the Medicare reimbursement system. Originally, HCPCS codes applied only to the services provided by physicians to Medicare patients. Since 1986, however, the federal government has required that physicians use HCPCS codes to report services provided to Medicaid patients as well. Moreover, with the passage of the Omnibus Reconciliation Act of 1986, hospitals are also required to report HCPCS codes on reimbursement claims for ambulatory surgery services as well as radiology and other diagnostic services provided to Medicare and Medicaid patients.

HCPCS codes enable providers and suppliers to accurately communicate information about the services they provide. Analysis of HCPCS data also helps Medicare carriers to establish financial controls that prevent expense escalation. Finally, the information from coded claims facilitates uniform application of Medicare and Medicaid coverage and reimbursement policies.

HCPCS includes two separate levels of codes. Level I is based on the current edition of CPT. Level II is made up of the National Codes that represent the medical supplies and services not included in CPT.

HCPCS Level I

Copyrighted and published by the AMA, Level I of HCPCS consists of five-digit Category I CPT codes. Level I HCPCS codes are used by physicians to report services such as hospital visits, surgical procedures, radiological procedures, supervisory services, and other medical services. Hospitals also use Level I codes to report hospital-based outpatient services, such as laboratory and radiological procedures and ambulatory surgeries, to Medicare and other third-party payers. Level I codes represent approximately 80 percent of the HCPCS codes submitted for reimbursement each year.

HCPCS Level II

Known as the National Codes, HCPCS Level II codes were developed by CMS for use in reporting medical services not covered in CPT. Level II codes are provided for injectable drugs, ambulance services, prosthetic devices, and selected provider services.

Level II codes are made up of five characters: The first character is a capital Arabic letter, and the following four characters are numbers. Examples of HCPCS Level II codes include the following:

    A4550   Surgical trays
    E1625   Water softening system, for hemodialysis
    J0475   Injection, baclofen, 10 mg
    L3260   Ambulatory surgical boot, each

Like Level I (CPT) codes, HCPCS Level II codes are updated annually on January 1. A list of current Level II codes can be requested from the U.S. Government Printing Office or any local Medicare carrier. Several commercial publishing companies distribute the National Codes in book form, which is more user-friendly than the government-issued lists owing to the addition of enhancements such as indexes and cross-references. In addition, an electronic file containing the most current version of the HCPCS Level II codes can be downloaded from the CMS Web site at Utilities/Miscellaneous, www.cms.gov/providers/pufdownload/. (HCPCS Level II codes are discussed in more detail in chapter 10 of this workbook.)

International Classification of Diseases, Ninth Revision, Clinical Modification

The *International Classification of Diseases, Ninth Revision, Clinical Modification* (ICD-9-CM), is based on an international classification system originally developed and maintained by the World Health Organization. The purpose of the international version of the ICD is the classification and reporting of morbidity data (illnesses and injuries) and mortality data (fatalities) from around the world. ICD-9 was modified for use in the United States and was first released as ICD-9-CM in 1979. The World Health Organization generally publishes revised editions of the ICD about every ten years, and the tenth revision of the international system is currently in use worldwide. However, the United States continues to use ICD-9-CM for diagnostic reporting, although U.S. providers currently use ICD-10 to code the content of death certificates for public health reporting. A draft version of a clinical modification of ICD-10 has been developed, but no dates for implementing ICD-10-CM in the United States have been established.

When federal legislation called for modifications in the Medicare reimbursement system in 1983, ICD-9-CM was adopted as part of the reporting requirements for the new Medicare prospective payment systems (PPSs). These systems have been gradually implemented in various healthcare settings over the past twenty years. Inpatient services were the first to be affected, but Medicare prospective payment systems have now been implemented in almost every setting. A PPS for inpatient psychiatric care was implemented in 2004. The difference between PPSs and older, cost-based reimbursement systems is that PPS reimbursement is based primarily on the patient's diagnosis rather than on the actual cost of providing specific services. For that reason, the accuracy of diagnostic coding has become extremely important for healthcare providers and third-party payers alike. (Note that the PPS for inpatient psychiatric services is somewhat different from the PPSs implemented for other types of care and treatment settings. The psychiatric PPS bases reimbursement on per diem rates, set rates paid for each day of hospital inpatient care.)

Today, CMS and private third-party payers require physicians and other medical providers to report ICD-9-CM diagnostic codes on virtually every reimbursement claim. The diagnostic information is used to assign cases to Medicare payment groups (for example, diagnosis-related groups for inpatient services) and to document the medical necessity and quality of the services provided to all patients.

The official version of ICD-9-CM is published in three volumes. Volume 1 contains the main list of diagnostic codes in tabular format. The codes are organized into chapters according to body system. For example, chapter 1 covers the codes for infectious and parasitic diseases. Volume 2 provides an alphabetic index of diseases and injuries that helps coders locate the appropriate code listings in the tabular list. Volume 3 includes procedural codes and an alphabetic index for procedures. Only inpatient acute care hospitals use ICD-9-CM volume 3 to report procedures for reimbursement. Therefore, hospital-based outpatient departments, physicians' offices, and other ambulatory facilities never use volume 3.

Like CPT and HCPCS, ICD-9-CM codes are reevaluated and appropriate revisions are implemented on a regular basis. ICD-9-CM code updates are now released by the federal government twice each year, on April 1 and October 1. The official version of ICD-9-CM is issued only in CD-ROM format by the Government Printing Office. Updated ICD-9-CM codes are also available electronically from the National Center for Health Statistics Web site. Several commercial publishers, however, offer enhanced print versions of the classification. The yearly editions of these codebooks are usually released during the summer and incorporate the official ICD-9-CM changes that will become effective on October 1 of the same year.

To ensure complete and accurate coding, healthcare providers must update or replace their ICD-9-CM codebooks as new codes are implemented and existing codes are amended or deleted. In addition, encoders and other coding software must also be updated at least yearly.

ICD-9-CM Diagnostic Codes

ICD-9-CM diagnostic codes represent the reasons why patients require and/or seek medical care. Each numerical code represents a specific symptom, condition, injury, or disease. ICD-9-CM diagnostic codes in the main classification (codes 001 through 999) consist of three, four, or five digits. The first three numbers represent a specific diagnosis, and one or two additional numbers may follow a decimal point after the three-number code to provide information that is more specific.

> **Example:** Code 562.13 represents a diagnosis of diverticulitis of the colon with intestinal hemorrhaging. The first three numbers (562) indicate a diagnosis of diverticula of the intestine; the number 1 after the decimal point represents the location of the diverticula, the colon; and the fifth digit represents the most specific diagnosis: diverticulitis of colon with hemorrhage.

Supplementary ICD-9-CM Codes

ICD-9-CM includes two supplementary classifications. Alphanumeric codes from the supplementary classifications provide additional information about the patient and/or the circumstances surrounding the patient's illness or injury. V codes (V01 through V85) represent the various factors that may influence the patient's health status and contact with health services. E codes (E800 through E999) represent the external factors that cause injuries and poisonings.

Diagnostic Coding

The Central Office on ICD-9-CM maintains the official coding guidelines for diagnostic coding. The guidelines require ICD-9-CM code assignments to be as specific as possible and to be supported by health record documentation. The guidelines also require the reporting of as many codes as necessary to completely describe the patient's condition. Guidelines also establish the order in which multiple codes are to be reported. The ICD-9-CM codebook also provides detailed advice on assigning codes correctly.

Every claim for outpatient services must contain at least one ICD-9-CM code, but care must be taken to report every applicable code in the sequence specified in the official coding guidelines. Medicare and most other third-party payers reject claims that report incomplete ICD-9-CM codes.

A set of *Official ICD-9-CM Coding Guidelines for Outpatient Services* was developed in 1990 and revised subsequently in 1995 and 2002. Coders must thoroughly understand and carefully follow these guidelines. Official ICD-9-CM coding advice is also published by the American Hospital Association (AHA) in its quarterly publication, *Coding Clinic*. The official coding guidelines for ICD-9-CM are available from the Central Office on ICD-9-CM of the American Hospital Association as well as from the CMS Web site.

The following examples illustrate correct and incorrect code assignments for a patient with a diagnosis of type II diabetes.

Example:

250.00	Diabetes mellitus without mention of complication, Type II or unspecified type, not stated as uncontrolled	**Correct**
250.0	Diabetes mellitus without mention of complication, Type II or unspecified type, not stated as uncontrolled	**Incorrect**
250	Diabetes mellitus without mention of complication, Type II or unspecified type, not stated as uncontrolled	**Incorrect**

(*Basic ICD-9-CM Coding*, by Lou Ann Schraffenberger, MBA, RHIA, CCS, CCS-P, provides a more detailed discussion of the basics of ICD-9-CM coding. The workbook also provides numerous practice exercises. A new edition of the workbook with updated codes is released by the American Health Information Management Association every summer.)

Documentation for Reimbursement

Health record documentation continues to play a pivotal role in the accurate and complete collection of health services data. The documentation records pertinent facts, findings, and observations about an individual's health history, including past and current illnesses, examinations, tests, treatments, and outcomes. By chronologically documenting the patient's care, the health record becomes an important element in the provision of high-quality healthcare and serves as the source document for code assignment.

The following general principles of health record documentation, developed jointly by the AMA and CMS, apply to the records maintained for all types of medical and surgical services:

- The health record should be complete and legible.

- The documentation of each patient encounter should include:

  —The reason for the encounter and the patient's relevant history, physical examination findings, and prior diagnostic test results

  —A patient assessment, clinical impression, or diagnosis

  —A plan for care

  —The date of the encounter and the identity of observer

- The rationale for ordering diagnostic and other ancillary services should be documented or easily inferred.

- Past and present diagnoses should be accessible to the treating and/or consulting physician.

- Appropriate health risk factors should be identified.

- The patient's progress and response to treatment and any revision in the treatment plan and diagnoses should be documented.

- The CPT and ICD-9-CM codes reported on health insurance claim forms or billing statements should be supported by documentation in the health record.

Additional documentation guidelines pertinent to evaluation and management (E/M) services are discussed in chapter 7 of this book. (Various links pertinent to the information discussed in this chapter are listed in the Web resources in appendix A of this workbook.)

Medicare Regulations

The Social Security Act of 1965 and its subsequent amendments establish the federal regulations that govern Medicare. Medicare regulations require the collection of several types of coded information on reimbursement claims for services provided to Medicare beneficiaries:

- ICD-9-CM diagnostic and procedural codes for inpatient hospital services

- ICD-9-CM diagnostic codes and HCPCS procedural codes for hospital outpatient services including laboratory and radiology procedures

- ICD-9-CM diagnostic codes and HCPCS procedural codes (regardless of the service location) for medical services provided by physicians and allied health professionals (psychologists, nurse practitioners, social workers, licensed therapists, and dietitians)

Health Insurance Portability and Accountability Act (HIPAA) Administrative Simplification

The intent of the federal government's simplification mandate is to streamline and standardize the electronic filing and processing of health insurance claims; to save money; and to provide better service to providers, insurers, and patients.

HIPAA Transaction and Code Set Standards

Before the implementation of HIPAA transaction and code set standards, healthcare providers and health plans used various formats when performing daily electronic transactions, which led to confusion. HIPAA requirements specify that all electronic data interchange formats be standardized. These standards apply to any health plan, clearinghouse, and any healthcare providers that transmit health information in electronic form in connection with defined transactions. HIPAA also required the standardization of the reporting of medical procedures with industry-established and -maintained codes. These are codes used by healthcare providers to identify what procedures, services, and diagnoses pertain to that encounter. The following code sets have been approved for use by HIPAA:

- International Classification of Diseases, 9th Edition, Clinical Modification (ICD-9-CM)
- Current Procedure Terminology (CPT)
- Healthcare Common Procedure Coding System (HCPCS)
- Current Dental Terminology (CDT)
- National Drug Codes (NDC)

Claims Submission

Reimbursement claims for medical services provided to beneficiaries of commercial and government-sponsored health insurance programs may be submitted in electronic or paper form. Electronic claims, however, must follow the standards developed by the Accredited Standards Committee (ASC) and mandated by the Health Insurance Portability and Accountability Act (HIPAA). ASC Standard X12 applies exclusively to electronic claims.

The CMS-1500 form shown in figure 1.1 is the standard billing document used for physician claims submitted on paper for Medicare Part B reimbursement. Providers also use this form for paper claims submitted to many private health insurance companies and Medicaid agencies. (CMS forms may be accessed on the Web by following the links and instructions at cms.hhs.gov/providers/edi/edi5.asp.)

Up to four diagnostic codes may be reported in field location 21 of this form; information on the service or procedure provided is reported in field location 24. Up to six HCPCS codes may be reported in column D of field location 24; in column E, the diagnostic codes are linked with the related HCPCS codes by placing a number (1, 2, 3, or 4) to show which diagnostic code is related to the procedure. Coders must be sure that any association of ICD-9-CM diagnostic codes with HCPCS procedure codes is logical and appropriate.

> **Example:** Patient's chief complaint is lower leg pain. The physician orders a lower leg x-ray and an EKG. The lower leg pain is linked with the x-ray, but there is no logical symptom or diagnosis to link with the EKG. Review of the health record may reveal an existing condition, such as premature ventricular contractions, or a symptom, such as tachycardia. Documentation must support the procedure or service provided; otherwise, the claim will be denied.

Medicare and many commercial third-party payers often establish coverage limits for certain services. Reimbursement claims for services with coverage limits (for example, inpatient psychiatric care) must include sufficient diagnostic information to support the medical necessity of the services provided. This diagnostic information is communicated in the form of ICD-9-CM codes.

Medicare policies include two types of coverage limits: national coverage decisions and local coverage determinations (LCD). CMS establishes contractual arrangements with the private insurance companies (referred to as carriers), intermediaries, and Program Safeguard Contractors who process Medicare claims in local geographic regions. These contractors are responsible for making coverage decisions for Medicare beneficiaries, and the contractors base their decisions on established national coverage requirements for specific medical supplies and services. For cases that are not covered by existing national policies, contractors may make local coverage determinations at their own discretion. A list of the Medicare coverage policies can be found on the CMS Web site. The following policy is an example of a LCD. (It was accessed on the Web site for the Ohio fiscal intermediary AdminaStar Federal.)

> **Example:** CPT codes 20974 and 20975 for electrical stimulation to aid bone healing are covered by Medicare only when one of the following ICD-9-CM diagnosis codes appears on the claim form:
>
> 733.82   Nonunion of Fracture
> 909.3   Late Effect of Complications of Surgical & Medical Care
> V45.4   Postsurgical Arthrodesis Status

The CMS-1450 form, better known as UB-92 (figure 1.2), is used primarily by hospitals for both outpatient and inpatient services. This form is used to submit claims for Medicare Part A services. It is also used by other third-party payers to report claims for outpatient and inpatient services provided by hospitals and ambulatory surgery centers (ASCs).

Figure 1.1. Sample CMS-1500 form

CARRIER

PLEASE
DO NOT
STAPLE
IN THIS
AREA

HEALTH INSURANCE CLAIM FORM

| PICA | | | | | | | PICA |

1. MEDICARE	MEDICAID	CHAMPUS	CHAMPVA	GROUP HEALTH PLAN	FECA BLK LUNG	OTHER	1a. INSURED'S I.D. NUMBER (FOR PROGRAM IN ITEM 1)
(Medicare #)	(Medicaid #)	(Sponsor's SSN)	(VA File #)	(SSN or ID)	(SSN)	(ID)	

2. PATIENT'S NAME (Last Name, First Name, Middle Initial)

3. PATIENT'S BIRTH DATE MM DD YY   SEX   M   F

4. INSURED'S NAME (Last Name, First Name, Middle Initial)

5. PATIENT'S ADDRESS (No., Street)

6. PATIENT RELATIONSHIP TO INSURED
Self   Spouse   Child   Other

7. INSURED'S ADDRESS (No., Street)

CITY   STATE

8. PATIENT STATUS
Single   Married   Other
Employed   Full-Time Student   Part-Time Student

CITY   STATE

ZIP CODE   TELEPHONE (Include Area Code)
(   )

ZIP CODE   TELEPHONE (INCLUDE AREA CODE)
(   )

9. OTHER INSURED'S NAME (Last Name, First Name, Middle Initial)

10. IS PATIENT'S CONDITION RELATED TO:

11. INSURED'S POLICY GROUP OR FECA NUMBER

a. OTHER INSURED'S POLICY OR GROUP NUMBER

a. EMPLOYMENT? (CURRENT OR PREVIOUS)
YES   NO

a. INSURED'S DATE OF BIRTH MM DD YY   SEX   M   F

b. OTHER INSURED'S DATE OF BIRTH MM DD YY   SEX   M   F

b. AUTO ACCIDENT?   PLACE (State)
YES   NO

b. EMPLOYER'S NAME OR SCHOOL NAME

c. EMPLOYER'S NAME OR SCHOOL NAME

c. OTHER ACCIDENT?
YES   NO

c. INSURANCE PLAN NAME OR PROGRAM NAME

d. INSURANCE PLAN NAME OR PROGRAM NAME

10d. RESERVED FOR LOCAL USE

d. IS THERE ANOTHER HEALTH BENEFIT PLAN?
YES   NO   *If yes*, return to and complete item 9 a-d.

READ BACK OF FORM BEFORE COMPLETING & SIGNING THIS FORM.

12. PATIENT'S OR AUTHORIZED PERSON'S SIGNATURE I authorize the release of any medical or other information necessary to process this claim. I also request payment of government benefits either to myself or to the party who accepts assignment below.

SIGNED _____ DATE _____

13. INSURED'S OR AUTHORIZED PERSON'S SIGNATURE I authorize payment of medical benefits to the undersigned physician or supplier for services described below.

SIGNED _____

PATIENT AND INSURED INFORMATION

14. DATE OF CURRENT: MM DD YY   ILLNESS (First symptom) OR INJURY (Accident) OR PREGNANCY(LMP)

15. IF PATIENT HAS HAD SAME OR SIMILAR ILLNESS. GIVE FIRST DATE MM DD YY

16. DATES PATIENT UNABLE TO WORK IN CURRENT OCCUPATION FROM MM DD YY   TO MM DD YY

17. NAME OF REFERRING PHYSICIAN OR OTHER SOURCE

17a. I.D. NUMBER OF REFERRING PHYSICIAN

18. HOSPITALIZATION DATES RELATED TO CURRENT SERVICES FROM MM DD YY   TO MM DD YY

19. RESERVED FOR LOCAL USE

20. OUTSIDE LAB? $ CHARGES
YES   NO

21. DIAGNOSIS OR NATURE OF ILLNESS OR INJURY. (RELATE ITEMS 1,2,3 OR 4 TO ITEM 24E BY LINE)
1. _____ . _____   3. _____ . _____
2. _____ . _____   4. _____ . _____

22. MEDICAID RESUBMISSION CODE   ORIGINAL REF. NO.

23. PRIOR AUTHORIZATION NUMBER

24.	A					B	C	D		E	F	G	H	I	J	K
	DATE(S) OF SERVICE					Place of Service	Type of Service	PROCEDURES, SERVICES, OR SUPPLIES (Explain Unusual Circumstances)		DIAGNOSIS CODE	$ CHARGES	DAYS OR UNITS	EPSDT Family Plan	EMG	COB	RESERVED FOR LOCAL USE
	From			To				CPT/HCPCS	MODIFIER							
	MM	DD	YY	MM	DD	YY										
1																
2																
3																
4																
5																
6																

PHYSICIAN OR SUPPLIER INFORMATION

25. FEDERAL TAX I.D. NUMBER   SSN   EIN

26. PATIENT'S ACCOUNT NO.

27. ACCEPT ASSIGNMENT? (For govt. claims, see back)
YES   NO

28. TOTAL CHARGE $

29. AMOUNT PAID $

30. BALANCE DUE $

31. SIGNATURE OF PHYSICIAN OR SUPPLIER INCLUDING DEGREES OR CREDENTIALS (I certify that the statements on the reverse apply to this bill and are made a part thereof.)

SIGNED _____ DATE _____

32. NAME AND ADDRESS OF FACILITY WHERE SERVICES WERE RENDERED (If other than home or office)

33. PHYSICIAN'S, SUPPLIER'S BILLING NAME, ADDRESS, ZIP CODE & PHONE #

PIN#   GRP#

(APPROVED BY AMA COUNCIL ON MEDICAL SERVICE 8/88)   *PLEASE PRINT OR TYPE*

APPROVED OMB-0938-0008 FORM CMS-1500 (12-90),   FORM RRB-1500,
APPROVED OMB-1215-0055 FORM OWCP-1500,   APPROVED OMB-0720-0001 (CHAMPUS)

Figure 1.2. Sample UB-92 (CMS-1450) form

Up to nine diagnostic codes can be reported in field locations 67 through 75 and six ICD-9-CM procedure codes in field locations 80 and 81. HCPCS codes (for outpatient services including surgery) are reported in field location 44. Required modifiers are appended to the HCPCS code in this field location. Up to two modifiers may be used to provide additional information about the HCPCS codes on the claim form for Medicare patients. Field locator 76 is for admitting diagnosis and 77 is for E-code reporting.

Exercise 1.1 Introduction

Review each of the following questions, and write the appropriate answers in the spaces provided.

1. What organizations are responsible for updating CPT codes and HCPCS Level II codes?

    _____

2. How many diagnostic codes may be submitted on the CMS-1500 form?

    _____

3. Which coding system(s) is (are) used for claims submitted by physicians?

    _____

4. Dr. Smith saw a Medicare patient with a diagnosis of rectal abscess in Central Hospital. She performed an incision and drainage in the outpatient surgery department.

    a. Which coding system(s) would Dr. Smith use to bill for her services?

        Diagnosis: _____

        Procedure: _____

    b. Which coding system(s) would Central Hospital use to bill for its services?

        Diagnosis: _____

        Procedure: _____

    c. Which form would Central Hospital use to submit a paper-based claim to Medicare for payment?

        _____

5. Which coding system describes the reason for the patient visit or encounter?

    _____

6. A patient was seen in a physician's office for excision of a 0.5-cm facial nevus (HCPCS Level I code 11440). The ICD-9-CM diagnostic code for the benign lesion is 216.3. During this encounter, the physician also evaluated the patient's hyperglycemia (ICD-9-CM code 790.6) and chronic simple anemia (ICD-9-CM code 281.9). A three-specimen glucose tolerance test (HCPCS Level I code 82951) was performed. Using the CMS-1500 form provided in figure 1.3, link the appropriate ICD-9-CM codes found in block 21 with HCPCS Level I codes found in block 24D. In column 24E, select the appropriate number (1, 2, or 3) to indicate which diagnostic code is related to the procedure.

    _____

Figure 1.3.   Information for question 6 of exercise 1.1

21. DIAGNOSIS OR NATURE OF ILLNESS OR INJURY, (RELATE ITEMS 1,2,3 OR 4 TO ITEM 24E BY LINE)		
1. ∟216.3	3. ∟790.6	
2. ∟281.9	4. ∟	

24.	A DATE(S) OF SERVICE From MM DD YY	To MM DD YY	B Place of Service	C Type of Service	D PROCEDURES, SERVICES, OR SUPPLIES (Explain Unusual Circumstances) CPT/HCPCS	MODIFIER	E DIAGNOSIS CODE
1	01-19				11440		
2	01-19				82951		
3							
4							
5							
6							

Chapter 1   Test

Choose or write the appropriate answers.

1. Which of the following statements is (are) true of CPT codes?
   a. They are numeric.
   b. They describe nonphysician services.
   c. They are updated annually by CMS.
   d. All of the above

2. CPT was developed and is maintained by:
   a. CMS
   b. AMA
   c. The Cooperating Parties
   d. WHO

3. CPT is updated:
   a. Annually for the main body of codes and every 6 months for category III codes
   b. Annually
   c. Every 6 months
   d. As often as required by new technology

4. There are six sections to CPT: evaluation and management, anesthesia, surgery, radiology, laboratory/pathology, and _____.

Chapter 2

Application of the CPT System

The American Medical Association (AMA) developed *Current Procedural Terminology* (CPT) to provide a uniform language that could be used to accurately designate medical, surgical, and diagnostic services. The CPT coding system is an effective means of facilitating communication among physicians, patients, and third-party payers nationwide. Published in 1966, the first edition of the CPT codebook consisted primarily of surgical procedures and limited codes for medicine, radiology, and laboratory procedures and services. The second edition, published in 1970, expanded the four-digit codes to five digits. And the last two editions, published in the late 1970s, reflected advances in medical technology and introduced a mechanism for updating the CPT codebook annually to keep it in step with changes in the medical field.

The AMA's CPT Editorial Panel, consisting of fifteen physicians and representatives from the Health Insurance Association of America, CMS, Blue Cross and Blue Shield, AHIMA, and the AHA, is responsible for the annual revision and modification of the codebook. The panel is assisted in this task by the CPT Advisory Committee, which is composed of physicians nominated by the National Medical Specialty Societies, and by the AMA Health Care Professionals Advisory Committee, which is composed of other healthcare professionals. (Links to the AMA and CMS Web sites pertinent to the discussion in this chapter are listed in the Web resources in appendix A of this workbook.)

Organization of CPT

To be included in the CPT codebook, a procedure or service must meet the following conditions: (1) It must be commonly performed by many physicians across the country, and (2) it must be consistent with contemporary medical practice. Consequently, a procedure's inclusion in, or exclusion from, the CPT codebook does not imply that the AMA does or does not endorse it. Nor does it mean that the procedure is or is not covered for reimbursement by insurance plans. For example, although codes exist in CPT to describe cosmetic surgery, most insurance carriers do not provide reimbursement for such procedures. Thus, patients would pay for such services out of pocket. Reimbursement rules and guidelines are not always consistent with CPT coding rules and guidelines. Just as insurance policies for healthcare services vary, so do the reporting requirements involving codes.

The listing of procedures or services and their codes by subsections does not restrict use of these codes to certain specialty groups. For example, when describing a service that has been rendered, a surgeon may use codes from any section, not just those from the surgery section.

Similarly, a family practice physician may use a code from the surgery section to describe office procedures or maternity care.

Each main section in the CPT codebook is divided into subsections, subcategories, headings, and procedures/services, as follows:

Surgery	Section
Integumentary system	Subsection
Skin, subcutaneous, and accessory structures	Subcategory
Incision and drainage	Heading
Incision and drainage of pilonidal cyst, simple	Procedure

The subsections, subcategories, and headings may identify any of the following:

- Services

- Procedures or therapies

- Examinations or tests

- Body systems

- Anatomic sites

Table 2.1 provides an example of each subdivision (when applicable) by section.

Exercise 2.1   Organization of CPT

Identify the CPT section and/or category (I, II, or III) in which the following codes are located.

1. 21300 _____

2. 99232 _____

3. 81000 _____

4. 0503F _____

5. 97001 _____

6. 70486 _____

7. 00918 _____

8. 0045T _____

9. 59510 _____

10. 99361 _____

11. 77261 _____

12. 88307 _____

Table 2.1.   Examples of CPT subdivisions

Section	Category/Subsection	Subcategory	Heading	Procedure/Service
E/M Services	Hospital Inpatient Services (99221–99239)	Initial Hospital Care (99221–99223)	New or Established Patient (99221–99223)	99223 Initial hospital care
Anesthesia	Head (00100–00222)	—	—	00104 Anesthesia for electroconvulsive therapy
Surgery	Respiratory System (30000–32999)	Nose (30000–30999)	Incision (30000–30020)	30020 Drainage abscess or hematoma, nasal septum
Radiology	Diagnostic Radiology (Diagnostic Imaging) (70010–76499)	Vascular Procedures (75600–75790)	Aorta and Arteries (75600–75790)	75600 Aortography, thoracic, without serialography, radiological supervision, and interpretation
Pathology and Laboratory	Anatomic Pathology (88000–88099)	Postmortem Exam (88000–88099)	—	88020 Necropsy (autopsy), gross and microscopic; without CNS
Medicine	Psychiatry (90801–90899)	Psychiatric Therapeutic Procedures (90804–90899)	Other Psychotherapy (90845–90857)	90845 Psychoanalysis
Category II Codes	Patient Management (0500F–0503F)	—	—	2000F Blood pressure, measured
Category III Codes	—	—	—	0003T Cervicography

Conventions and Characteristics of CPT

The CPT codebook follows several conventions, including the use of the following symbols:

- Semicolons ;
- Bullets •
- Triangles ▲
- Facing triangles ►◄
- Plus symbols +
- Circled bullets ⊙
- Null Symbol ⊘
- Pending Symbol ∿

The meanings of these symbols are explained in an introduction section at the beginning of the CPT book.

Semicolons

The format of the CPT codebook is designed to provide descriptions of procedures that can stand alone without additional explanation. To conserve space, many descriptions refer to a common portion of the procedure listed in a preceding entry rather than repeating the procedure in its entirety. When this occurs, the incomplete procedural description or descriptions are indented under the main entry, and the common portion of the main entry is followed by a semicolon (;). This signifies that the main entry applies to, and is part of, all indented entries that follow with their codes. The indented entries can yield different kinds of information, as illustrated in the following examples:

- The indented information may provide diagnostic data.

49520	Repair recurrent inguinal hernia, any age; reducible	
49521	incarcerated or strangulated	

The common portion of the description for code 49520 (the part before the semicolon) should be considered part of code 49521. Therefore, the full description of code 49521 reads: Repair recurrent inguinal hernia, any age; incarcerated or strangulated.

- The indented entries may describe alternate anatomical sites.

27705	Osteotomy; tibia	
27707	fibula	
27709	tibia and fibula	
27712	multiple, with realignment on intramedullary rod (eg, Sofield-type procedure)	

The full description of code 27707 reads: Osteotomy; fibula.

- The indented entries may designate specific procedures.

44150	Colectomy, total, abdominal, without proctectomy; with ileostomy or ileoproctostomy
44151	with continent ileostomy
44152	with rectal mucosectomy, ileoanal anastomosis, with or without loop ileostomy
44153	with rectal mucosectomy, ileoanal anastomosis, creation of ileal reservoir (S or J), with or without loop ileostomy

The full description of code 44153 reads: Colectomy, total, abdominal, without proctectomy; with rectal mucosectomy, ileoanal anastomosis, creation of ileal reservoir (S or J), with or without loop ileostomy.

- The indented entries also may describe extensive procedures requiring the assignment of two codes. CPT often designates more extensive procedures by using the code for a stand-alone procedure and the code for an indented procedure to fully describe the extent of the surgery. When both codes are appropriate, the code for the indented description is preceded by the plus symbol (+) for add-on code.

15200	Full-thickness graft, free, including direct closure of donor site, trunk; 20 sq cm or less
+ 15201	each additional 20 sq cm (List separately in addition to code for primary procedure)

- When a 40-cm^2 graft is performed on a patient, both codes 15200 and 15201 are assigned. The performance of a 60-cm^2 graft requires the following codes to be reported: 15200, 15201, and 15201.

Bullets and Triangles

CPT uses bullets (•) and triangles (▲) to identify changes in the current codebook. A bullet before a code identifies that code as a new addition, and a triangle before a code identifies a revision to the narrative description accompanying that code. Appendix B of the CPT codebook contains a comprehensive list of all revisions, including deletions and additions in code order. The following entry is an example of a new code found in CPT 2006:

• 37718	Ligation, division, and stripping, short saphenous vein

The next is an example of a code that has been changed in CPT 2006:

▲ 45540	Proctopexy (eg, for prolapse); abdominal approach

Facing Triangles

The facing triangle symbols (►◄) are used to indicate the beginning and ending of new and/or revised text within the guidelines and instruction notes. The coder should carefully review the information identified within facing triangles to ensure correct code assignment. An example of new text found in CPT 2006 can be found in the note that appears before code 45990.

> ► Surgical diagnostic anorectal exam (45990) includes the following elements: external perineal exam, digital rectal exam, pelvic exam (when performed), diagnostic anoscopy, and diagnostic rigid proctoscopy◄

Plus Symbols

When a procedure is commonly carried out with another procedure, it may be designated as an add-on code. Therefore, it should not be used alone. CPT identifies add-on codes with plus symbols. For example:

> 11000   Debridement of extensive eczematous or infected skin; up to 10% of body surface
>
> + 11001   each additional 10% of body surface (List separately in addition to code for primary procedure)

The plus symbol (+) indicates that 11001 is an add-on code and must be used with code 11000. It may not be reported alone. Notes reinforce the correct use of add-on codes. For example, after code 11001, the following instructional note appears:

> (Use 11001 in conjunction with code 11000)

Appendix D of CPT 2006 contains a complete list of add-on codes.

Circled Bullets

A circled bullet symbol (⊙) before a CPT code indicates that the use of moderate (conscious) sedation is an inherent part of the procedure. Moderate sedation is often used for procedures that do not require general anesthesia, which causes complete unconsciousness. Moderate sedation works by inducing an altered state of consciousness that minimizes pain and discomfort by administering pain relievers and sedatives. The patients who receive moderate sedation are usually able to speak and respond to verbal cues throughout the procedure, and so they are able to communicate any discomfort to the provider.

According to CPT coding guidelines, it is not appropriate for the same physician to report both the service codes and moderate sedation codes (99143–99145) when it is included in the service code. It is important to note that the inclusion of a procedure from the moderate (conscious) sedation list does not prevent separate reporting of an associated anesthesia procedure or service (CPT codes 00100–01999) when the service was performed by a physician other than the healthcare professional performing the diagnostic or therapeutic procedure. Appendix G of CPT 2006 provides a complete list of the codes that include moderate (conscious) sedation and guidelines on the use of these codes.

Null Symbol

The null symbol (⊘) indicates codes that may not be appended with modifier –51, Multiple Procedures. For example, code 32000 (Thoracentesis, puncture of pleural cavity for aspiration, initial or subsequent) may not be used with modifier –51. Appendix E of CPT 2006 provides a complete list of codes that are exempt from the use of modifier –51. (For a more detailed discussion of modifiers, see chapter 3 of this workbook.)

Pending Symbol

The pending symbol (Ν) indicates that the CPT code is for a vaccine that is pending approval from the Food and Drug Administration (FDA). For example:

> Ν⊘•90736   Zoster (shingles) vaccine, live, for subcutaneous injection

---

Exercise 2.2   CPT Conventions

Review each of the following questions, and write the appropriate answers in the spaces provided.

1. What is the full description of code 35207?

2. The reporting of CPT codes 28150 and 28150 indicates the removal of how many toes?

3. Is code 30130 identified as a code with a new descriptor or a revised descriptor?

4. What is the full description for code 43219?

5. Is code 50250 identified as a code with a new descriptor or a revised descriptor?

6. Can code 15401 be used alone?

7. Can code 31500 be appended with modifier –51?

8. Review the range of CPT codes 13150 through 13153. What is the correct code assignment for a 7.8-cm complex wound repair of the ear?

9. Review the range of CPT codes 40810 through 40816. What is the correct code assignment for an excision of a mucosal lesion of the vestibule of mouth with a complex repair?

10. Review the range of CPT codes 31575 through 31578. What is the correct code assignment for a flexible fiberoptic laryngoscopy for removal of a lesion and a separate biopsy of inflamed tissue?

Category I, II, and III Codes

In 2000, the AMA completed its CPT-5 project, which was an initiative to make improvements in the structure and processes of CPT. As a result, three categories of CPT codes were established.

Category I codes include the traditional, five-digit numeric codes that identify procedures and services. Code 10021 (Fine needle aspiration; without imaging guidance) is an example of a category I CPT code.

Category II codes include alphanumeric codes that are used for tracking purposes to represent performance measurements. Category II codes are located in a section after the Medicine codes in the CPT codebook. The use of tracking codes for performance measurement facilitates data collection and minimizes administrative burden. The five-digit alphanumeric codes can be identified by adding the letter F at the end of the code. Code 4000F (Tobacco use cessation intervention, counseling) is an example of a category II code.

The use of category II codes is optional. The tracking codes are reviewed as part of healthcare quality tracking by the American Medical Association (AMA), the Joint Commission on Accreditation of Healthcare Organizations (JCAHO), and the National Committee for Quality Assurance (NCQA), among others. Appendix H of the CPT 2006 codebook contains an alphabetic index of performance measures arranged by clinical condition or topic.

Category III codes are temporary codes used to represent emerging technology services and procedures. These codes were developed to allow researchers to track the use of emerging technology services. The codes are included in a section of the codebook that falls after the category II codes and the Medicine section.

Category III codes are assigned an alphanumeric identifier (for example, 0017T). After they have been approved by the CPT Editorial Panel, new category III codes are added on a semiannual (twice-yearly) basis and made available through the AMA Web site. Category III codes are archived when they have not been moved to the category I section after five years unless it can be demonstrated that the codes are still useful. Payment for category III services and procedures depends on the reimbursement policies of individual payers.

Unlisted Procedures

Because of rapid advances in medical research and technology, new services or procedures may be performed before codes have been added to the CPT system to represent them. In these rare instances, an unlisted code should be reported along with a written report describing the procedure or service. The operative report is usually sufficient when reporting an unlisted surgical code. The introduction to each section of the CPT codebook includes a complete list of the unlisted service/procedure codes available for that section. Unlisted codes for various subsections can be found in the alphabetic index of the CPT codebook under the main heading Unlisted Services and Procedures. Before any unlisted code is assigned, the coder should review HCPCS Level II (National) codes to confirm that CMS has not developed a specific code for the procedure or service in question. CPT category III codes, which are developed specifically for reporting new technology, should also be reviewed.

Notes

Coders using the CPT codebook should pay special attention to the notes located at various levels within the text. Notes may appear at the beginning of a heading, within parentheses before or after a code, or within parentheses in the code description.

Notes placed at the beginning of a heading provide additional information about the services or procedures that follow. For example:

- Integral components of a service or procedure

    Example: A note under the heading Endoscopy (31231–31294) states that a surgical sinus endoscopy always includes a sinusotomy (when appropriate) and a diagnostic endoscopy.

- Definitions of terms and/or codes

    Example: Under the heading Shaving of Epidermal or Dermal Lesions (11300–11313), a note defines shaving as "the sharp removal by transverse incision or horizontal slicing to remove epidermal and dermal lesions without a full-thickness dermal excision."

- Directions to assign additional codes

    Example: Under the heading Combined Arterial–Venous Grafting for Coronary Bypass (33517–33530), the note reminds the coder that two codes are required to identify coronary artery bypass grafting using both arterial and venous grafts.

Notes that appear before or after individual codes provide additional coding guidelines. For example:

- Alternative codes

    Example: The note appearing after code 11772 directs the coder to use 10080 or 10081 for an incision of a pilonidal cyst.

- Deleted codes

    Example: The note appearing after code 36522 advises the coder that 36530 has been deleted. To report the procedure previously identified by code 36530, the coder should assign code 36563.

- Add-on codes

    Example: The note appearing after code 19001 instructs the coder not to assign code 19001 as a single code. It must be used with code 19000.

- Other instructional information

    Example: The note appearing before code 35480 instructs the coder to use modifier –51 or –52 when the procedures are performed as part of another operation.

Notes also appear within the text of some codes to provide additional explanation. For example:

    Example: Within code 10040, the coder is provided with the example of acne surgery.

Alphabetic Index

At the back of the CPT codebook, an index provides a list of specific codes organized by main entries such as:

. . .Replantation
Report preparation
Reposition
Repositioning
Reproductive tissue
Reprogramming. . .
Resection. . .

The main entries are printed in boldface type and arranged in alphabetic order. The main entries are based on:

- Procedures, services, or examinations such as coccygectomy, mastopexy, preventive medicine, physical therapy, nuclear medicine, and organ- or disease-oriented panel

- Organs or other anatomic sites such as bladder, blood vessels, ethmoid, ganglion, muscle, and sweat glands

- Conditions or diagnoses such as abrasion, hematoma, heel spur, meningioma, mumps, omphalocele, and septal defect

- Synonyms, eponyms, or abbreviations such as Ewart procedure, FAST, LHR, Pereyra procedure, Pomeroy's operation, TLC screen, and HLA typing

Some of the main entries include subterms that provide additional information that must be reviewed before a code can be selected. For example:

Laryngoscopy	
Diagnostic	31505
Direct	31515–31571
Exploration	31505, 31520–31526, 31575
Fiberoptic	31575–31579
with Stroboscopy	31579
Indirect	31505–31513
Newborn	31520
Operative	31530–31561

The CPT alphabetic index also uses cross-references to help coders identify the most appropriate code. *See* cross-references appear most frequently with eponyms, synonyms, and abbreviations and refer coders to other main terms. For example, the entry for AHG includes a cross-reference that refers the coder to the main entry for clotting factor.

See cross-references can also direct the coder to another main term, but only when the information sought did not follow the first main term. For example:

Sweat Test	82435
See Chloride, Blood	

These examples illustrate the importance of referring to the additional main entries as directed by the cross-references to ensure the highest level of specificity in code selection.

The alphabetic index offers at least one code under each entry, although in some cases more than one code or a range of codes is provided. Every code and its description must be reviewed carefully to ensure accurate code assignment and appropriate payment. Consider the following example:

Mastectomy
    Gynecomastia 19140
    Modified Radical .19240
    Partial 19160–19162
    Radical 19200–19220
    Simple, Complete .19180
    Subcutaneous 19182

When coding a partial mastectomy, the coder must review the descriptions for all of the codes in the range 19160 through 19162 before assigning a final code.

The first step in locating a code in the alphabetic index is to find the procedure or service performed, such as jejunostomy or peritoneocentesis. If the service or procedure is not listed, the coder should locate the organ or anatomic site involved; the condition or diagnosis; or the synonym or eponym, such as phalanx, Epstein-Barr virus, or Dandy operation. The subterms should be reviewed and any cross-references followed. Each code listed in the index should be noted and each description reviewed until a match is established.

Becoming familiar with the CPT codebook will expedite the coding process. For example, a comprehensive knowledge of the codebook would show that correct codes often are found under several main terms.

Consider these procedures: hallux valgus correction and Mayo bunionectomy. Review of the alphabetic index will yield the following entries and codes:

Bunion Repair 28296–28299
    Mayo Procedure. 28292

Mayo Procedure. 28292

Repair
    Hallux Valgus. 28290–28299

Repair
    Toe
        Bunion 28290–28299

Repair
    Bunion 28290–28299

Note: The terms *Hallux valgus* and *Correction, hallux valgus* do not appear in the alphabetic index.

General Rules for CPT Coding

Here are some general rules to consider when applying CPT codes:

- Analyze the note or procedural statement provided by the physician or other healthcare provider and/or included in the health record.

- Determine the procedure, test, or service to be coded.

- Locate the main term in the index by checking under the procedure, anatomic site, condition, synonym, eponym, service, or abbreviation, as necessary.

- Review and select the subterms indented below the main term.

- Note the code number(s) found opposite the selected main term or subterm:

  —If a single code number is provided, locate the code in the body of the CPT codebook. Verify the code and its description against the procedural statement to make sure they match.

  —If two or more codes separated by a comma are shown, locate each code in the body of the CPT codebook. Read the description of each code before selecting the appropriate one to match the procedural statement.

  —If a range of codes is shown, locate that range in the body of the CPT codebook. Review the description of each entry before selecting a code. The code description should always match the procedural statement.

- If applicable, follow cross-references.

- Never code directly from the index.

- Read all notes that apply to the code selected. They can appear at the beginning of a section or subsection, directly under, or within the code description.

- Select the appropriate modifier, when applicable, to complete the code description. Modifiers may not always apply to hospital reporting of outpatient hospital procedures. Individual health plans may have specific guidelines for the use of modifiers and for the acceptance of Level II modifiers. For accurate reporting, the coding professional must be familiar with the specific reporting requirements for the circumstances.

- Continue coding all components of the procedure/service according to the directions in the CPT codebook.

Exercise 2.3   Use of the Alphabetical Index

Assign the appropriate CPT codes and provide the corresponding index entries for the following terms.

1. Green operation

    Code: _____

    Index entry: _____

2. Fine needle aspiration of cyst of thyroid, without imaging guidance

    Code: _____

    Index entry: _____

3. Femoral–popliteal bypass graft with vein

    Code: _____

    Index entry: _____

4. Repair of reducible recurrent femoral hernia

    Code: _____

    Index entry: _____

5. Incision and drainage of infected bursa, left hip

    Code: _____

    Index entry: _____

6. Anesthesia provided for application of shoulder cast (assign only the code for the anesthesia services)

    Code: _____

    Index entry: _____

7. Direct diagnostic laryngoscopy for 45-year-old patient

    Code: _____

    Index entry: _____

8. MRI of lumbar spine with contrast material

    Code: _____

    Index entry: _____

9. Paring of a single corn of the right foot

    Code: _____

    Index entry: _____

10. HIV-1 antibody testing

    Code: _____

    Index entry: _____

(Continued on next page)

Exercise 2.3 (Continued)

11. Biopsy of posterior one-third of tongue

    Code: _____

    Index entry: _____

12. Esophagogastroduodenoscopy (EGD) with biopsy

    Code: _____

    Index entry: _____

13. Arthroscopic medial meniscectomy

    Code: _____

    Index entry: _____

14. All-night recording EEG

    Code: _____

    Index entry: _____

15. Removal of metal shaving from cornea without use of slit lamp

    Code: _____

    Index entry: _____

16. Endometrial ablation with ultrasound guidance

    Code: _____

    Index entry: _____

17. Beta-blocker therapy prescribed

    Code: _____

    Index entry: _____

18. Ocular photoscreening

    Code: _____

    Index entry: _____

19. DXA, vertebral fracture assessment

    Code: _____

    Index entry: _____

20. Excision of recurrent ganglion of wrist

    Code: _____

    Index entry: _____

Abstracting Documentation

This workbook provides two types of exercises: one-line procedure coding and operative narratives. The one-line procedures offer students the opportunity to use the index to locate the coding selection and apply the guidelines introduced in the chapter. Coding from operative notes found in office records, operative reports, and/or emergency department notes allows students to practice the skill of abstracting needed information to assign a code successfully. When reviewing the documentation in an operative report, students are encouraged to scan the report for procedures performed (action types of words: excision, incision, aspiration, endoscopy, and so forth) and associated diagnoses.

After looking in the index and, subsequently, in the main body portion of the CPT codebook to locate coding selections, it will be necessary to note the types of information that may influence the choice of codes and then to read the operative report again for information that will help determine the correct answer.

Exercise 2.4   CPT Coding Process

Operative Report

Preoperative Diagnosis:	History of colon cancer	→ Reason for encounter
Postoperative Diagnosis:	Rectosigmoid polyp	
Procedure:	Colonoscopy and polypectomy	→ Procedure performed

Indications: The patient has had three previous resections of three different primary carcinomas of the colon. His last resection of carcinoma was in 2000. He has been doing well in general.

Premedications: Demerol 50 mg IV and Versed 2.5 mg IV

Procedure: The CF100-L video colonoscope was passed without difficulty from the anus up through the anastomosis, which appears to be in the distal transverse colon. The instrument was advanced into the distal small bowel and then slowly withdrawn with good view obtained throughout. A small, 3-mm polyp near the rectosigmoid junction was removed with hot biopsy forceps and retrieved. Otherwise, the patient has a satisfactory postoperative appearance of the colon. It is shortened due to previous resections, but there is no other evidence of neoplasm. The instrument was completely withdrawn without other findings.

Read the preceding operative report. Then perform the steps in the coding process as listed below. Show your results in the spaces provided.

1. Scan the documentation to identify the procedure performed.

   _____

2. Search the index for Colonoscopy, Removal, Polyp, and identify the code range for the procedure.

   _____

3. Review the coding descriptions to determine what additional documentation is needed before you can accurately select a code.

   _____

4. Read the operative report again to determine the method of removal utilized.

   _____

5. Choose the code that reflects this documentation.

   _____

Exercise 2.5 CPT Coding Process

Operative Report

Preoperative Diagnosis: Subepidermal nodular lesion of the forearm ⟶ | Reason for encounter |

Operation: Excision of 2.0-cm lesion of the forearm

Procedure: Under local anesthesia, the 2.0-cm lesion was removed with 0.5-cm margins. The lesion was submitted to pathology. Bleeding was controlled with electro-cautery, and the wound was closed with five vertical mattress sutures of 5-0 nylon. Polysporin and dressing were applied to the wound.

Pathological Diagnosis: Well-organized basal cell carcinoma

Review the preceding operative report and note the pathological diagnosis. Then perform the steps in the coding process as listed below. Record your results in the spaces provided. (Hint: Be sure to abstract the following information from the operative report: size of lesion and margins; morphology, benign or malignant; location; and method of removal.)

1. Scan the documentation and record the main procedure to be located in the alphabetic index.

   _____

2. Search the index for the main terms/subterms and record the code selections.

   _____

3. Review the code descriptions to determine what additional documentation is needed before you can accurately select a code.

   _____

4. Read the operative report and pathological diagnosis again to determine the additional documentation to clarify the selection.

   _____

5. Choose the code that reflects this documentation.

   _____

Exercise 2.6 CPT Coding Process

Operative Report

Preoperative Diagnosis: Umbilical hernia

Postoperative Diagnosis: Same

This is a 38-year-old male who presents with an umbilical hernia. He has been experiencing flu-like symptoms, which he describes as crampy abdominal pain. Risks versus benefits including bleeding, infection, and the high recurrence rate because of his obesity were discussed. The patient states he understands and elects to proceed.

After adequate general endotracheal anesthesia had been induced, the patient was placed in the supine position, and prepped and draped in the usual sterile manner. A curvilinear incision was made just inferior to the umbilicus. This was extended down through adipose tissue to the level of the rectus fascia. The herniosac was amputated and sent to pathology. The fascia was then reapproximated transversely using interrupted 0 prolene sutures. The skin was reapproximated using 4-0 nylon. Sponge and needle counts were accurate. The patient tolerated the procedure well and left the operating room in stable condition.

Review the preceding operative report, and abstract the information that is needed for a correct code assignment. Answer the following questions in the spaces provided.

1.   What procedure was performed?

_____

2.   What code selections were listed in the index entry for the main terms describing the procedure?

_____

3.   What additional documentation is needed before an accurate code can be assigned?.

_____

4.   What is the correct code for the procedure?

_____

5.   Should a CPT code also be assigned for the suturing of the wound at the conclusion of the procedure?

_____

Identification of Operative Procedures for Coding

New coders often have difficulty determining whether a procedure is an integral part of the main operative procedure or a separately identifiable procedure. For example, when a patient has a breast mass removed, a code for the wound closure would not be assigned because it is an integral part of the main procedure. The ability to discriminate between reportable and nonreportable procedures is a skill that must be developed and one that significantly affects accurate code selection. Coders need to have surgical references to help them understand procedures and techniques. The references section of this book provides a list of helpful resources. In addition to understanding surgical techniques, coders must know when to assign additional codes and will find instructions on doing so in the CPT guidelines. Various types of notes and descriptions located throughout CPT guidelines are illustrated below.

52601	Transurethral electrosurgical resection of prostate, including control of postoperative bleeding, complete (Vasectomy, meatotomy, cystourethroscopy, urethral calibration and/or dilation, and internal urethrotomy are included)

Many CPT codes combine the main procedure with minor procedures that do not warrant additional codes. In these cases, the code description contains a note specifying the secondary procedures that are to be included in the primary code. In the preceding example, if the surgeon performs a transurethral electrosurgical resection of prostate (TURP) with vasectomy, the correct code assignment is 52601. Because the code description states that vasectomy is included in the code for the TURP procedure, the vasectomy is not assigned a separate code.

58150	Total abdominal hysterectomy (corpus and cervix), with or without removal of tube(s), with or without removal of ovary(s)

If the surgeon performs a total abdominal hysterectomy with salpingo-oophorectomy, the only code submitted would be 58150. The code description explains that no additional code would be submitted for the salpingo-oophorectomy.

Some notes in the CPT codebook offer guidance on multiple code assignment for an entire section. For example, look at the note before code 14000 in the Adjacent Tissue Transfer or Rearrangement portion of the integumentary system subsection of the surgery section. The second paragraph includes the following clause: "Excision (including lesion) and/or repair by adjacent tissue transfer or rearrangement." According to this note, when a surgeon removes a skin lesion and the defect is repaired with an adjacent tissue transfer, only the tissue transfer should be coded. The excision of lesion is not identified with an additional code.

Some notes provide instructions for use of add-on codes. For example, code 69990, Operating microscope, is reported only as an additional code. In some procedures, physicians utilize an operating microscope during the surgical episode. CPT provides specific instructions in the note before code 69990 to help the coder determine whether this add-on code is to be used with a particular primary procedure code.

Instruction is often given in the form of a note under a specific code, for example, the note under CPT code 63078 that instructs the coder not to report code 69990 in addition to codes 63075 through 63078.

Coding References

Both the American Medical Association (AMA) and the Centers for Medicare and Medicaid Services (CMS) are resources for CPT coding guidelines.

American Medical Association

The AMA is the primary, authoritative reference for CPT guidelines and changes. The AMA publishes *CPT Assistant,* a monthly newsletter that provides information on the correct application of CPT codes. The newsletter includes a question-and-answer section that provides answers to coders' questions. The AMA also offers a subscription service for assistance with coding questions. Most large healthcare facilities subscribe to an online version of *CPT Assistant.* Exercises 2.7 and 2.8 require access to *CPT Assistant.*

Exercise 2.7   Coding References

Exercise 2.4 asked you to analyze documentation and assign the correct code for a colonoscopy with a polypectomy procedure. For correct CPT assignment, you needed to know what method was used to remove the polyp. In the operative report for that exercise, the surgeon used hot biopsy forceps. For this exercise, assume that the surgeon removed the small polyp by using a cold biopsy forceps.

1.   What is the correct coding assignment for this procedure?

   _____

2.   What volume of *CPT Assistant* provided the information needed to arrive at this code assignment?

   _____

Centers for Medicare and Medicaid Services

The federal government provides some interpretative guidance on the use of CPT codes and modifiers as an element of HCPCS. The HCPCS guidelines are published in the form of transmittals, manuals, and other documents. Most of the Medicare and Medicaid manuals are available for downloading from the CMS Web site.

Exercise 2.8   Coding References

In exercise 2.5, the surgeon excised a lesion of the forearm. Suppose that the surgeon took a biopsy of the lesion before removing it. The following exercise requires reference to *CPT Assistant* and a CMS Regional PRO letter (No. 91-18, Regional Office VI, Dallas).

1.   Should both the biopsy and the excision be coded or just the excision?

   _____

2.   Which volume of *CPT Assistant* provided the information needed to answer this question?

   _____

Exercise 2.9   Chapter 2 Review

Answer the following questions in the spaces provided.

1.   Which symbol indicates that a procedure code is new in CPT?

   _____

2.   Refer to CPT codes 11100 and 11101. Assume that a surgeon performed a biopsy of two different skin lesions during the same procedure. Which code should be assigned?

   _____

3.   Which category of CPT codes is reserved for emerging technology?

   _____

4.   Refer to CPT codes 42310 and 42320. Assume that a surgeon drained an external submaxillary abscess. Which code should be assigned?

   _____

5.   Refer to CPT codes 40840 through 40844. Assume that a surgeon performed a bilateral, posterior vestibuloplasty. Which code should be assigned?

   _____

6.   Refer to CPT code 56630. What documentation in the operative report would be needed to support the use of this code?

   _____

7.   Refer to CPT codes 54050 through 54060. Assume a surgeon removed condylomas of the penis. What medical record documentation would be needed to assign one of the codes accurately?

   _____

8.   Assume that a gastroenterologist performed an EGD (CPT code 43235) and administered Versed during the procedure. Would the physician submit codes to reflect both the procedure (43235) and the administration of anesthesia?

   _____

9.   Refer to CPT codes 76856 through 76857. Documentation indicates that a radiologist examined the fallopian tubes and ovaries to compare the abnormal surgical findings to an ultrasound performed the preceding month. What would be the correct code assignment?

   _____

10.   Refer to CPT codes 11730 through 11732. Assume that a physician performed a complete avulsion of the nail plate of the thumb and index and ring fingers. What would be the correct code assignment?

   _____

Chapter 2 Test

Choose the appropriate answers.

1. Per CPT guidelines, a separate procedure:
   a. Is coded when it is performed as a part of another, larger procedure
   b. Is considered to be an integral part of another, larger service
   c. Is never coded under any circumstance
   d. Both a and b above

2. What does the symbol ▲ before a code in the CPT manual signify?
   a. The code is new for this year.
   b. The code is exempt from bundling requirements.
   c. The code can only be used as an add-on code, never reported alone or first.
   d. The code has been revised in some way this year.

3. The Alphabetic Index to CPT includes listings for:
   a. Procedures/services
   b. Examinations/tests
   c. Anatomic sites
   d. All of the above

4. The symbol + before a code in CPT means that:
   a. This code can never be reported alone.
   b. This code can never be reported first.
   c. This is an add-on code.
   d. All of the above

5. A listing of all current modifiers is found in which appendix of CPT?
   a. Appendix A
   b. Appendix B
   c. Appendix C
   d. Appendix D

Chapter 3

Modifiers

Modifiers may be reported along with a CPT code to indicate that a particular event modified the service/procedure, but with no change to its basic definition. Modifiers may indicate any of the following situations:

- A service/procedure has both a professional component and a technical component.

- A service/procedure was performed by more than one physician and/or in more than one location.

- A service/procedure has been increased or reduced in scope.

- A service was performed only partially.

- An adjunctive service was performed.

- A bilateral procedure was performed.

- A service/procedure was performed more than once.

- An unusual event occurred during the service/procedure.

There is a distinct advantage to conveying as much information as possible to the third-party payer to ensure appropriate payment when billing for professional physician services or services provided by an ambulatory surgery or service center. Use of a modifier, in selected cases, allows the healthcare provider to explain special circumstances that surround the charge for the service and may affect claim payment. Use of an appropriate modifier also can prevent a claim from being denied.

Appendix A of the CPT codebook includes a complete list of currently accepted modifiers and their descriptions. Coders should examine modifier descriptions carefully for conditions that may limit use of a modifier to a specific section of CPT. For example, modifier –25 is limited by definition to evaluation and management codes and would not be appended to a code from the surgery section. Modifier –78 (Return to Operating Room for a Related Procedure During the Postoperative Period) would only be appended to a CPT surgical code. (Links to the Centers for Medicare and Medicaid Services Web site pertinent to the discussion in this chapter are in the Web resources at the back of this book.)

Use of Modifiers

The CPT and HCPCS systems for describing and reporting medical procedures and services include the use of special supplementary codes called modifiers. Modifiers are two-character codes that can be appended to some of the CPT Level I codes and the HCPCS Level II codes to provide additional information.

Different sets of modifiers apply to different services and settings. For example, two-digit numerical modifiers can be appended to CPT codes for reporting additional information relevant to physician and outpatient hospital services. In addition, two-digit alphabetic or alphanumeric modifiers permit more concise reporting of services in Level II (National) HCPCS codes.

Modifiers have been used by physicians and other Medicare Part B professional service providers for a number of years. Modifiers have also been used for reporting Medicare hospital outpatient services since the implementation of the ambulatory patient classification prospective payment system (APC PPS) in 2000. Several specific CPT modifiers are required for reporting hospital outpatient services and are designated for hospital use only.

(Please note that for purposes of instruction, this book uses a dash to separate each five-character CPT code from its two-character modifier. However, dashes are not used in actual code assignments and reimbursement claims, which report seven-character codes with no spaces between the characters when the assignment of modifiers is appropriate.)

Use of Modifiers for Physician Services

In most cases, modifiers applicable to the codes for physician services are simply appended to the appropriate CPT code, as in the following example:

> **Example:** 35840–78
>
> Postoperatively, a patient is taken to the operative room for exploration of postop hemorrhage.

Some third-party payers have special reporting requirements that affect the assignment of modifiers. For example, they may ask that claims for surgical procedures performed bilaterally include the appropriate surgical code twice, with modifier –50 assigned only on the second listing of the code to indicate that the same procedure was performed twice. This practice does not follow the AMA's guidelines for reporting bilateral procedures, and CMS requires a one-line method of reporting bilateral procedures for Medicare claims.

> **Example:** 49500
> 49500–50   Required reporting by some payers
> 49500–50   AMA and CMS method of reporting

In addition to the CPT modifiers, HCPCS Level II National Codes include many modifiers for more concise reporting of procedures performed by physicians. These two-digit alphanumeric modifiers can be used to identify:

- The specific finger or toe involved

- A visit for a second or third opinion

- A service provided by someone other than a physician

- Right- or left-side involvement

The CPT codebook lists the required HCPCS modifiers for outpatient services in appendix A. Additional HCPCS modifiers can be found in the national HCPCS codebook.

Example: RT Right side
TA Left foot, great toe
AH Clinical psychologist
F9 Right hand, fifth digit
QW CLIA-waived test

Use of Modifiers for Hospital Services

The following CPT modifiers are available for use by hospitals for outpatient Medicare services. The modifiers should be reported as two digits appended to the appropriate CPT code in field location 44 of the CMS-1450 form (UB-92). (See figure 1.2 on p. 11.)

25 Significant, Separately Identifiable Evaluation and Management Service by the Same Physician on the Same Day of a Procedure or Other Service
27 Multiple Outpatient Hospital E/M Encounters
50 Bilateral Procedure
52 Reduced Services
58 Staged or Related Procedure or Service by the Same Physician During the Postoperative Period
59 Distinct Procedural Service
73 Discontinued Outpatient Hospital/Ambulatory Surgery Center (ASC) Procedure Prior to the Administration of Anesthesia
74 Discontinued Outpatient Hospital/Ambulatory Surgery Center (ASC) Procedure after Administration of Anesthesia
76 Repeat Procedure by Same Physician
77 Repeat Procedure by Another Physician
78 Return to Operating Room for a Related Procedure During the Postoperative Procedure
79 Unrelated Procedure or Service by the Same Physician During the Postoperative Period
91 Repeat Clinical Diagnostic Laboratory Test

Example: 49505–50 Repair initial inguinal hernia, age 5 years or over; reducible

By adding modifier –50, the coder has identified a left-sided and right-sided (bilateral) hernia repair.

In addition, the following Level II modifiers are acceptable for hospital use:

LT Left Side
RT Right Side
E1 Upper Left, Eyelid
E2 Lower Left, Eyelid
E3 Upper Right, Eyelid
E4 Lower Right, Eyelid

FA   Left Hand, Thumb
F1   Left Hand, Second Digit
F2   Left Hand, Third Digit
F3   Left Hand, Fourth Digit
F4   Left Hand, Fifth Digit
F5   Right Hand, Thumb
F6   Right Hand, Second Digit
F7   Right Hand, Third Digit
F8   Right Hand, Fourth Digit
F9   Right Hand, Fifth Digit
TA   Left Foot, Great Toe
T1   Left Foot, Second Digit
T2   Left Foot, Third Digit
T3   Left Foot, Fourth Digit
T4   Left Foot, Fifth Digit
T5   Right Foot, Great Toe
T6   Right Foot, Second Digit
T7   Right Foot, Third Digit
T8   Right Foot, Fourth Digit
T9   Right Foot, Fifth Digit
LC   Left Circumflex Coronary Artery
LD   Left Anterior Descending Coronary Artery
RC   Right Coronary Artery
CA   Procedure payable only in the inpatient setting when performed emergently on an outpatient who dies prior to admission
GA   Waiver of liability statement on file
GG   Performance and payment of a screening mammogram and diagnostic mammogram on the same patient, same day
GH   Diagnostic mammogram converted from screening mammogram on same day
QM   Ambulance Service Provided under Arrangement by a Provider of Services
QN   Ambulance Service Furnished Directly by a Provider of Services

Category II Modifiers

Introduced in 2006, Category II performance measurement modifiers indicate that a service specified in the measure(s) was considered but, due to either medical or patient circumstances(s), was not provided. The new modifiers are as follows:

1P   Performance Measure Exclusion Modifier due to Medical Reasons
2P   Performance Measure Exclusion Modifier due to Patient Choice

Category II modifiers should only be reported with Category II codes and the circumstances must be documented in the medical record.

Medicare Transmittals

Periodically, Medicare issues its own guidelines or clarification memos pertaining to coding issues. Whenever CMS sees the need to alter or provide additional clarification on the correct usage of CPT codes or modifiers for Medicare reimbursement, it issues one of these memorandums. Several transmittals related to the use of modifiers have been issued, including:

- Transmittal 726, January 1998 (Use of Modifiers in Reporting Hospital Outpatient Services)

- Transmittal A-99-41, September 1999 (Clarification of Modifier Usage in Reporting Outpatient Hospital Services)

- Transmittal A-00-07, February 2000 (Addition of Modifiers 25, 58, 78, and 79 to the List of Modifiers Approved for Hospital Outpatient Use and Correction to Program Memorandum A-99-41)

- Transmittal A-00-40, July 2000 (Further Information on the Use of Modifier 25 in Reporting Hospital Outpatient Services)

- Transmittal A-00-73, October 2000 (Clarification of Modifier Usage in Reporting Outpatient Hospital Services)

- Transmittal A-02-129, January 2003 (Update of the Hospital Outpatient Prospective Payment System)

The most current transmittal information is available on the CMS Web site (www.cms.gov).

Use of Modifiers with Surgery Codes

The modifiers described in Figure 3.1 may be appended to surgery codes for professional services. Other modifiers are described in other chapters of this workbook. Note that a complete list of CPT modifiers and modifiers approved for ambulatory surgery center (ASC) hospital outpatient use can be found in appendix A of CPT 2006.

Use of Modifiers for Genetic Testing Codes

CPT/HCPCS also includes a list of alphanumeric modifiers to be used for reporting the molecular laboratory procedures performed for the purpose of genetic testing. (The list is provided in appendix I of CPT 2006.) The modifiers report additional information without altering the CPT/HCPCS code descriptions for the laboratory procedures. Coding guidelines for applying these modifiers are provided in the molecular diagnostic and molecular cytogenetic code sections in CPT.

The first character of these modifiers is numeric, and it indicates the disease category, and the second (alphabetic) character identifies the gene type. The modifiers for genetic testing are categorized according to the type of genetic mutation being tested for, specifically:

- Neoplasia (solid tumors or lymphoid/hematopoietic conditions)

- Nonneoplastic hematology/coagulation

- Histocompatibility/blood typing

- Neurologic, nonneoplastic

- Muscular, nonneoplastic

- Metabolic, other

- Metabolic, transport

- Metabolic, pharmacogenetics

- Dysmorphology

Figure 3.1.   Modifiers for use with surgical codes

---

22   Unusual Procedural Services

Modifier –22 is intended only for use by physicians. It may be reported to identify that the service provided was greater than that usually required for a particular procedure. It may be necessary to submit supportive documentation to the third-party payer to justify use of modifier –22.

Example: Because of the patient's extreme obesity, a physician required an additional 30 minutes to perform a chole-cystectomy. He should report 47600–22.

47   Anesthesia by Surgeon

Modifier –47, also for physician use only, may be reported to indicate that the surgeon provided regional or general (not local) anesthesia for a surgical procedure. This modifier should not be reported with the anesthesia codes (00100–01999).

Example: Obstetrician performs emergency Cesarean delivery for an out-of-town patient visiting relatives. He also administers a pudendal block (regional anesthesia). Moreover, he will provide postpartum care for the patient until she is able to return home. The physician should report 59515–47 and 64430.

50   Bilateral Procedure

Modifier –50 may be reported by both physicians or hospitals to identify bilateral procedures that are performed during the same operative episode. However, if the code describes the procedure as bilateral, modifier –50 should not be reported.

Example: Physician performs a complex anterior packing of both nares for a nosebleed. Both physicians and hospitals providing this service for Medicare patients should report 30903–50.

51   Multiple Procedures

Modifier –51 may be reported to identify that multiple procedures were performed on the same day or during the same operative episode. The first procedure listed should identify the major or most resource-intensive procedure, which usually is paid at 100 percent of the allowed reimbursement. Subsequent or secondary procedures should be appended by modifier –51, and payment should be reduced according to the terms of the health plan. Policies on payment of multiple procedures vary depending on the third-party payer, so a complete understanding of the individual payer's policies is required to ensure appropriate reimbursement. This is a physician-only modifier and is not used in the hospital setting.

Example: Physician performed an excision of a chalazion and a dacryolith from the lacrimal passage. She should report 67800 and 68530–51.

Some procedures in the CPT codebook are not intended to stand alone, so they are reported as add-on codes to describe a more extensive procedure. Modifier –51 should not be appended to these codes.

Example: Percutaneous transluminal coronary angioplasty is performed on two coronary arteries. The physician should report 92982 and 92984. Modifier –51 should not be reported in this situation because code 92984 is considered an add-on code and thus must be reported with code 92982.

52   Reduced Services

Modifier –52 may be reported by physicians and hospitals to indicate that a service/procedure is partially reduced in scope or eliminated at the discretion of the physician.

Although this modifier serves the purpose of identifying a reduction in the procedure/service, many physicians also use it to report a reduction in the charge for a particular procedure because the complete procedure was not performed. However, CMS directs hospitals to use modifier –73 instead of –52 when a procedure is partially reduced or eliminated at the physician's election before anesthesia is induced. This would apply when the patient has been prepared and taken to the room for surgery, but the surgery is not carried out due to specified circumstances. In 1999, modifier –73 was added to differentiate the definitions between physicians and hospitals for this situation.

Example: Patient was taken to the operating room (OR) for excisional debridement of a decubitus ulcer. However, before anesthesia was administered, the physician was called for emergency surgery of a trauma patient, and the ulcer surgery was postponed until a later date. In this case, the hospital would report the appropriate code for the excisional debridement, along with modifier –73 to indicate that, at the discretion of the physician, the surgery was not performed. The physician would not report a procedure code because no professional services were rendered.

Figure 3.1. (Continued)

53 Discontinued Procedure

Modifier –53 is appropriate in circumstances where the physician elects to terminate or discontinue a surgical or diagnostic procedure, usually because of a risk to the patient's well-being. However, this modifier should not be used to report the elective cancellation of a procedure prior to the patient's surgical preparation or prior to the induction of anesthesia. Also, the appropriate ICD-9-CM code should be assigned to identify the reason for the procedure's termination or discontinuation.

For hospital reporting, the CMS guidelines state that modifier –74, not –53, should be used when a procedure must be discontinued at the physician's election after the induction of anesthesia or after the procedure is under way. Elective cancellation of a procedure by the patient is not reported in this way.

Example: Patient was admitted for a cystourethroscopy with bladder biopsy. Twenty minutes into the procedure, the patient developed some arrhythmia and the surgery was stopped. The physician should report 52204–53. The hospital should report 52204–74

54 Surgical Care Only

Modifier –54 may be reported by physicians only to indicate that one physician performed the surgical procedure and another provided the pre- and postoperative care.

Example: Dr. Reynolds is asked to perform an extracapsular cataract extraction for his partner, Dr. Owens, who is detained out of town. Dr. Owens provided the preoperative care and will provide postoperative care for his patient. Dr. Reynolds should report 66940–54.

55 Postoperative Management Only *(for physician use only):* **Modifier –55 may be reported to identify that the physician provided only postoperative care services for a particular procedure.**

Example: Patient sustains a fracture of the distal femur while skiing in Colorado. The physician in Colorado performed a closed treatment of the fracture with manipulation. However, the patient's postoperative care will be provided by his hometown physician, Dr. Rogers. Dr. Rogers should report 27510–55.

56 Preoperative Management Only

Modifier –56 may be reported by physicians to indicate that the physician provided only preoperative care services for a particular procedure.

Example: Dr. Smith provides preoperative care services for his patient, who will be transferred later the same day to another hospital to undergo a lower lobectomy of the right lung. The physician should report 32480–56.

58 Staged or Related Procedure or Service by the Same Physician During the Postoperative Period

Both hospitals and physicians may report modifier –58 to indicate that a staged or related procedure performed by the same physician is provided during the postoperative period. This procedure may have been planned (staged) prospectively at the time of the original procedure, it may be more extensive than the original procedure, or it may be for therapy following a diagnostic surgical procedure.

Example: Physician performed the first stage of a hypospadias repair one month ago. The patient now returns for the second-stage repair, which includes a urethroplasty with a free skin graft obtained from a site other than genitalia. The physician should report the following for the second-stage procedure: 54316–58.

59 Distinct Procedural Service

Modifier –59 may be used by physicians and hospitals to identify that a procedure/service was distinct or independent from other services provided on the same day. Furthermore, modifier –59 is useful when circumstances require that certain procedures/services be reported together, even though they usually are not. Use of this modifier often signifies a different session or patient encounter, a different procedure or surgery, a different site or organ system, a separate incision/excision, or a separate lesion or injury not ordinarily encountered or performed on the same day by the same physician. Modifier –59 should not be reported if another modifier can more appropriately describe the circumstance.

Example: Procedures 23030 (Incision and drainage of shoulder area; deep abscess or hematoma) and 20103 (Exploration of penetrating wound; extremity) are performed on the same patient during the same operative session. Ordinarily, if these codes were reported together without a modifier, code 20103 would be denied as integral to code 23030. Because incision and drainage of the shoulder is the definitive procedure, any exploration of the area (code 20103) preceding this would be considered an inherent part of the more comprehensive service. If the exploration procedure were performed on the other limb, modifier –59 explains that the codes are distinct from each other and both services are eligible for reimbursement from the health plan.

(Continued on next page)

Figure 3.1.   (Continued)

62	**Two Surgeons**

Physicians may report modifier –62 to identify that two surgeons were required to perform a particular procedure. Each surgeon should report his or her distinct operative work by adding the modifier to the procedure code and any associated add-on code(s) for that procedure as long as both surgeons continue to work together as primary surgeons. To expedite payment, the operative note dictated by each physician should be sent to the third-party payer.

63   Procedure Performed on Infants Less than 4 kg

Modifier –63 may be appended to codes in the 20000 through 69999 series when a procedure or service is performed on a neonate or infant with a body weight of up to 4 kg. Use of this modifier indicates that the procedure involved significantly increased complexity of physician work, which is commonly associated with these patients. Modifier –63 should only be assigned by physicians and should not be appended to any CPT code listed in the evaluation and management services, anesthesia, radiology, pathology and laboratory, or medicine sections.

66   Surgical Team

Modifier –66 may be reported by physicians only to identify a complex procedure performed by a team of physicians and other highly skilled personnel.

Example: Patient is admitted for a liver transplant. All the physicians involved in performing this complex procedure should report 47135–66.

73   Discontinued Outpatient Procedure Prior to Anesthesia Administration

Modifier –73 is approved for hospital use only. If a surgical patient is taken to the operating room (or cystoscopy suite, gastrointestinal lab, and so on) and is prepared for surgery, but the surgery is cancelled before anesthesia is administered, the intended procedure code, along with modifier –73, is assigned. This modifier is not to be reported for an elective cancellation of a procedure. The medical record documentation should reflect the circumstances surrounding the cancellation.

Example: Patient is scheduled for a knee arthroscopy for a lateral meniscus repair. The patient is taken to the OR and prepped, but it was noted that before anesthesia was administered, the patient was experiencing severe hypotension. The procedure was cancelled. The correct code assignment would be 29882–73.

74   Discontinued Outpatient Procedure after Anesthesia Administration

Modifier –74 is reported by hospitals only when a patient's surgery is cancelled after administration of anesthesia or after the procedure was begun (for example, after an incision was made or after an endoscope was inserted). The procedure in progress at the time of cancellation should be reported, not all intended procedures.

Example: Patient is scheduled for a knee arthroscopy for a lateral meniscus repair. The patient is taken to OR, prepped, and anesthesia is administered. Ten minutes into the procedure, the patient develops cardiac arrhythmia and the surgery is cancelled. The correct code assignment would be 29882–74.

76   Repeat Procedure by Same Physician

Modifier –76 may be reported by hospitals and physicians to identify a procedure that was repeated by the physician who performed the original procedure. Some third-party payers may require supportive documentation. Hospitals also may report this modifier.

Example: Patient is admitted with significant pleural effusion and congestive heart failure, and the physician performs a thoracentesis. Later in the day, the lungs again fill up with fluid and the same physician performs a second thoracentesis. The physician or hospital should report the following: 32000 (first thoracentesis); 32000–76 (second thoracentesis identified as a repeat procedure with modifier –76).

77   Repeat Procedure by Another Physician

Modifier –77 may be reported by hospitals and physicians to identify a procedure that was repeated by a physician other than the one who performed the original procedure. As with modifier –76, some third-party payers may require supportive documentation. Hospitals also may report this modifier as appropriate.

Example: Dr. Reynolds performs a percutaneous transluminal balloon angioplasty of the renal artery. Later in the day, a diagnostic evaluation determines that the artery has occluded again. Because Dr. Reynolds cannot be reached, Dr. Smith repeats the earlier procedure. Dr. Reynolds should report 35471 to identify the first angioplasty performed, and Dr. Smith should report 35471–77 to identify the repeat angioplasty.

Figure 3.1. (Continued)

78 Return to the Operating Room for a Related Procedure During the Postoperative Period

Modifier –78 may be used by hospitals and physicians to report a related procedure performed during the postoperative period of the initial procedure. However, procedures repeated on the same day as the original procedure should be reported with modifier –76.

Example: Patient has a fracture of the tibia and fibula that has not healed properly. The physician who repairs the malunion should report 27720–78. Reporting modifier –78 indicates to the third-party payer that the second procedure was performed during the postoperative period of the first procedure and is related to it in some way.

79 Unrelated Procedure or Service by the Same Physician During the Postoperative Period

Modifier –79 may be used by hospitals and physicians to report an unrelated procedure performed during the postoperative period of the initial procedure. However, procedures repeated the same day as the original procedure should be reported with modifier –76.

Example: Patient had a hernia repair two weeks ago. He now returns to the hospital complaining of chills, fever, and right quadrant abdominal pain. Suspecting appendicitis, the physician admits the patient for an emergency appendectomy. To describe the appendectomy admission, the physician should report 44950–79. The appendectomy is unrelated to the initial procedure performed (hernia repair), so modifier –79 is reported to indicate that the procedure was performed during the postoperative period but is unrelated to the initial surgery.

80 Assistant Surgeon

Modifier –80 may be reported by physicians only to indicate that the physician provided surgical assistant services for a particular procedure. The surgeon who assists another physician reports the code for the procedure that was performed along with modifier –80. The operating surgeon should not report modifier –80. (Assistant surgeons are usually assumed to have been present throughout the entire surgical procedure.)

Example: Dr. Reynolds performs a total abdominal hysterectomy with removal of fallopian tubes and ovaries. Dr. Jones provides surgical assistance. Dr. Reynolds should report 58150, and Dr. Jones should report 58150–80.

81 Minimum Assistant Surgeon

Modifier –81 may be reported by physicians only to indicate that a physician provided minimal surgical assistance when another surgeon's presence typically is not required throughout the entire procedure. The physician who provided minimal assistance reports the code for the procedure performed, along with modifier –81. As in the case of modifier –80, the operating surgeon should not report modifier –81.

82 Assistant Surgeon (when qualified resident surgeon not available)

Modifier –82 may be reported by physicians only when a physician provides surgical assistance to another surgeon and a resident surgeon is unavailable. This situation occurs primarily in teaching facilities where resident surgeons typically assume the role of assistant surgeon. When a qualified resident surgeon is unavailable, another physician may serve as an assistant surgeon and report the appropriate procedure code along with modifier –82. As in the case of modifiers –80 and –81, the operating surgeon should not report modifier –82.

99 Multiple Modifiers

Modifier –99 may be reported by physicians only to alert third-party payers that more than one modifier is being submitted on a claim. Many health plans have limitations on the number of modifiers recognized.

Exercise 3.1   Chapter 3 Review

Refer to appendix A of the CPT 2006 codebook to identify the appropriate modifiers to be reported for the procedures in items 1 through 5. For items 6 through 11, assign the correct CPT code(s) and the appropriate modifiers (CPT and HCPCS National).

1. The modifier that is to be assigned to indicate that a physician provided only postoperative care.

    _____

2. The modifier that is to be used when a different physician repeated a procedure on the same date.

    _____

3. The modifier that is to be used when more than one procedure is performed on a patient during the same operative episode.

    _____

4. The modifier that can be appended to a code to indicate that two surgeons were required to perform the procedure.

    _____

5. The modifier that is to be used when a procedure was begun but had to be discontinued because of deterioration in the patient's condition (coding is for physician services, not hospital).

    _____

6. A patient undergoes carpal tunnel releases on both the left and right wrists.

    _____

7. The physician performed a partial avulsion of the nail plate of the left thumb.

    _____

8. A patient was taken to the outpatient surgery suite for an excisional debridement of the skin that extended into the muscle. The patient was prepped, but before anesthesia was administered, the physician was called for an emergency surgery of a trauma patient and the outpatient surgery was cancelled. (Assign code[s] to be reported by the hospital.)

    _____

9. A patient who had previously undergone a left leg amputation was seen in the hospital for a Doppler scan arterial study of the right leg.

    _____

10. The patient underwent a percutaneous needle core biopsy of the left breast with the use of imaging.

    _____

11. The surgeon performed an open reduction with internal fixation for a right, fifth metatarsal fracture.

    _____

Chapter 3 Test

Choose or write the appropriate answers.

1. The modifier used to report therapeutic interventional procedures on the right coronary artery is

   _____

2. Which of the following circumstances can be described by the use of a HCPCS modifier?

   _____

   a. A service has been increased or reduced.
   b. Only part of a service was performed.
   c. A service was provided more than once.
   d. All of the above

3. A radiologist interprets x-rays for a community hospital. The equipment belongs to the hospital. What modifier should the radiologist append to his CPT codes?

   _____

4. A pediatric thoracic and cardiovascular surgeon performs a curative procedure on an infant but does not see the child again. Instead, a pediatric cardiologist does all follow-up. What modifier should the surgeon append to his CPT procedure code?

   _____

5. When clinical laboratory tests are repeated on the same day, what modifier should be assigned?

   _____

6. When absolutely identical procedures are performed on both members of a set of paired organs, such as kidneys, what modifier is assigned?

   _____

7. When a patient is seen in two hospital outpatient departments in one day, what modifier should be appended to the second evaluation and management code to ensure appropriate reimbursement?

   _____

8. In addition to the claim submitted by the surgeon, the assistant surgeon bills for his or her services. What modifier does the assistant surgeon attach to the procedure code?

   _____

9. Sex reassignment surgery (55980 or 55970) is a complex procedure that requires a team of surgeons. What modifier should each participating surgeon attach to the surgery code?

   _____

10. Some reconstructive plastic surgical procedures are performed in multiple stages. What modifier should the surgeon report when the patient is returned to surgery for a planned staged procedure?

   _____

Chapter 4

Surgery

To assign codes accurately from the surgery section, physicians and coders must work together to ensure that the documentation in the health record supports the code(s) selected. In the hospital setting, as in the office setting, the operative or procedure report serves as the source document when identifying the type of procedure that has been performed.

The surgery section provides codes for procedures performed by physicians of any specialty type (general surgeons, ophthalmologists, cardiovascular surgeons, neurosurgeons, and so on). It is further divided into the following subsections:

Subsection	Code Range
General	10021–10022
Integumentary System	10040–19499
Musculoskeletal System	20000–29999
Respiratory System	30000–32999
Cardiovascular System	33010–37799
Hemic and Lymphatic Systems	38100–38999
Mediastinum and Diaphragm	39000–39599
Digestive System	40490–49999
Urinary System	50010–53899
Male Genital System	54000–55899
Intersex Surgery	55970–55980
Female Genital System	56405–58999
Maternity Care and Delivery	59000–59899
Endocrine System	60000–60699
Nervous System	61000–64999
Eye and Ocular Adnexa	65091–68899
Auditory System	69000–69979
Operating Microscope	69990

This chapter reviews the guidelines and conventions specific to surgical coding and introduces specific subsections. (Links to various Web sites pertinent to the discussion in this chapter are located in the Web resources at the back of this book.)

Surgical Packages

The term *surgical procedure* refers to any single, separate, systemic process upon or within the body that is complete in itself. Surgical procedures are performed for a number of purposes, including:

- To restore disunited or deficient parts
- To remove diseased or injured tissues
- To extract foreign matter from the body
- To assist in obstetrical delivery
- To provide diagnostic information

Each individual *surgical operation* includes one or more surgical procedures performed at one time for one patient via a common approach or for a common purpose.

The term *surgical package* refers to a combination of individual services provided during one surgical operation. A surgical package is treated as one single service for purposes of reimbursement, and a single payment is issued for each package of related surgical services. The services covered in each surgical package include the following:

- The actual surgical procedure(s)
- Local infiltration, metacarpal/metatarsal/digital block, or topical anesthesia
- After the decision to perform surgery has been made, one related E/M encounter on the date of, or immediately prior to, the date of the procedure (including history and physical)
- Immediate postoperative care, including dictation of operative notes and meetings with the family and other physicians
- Preparation of orders
- Evaluation of the patient in the postanesthesia recovery area
- Typical postoperative follow-up care

This reimbursement concept is sometimes referred to as global surgery payment.

For example, if a physician performed a surgical operation and a few days later saw the patient in her office for standard follow-up care (for example, removal of sutures), the follow-up visit provided by the physician would not be reported separately. It would be included under the code(s) for the surgical procedure(s) performed during the first encounter, and both encounters would be submitted as a single reimbursement claim. In some cases, however, the code for the postoperative follow-up visit (99024) might also be reported for documentation purposes.

> **Example:** Four weeks ago, Dr. Smith repaired a closed tibial shaft fracture without manipulation. Today, the patient has returned to Dr. Smith's office to have his cast removed. Dr. Smith may bill only for the repair of the fracture, which includes the normal, uncomplicated follow-up care, including cast removal. Thus, only code 27750 is reported on his claim. The subsequent visit for removal of the cast is not billed separately; however, for tracking purposes only, code 99024 may be assigned for that encounter.

Services other than standard postoperative care, however, would not be included in the same surgical package. Follow-up visits for the treatment of complications resulting from the surgical procedure (for example, wound infection at operative site) would be reported with codes for the appropriate E/M level of service, along with the appropriate ICD-9-CM code, to describe the complication.

Example: Two weeks ago, Dr. Smith performed a cholecystectomy. Today, the patient returns with complaints of redness, inflammation, and oozing from the wound site. Dr. Smith determines that the patient has developed an infection at the operative wound site and treats it appropriately. For the second office visit, Dr. Smith should report the appropriate E/M level of service code and assign ICD-9-CM code 998.59 to describe the wound infection.

Medicare guidelines for reimbursement for services involving complications are slightly different from CPT. These guidelines can be referenced in the *Medicare Providers Manual* published by the Centers for Medicare and Medicaid Services (CMS).

The surgical package or global surgery concept does not apply in the hospital outpatient settings. Hospitals may report postoperative visits that occur on subsequent days by using standard billing procedures, such as assigning the appropriate ICD-9-CM diagnosis code to describe the reason for the visit.

Example: Patient returns to the outpatient department of Central Hospital for a change of surgical dressing. The hospital assigns ICD-9-CM code V58.3 (Attention to surgical dressings) to identify the reason for the visit. The E/M code appropriate to the circumstance (new or established) reflects the service rendered.

The services included in a surgical package may vary depending on individual third-party payer requirements. The Medicare global surgery definition for major surgeries includes the following types of services:

- The actual surgical procedure

- Preoperative services provided one day prior to surgery or the day of surgery, except when modifier –57 or modifier –25 applies

- Postoperative services provided within 90 days of the surgical procedure, except when modifier –24 applies

- Insignificant surgical procedures not performed in the operating room, including dressing changes, removal of operative packs, and care of the operative incision site; removal of sutures, staples, wires, lines, tubes, drains, casts, and splints; insertion, irrigation, and removal of urinary catheters; routine peripheral intravenous lines; removal of nasogastric tubes and rectal tubes; care of tracheostomy tubes

The Medicare global surgery definition for minor and endoscopic surgeries includes the following types of services:

- The actual surgical procedure

- Preoperative services provided one day prior to surgery or the day of surgery, except when modifier –57 or modifier –25 applies

- Postoperative services provided within 0 to 10 days of the surgical procedure, except when modifier –24 applies

Follow-up Care for Diagnostic and Therapeutic Procedures

Follow-up care for diagnostic or therapeutic procedures includes only that care related to recovery from the diagnostic procedure itself or care that is usually part of the surgical service. When follow-up care involves the initiation of treatment for the condition that has been diagnosed or for a complication, the treatment should be coded and reported separately. Complication, exacerbation, or recurrence, or the presence of other diseases or injuries requiring additional services should be reported with the appropriate code for that procedure.

Separate Procedures

The CPT codebook defines a separate procedure as one that, when performed in conjunction with another service, is considered an integral part of the major service; therefore, it should not be coded separately. In normal circumstances, it is fraudulent to report the codes separately and charge separate fees for each procedure.

However, the separate procedure may be coded when it is performed independently and not in conjunction with the so-called larger or major procedure. A modifier, such as modifier 59 (Distinct Services), may be added to explain special circumstances where the separate procedure was not performed integral to the larger procedure. For example, assume that the following procedures were performed on a patient:

Example: 58720   Salpingo-oophorectomy, complete or partial, unilateral or bilateral (separate procedure)

58150   Total abdominal hysterectomy (corpus and cervix), with or without removal of tube(s), with or without removal of ovary(s)

58180   Supracervical abdominal hysterectomy (subtotal hysterectomy), with or without removal of tube(s), with or without removal of ovary(s)

Assignment of code 58720 would be appropriate in circumstances where *only* a salpingo-oophorectomy was performed. If the salpingo-oophorectomy was done as part of a larger procedure, as described in code 58150 or 58180, an additional code of 58720 is inappropriate and would be considered unbundling of services.

In another example, assume the physician performed a flexible bronchoscopy with cell washings (CPT code 31622) and a transbronchial lung biopsy (CPT code 31628). In this example, only CPT code 31628 is reported. CPT code 31622 is a "separate procedure" code and would not be assigned with 31628.

Correct Coding Initiative

A list of coding edits has been developed by CMS in an effort to promote correct coding nationwide and to prevent the inappropriate unbundling of related services. The National Correct Coding Initiative (NCCI) edits help CMS to detect inappropriate codes submitted on claims and are based on CPT coding guidelines, current standards of medical/surgical coding practice, and advice from specialty societies. There are two major types of coding edits: the comprehensive/component edit and the mutually exclusive edit.

Comprehensive/Component Edit

The comprehensive/component edit pertains to HCPCS codes that should not be used together. Note the following table as an example of a NCCI listing. Under the NCCI, if bills contain a procedure in both the comprehensive code column and the component code column for the same patient on the same date of service, only the comprehensive code column code is covered (provided that code is on the list as an approved procedure for reimbursement). For example:

Comprehensive Code   **Components Code(s)**
20912   12014, 13152

In the preceding example, code 20912 describes a cartilage graft of nasal septum. During the procedure, the surgeon may mention that a wound repair (12014, 13152) was performed, but it is considered part of the more involved procedure (20912) and should not be coded. If the coder assigned the additional wound repair codes, it would be considered unbundling.

Mutually Exclusive Edit

The mutually exclusive edit applies to improbable or impossible combinations of codes. For example, code 69601, Revision mastoidectomy; resulting in complete mastoidectomy, would never be performed with code 69604, Revision mastoidectomy; resulting in tympanoplasty.

CCI edits are included in most encoding software packages. The software vendors are responsible for maintaining up-to-date edits to support the coding/billing function. More information about CCI edits can be found on the CMS Web site.

Integumentary System

The integumentary system subsection includes codes for procedures performed on the following body parts:

- Skin and subcutaneous structures, including excision of skin lesions, wound closure, skin grafting, burn treatment, Mohs chemosurgery, incision and drainage, and debridement

- Nails, including debridement, excision, and reconstruction of nail bed

- Breast, including needle, incisional, and excisional biopsies, and all types of mastectomies

Figure 4.1 shows the skin and its components.

The integumentary system subsection includes many definitions that are located at various levels within the subsection. A careful review of each definition is necessary before codes are assigned.

Excision of Lesions

Two separate code ranges can be found in this subsection to describe the excised site of benign (11400–11471) and malignant (11600–11646) lesions. Both series of codes are further subdivided, first by body part and then by lesion size. To accurately code excision of lesions, the coder must be able to answer the following questions:

- *Is the lesion malignant or benign?* Careful review of the operative report and, more important, the pathology report is required to determine the lesion type. Coding from

Figure 4.1. The skin and its components

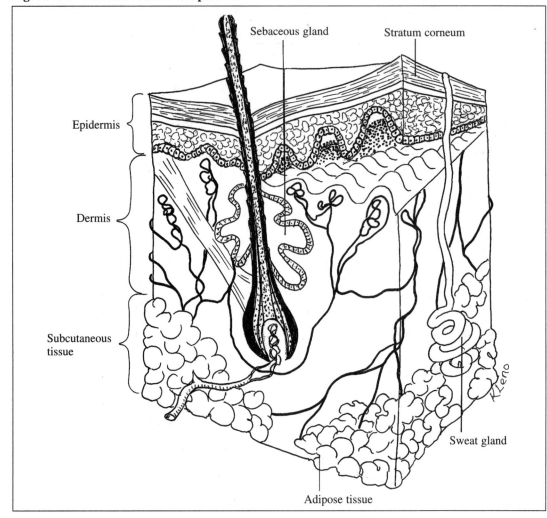

superbills or encounter forms, which do not reveal pathology results, often leads to inappropriate code assignment.

- *What site or body part is involved with the lesion?* The operative report should be reviewed for this information.

- *How large is the excised area (in centimeters, including margins, if applicable)?* The total size of the excised area is needed for accurate coding. Usually, this information is provided in the operative report. It is very important that surgeons be educated and trained to provide lesion size information. The pathology report typically provides the specimen size rather than the lesion or excised size. Because the specimen tends to shrink, this is not an accurate measurement according to the intent of the code assignment. Inches should be converted to centimeters, when necessary.

  1 mm = 0.1 cm
  10 mm = 1.0 cm
  1 inch = approximately 2.54 cm
  1 cm = 0.4 inch

- *What type of wound closure was performed?* Both series of codes (11400–11471 and 11600–11646) include simple closure. Separate codes should be reported when the excision requires more than simple closure, such as an intermediate repair.

When more than one dimension for an excised area is provided, the size is equal to the largest dimension of the excision, including margins.

> **Example:** The physician excised a benign lesion of the hand that was reported as 3.0 cm × 2.0 cm. Documentation in the operative report states that 0.5-cm margins were excised around the lesion. For coding purposes, the size of the excision was 3.0 cm + 0.5 cm + 0.5 cm = 4.0 cm in total. The correct code assignment would be 11424. (See figure 4.2.)

When excision of a malignant or benign lesion involves repair by adjacent tissue transfer—such as Z-plasty, W-plasty, V-Y plasty, rotation, advancement, or double pedicle flap—codes 14000–14350 should be reported. It should be noted that these codes include both the excision and the tissue transfer or rearrangement. A separate code should not be reported for the lesion excision.

The preceding information describes excision of a skin lesion involving full-thickness removal. The CPT codebook identifies other methods of skin lesion removal in the following code series:

- Shaving (11300–11313) is the sharp removal by a horizontal slicing to remove epidermal and dermal lesions.

- Destruction (17000–17286) is the eradication, ablation, or obliteration of benign, premalignant, or malignant lesions by any method including electrocautery, electrodesiccation, cryosurgery, laser, or chemical treatment.

Every excised lesion should be reported individually with the correct CPT code. Multiple lesion excisions are not treated as a single excision.

Figure 4.2. Depth of split-thickness and full-thickness grafts

Epidermis

Dermis

Subcutaneous tissue

Split-thickness graft

Full-thickness graft

Exercise 4.1 Integumentary System

Assign appropriate CPT code(s) to the following procedures and indicate the index entries that were used to identify the codes. Assign only CPT surgical codes (no E/M codes) and append any applicable modifiers.

1. Physician excises two benign skin lesions. The excised areas are 2.0 cm from arm and 1.0 cm from neck.

   Code(s): _____

   Index entries: _____

   _____

2. Laser removal of four benign skin lesions from the back.

   Code(s): _____

   Index entries: _____

   _____

3. Physician excises a lesion from the chin. The excised dimension is 1.5 cm. Pathology report reveals malignant melanoma.

   Code(s): _____

   Index entries: _____

   _____

4. In the physician's office, the patient has seven skin tags removed.

   Code(s): _____

   Index entries: _____

   _____

5. Physician excised an area 3.0 cm × 2.0 cm × 1.5 cm from the patient's back. The pathology report shows a lipoma in the subcutaneous layer of skin.

   Code(s): _____

   Index entries: _____

   _____

6. Physician excised a 2.0-cm squamous cell carcinoma from the forehead. The total excision, including margins, was 3.5 cm in diameter.

   Code(s): _____

   Index entries: _____

   _____

7. Excision of malignant melanoma of the forehead (1.0 cm) and nose (0.5 cm).

   Code(s): _____

   Index entries: _____

   _____

Exercise 4.2 Integumentary System

Operative Report

Preoperative Diagnosis: Sebaceous cyst, left face

Postoperative Diagnosis: Same

Procedure: Excision of left-face sebaceous cyst

Anesthesia: Local with IV sedation

The patient is a 69-year-old female who has a sebaceous cyst on the left side of her face that has started to get larger. She presents now for excision of the cyst.

The patient was brought to the OR and placed on the operating table in the supine position. She was given 50 mg of Demerol and 1 mg of Versed IV. The left face was prepped and draped in the usual sterile fashion. The area overlying the cyst was anesthetized with 1% lidocaine with epinephrine. An elliptical incision was made of the cyst in the direction of the facial wrinkles. The cyst itself was 1 cm in diameter. The underlying cyst was dissected away from the surrounding tissues, taking care to remove the entire cyst, with an excised area of 2.0 cm × 0.5 cm. Hemostasis was obtained using electrocautery. The wound was then closed with 3-0 Vicryl. It was then dressed with Masticel and Steri-Strips. The patient tolerated the procedure well and was taken to the recovery room in stable condition.

Pathology Report

Clinical Diagnosis: Cyst of the face

Specimen: Ellipse of skin measuring 2.0 × 0.5 × 0.2 cm

Pathological Diagnosis: Epidermal inclusion cyst with rupture, marked acute and chronic inflammation

Assign appropriate CPT code(s) for the preceding procedure and indicate the index entries that were used to identify the code(s). Assign only CPT surgical codes (no E/M codes) and append any applicable modifiers.

1. Code(s): _____

    Index entries: _____

    _____

Exercise 4.3   Integumentary System

Operative Report

Preoperative Diagnosis: Epidermoid nevus of scalp

Postoperative Diagnosis: Same

Procedure: Shave excision of 4.0-cm benign scalp lesion

This patient is a gentleman on chronic anticoagulation, from whom we have previously removed a sub-galeal lipoma. At that time he was not interested in having his seborrheic keratosis removed from his scalp, although it was offered. He has had a very nice result from his original surgery and is now willing and wishing to undergo removal of what I believe is a seborrheic keratosis. Although, according to the history, it has been there as long as he can remember, it may be an epidermal nevus. A small portion is sent for biopsy to create the definitive diagnosis. The patient understands the risks of bleeding.

The patient was brought to the operating room and made comfortable in a supine position on the table. The area to be worked up was infiltrated with 1% lidocaine with 1:100,000 parts epinephrine. The area was then prepped and draped in the usual sterile fashion. A #15 blade was used to remove a small portion of the lesion, which was carefully labeled and sent to pathology for exam. The rest was then shaved off at the level of the dermis, where there was punctate bleeding. Hemostasis was achieved with cautery. A dressing of Gel-foam soaked in thrombin was placed over this, and the patient was allowed to return to the recovery room with stable vital signs. The estimated blood loss was less than 15 cc, which was replaced with crystalloid solution only. Sponge, needle, and instrument counts were reported as correct.

Assign appropriate CPT code(s) for the preceding procedure and indicate the index entries that were used to identify the code(s). Assign only CPT surgical codes (no E/M codes) and append any applicable modifiers.

1. Code(s): _____

    Index entries: _____

    _____

Wound Repair/Closure

The CPT codebook describes three types of wound repair/closure, as follows:

- A simple repair is a superficial repair that primarily involves the epidermis, dermis, or subcutaneous tissues without involvement of deeper structures. This repair usually requires simple suturing of only one layer of skin.

- An intermediate repair, like a simple wound repair, is considered a superficial repair, requiring that one or more of the deeper layers of the subcutaneous tissue and superficial fascia, as well as the skin, be closed in layers. Wounds that are closed with only one layer, but which are so heavily contaminated that they require extensive cleaning or removal of foreign material such as gravel or glass, also may be classified as an intermediate repair.

- A complex repair of a wound goes beyond a layer closure and requires scar revision, debridement, extensive undermining, stents, or retention sutures. Wounds described as angular, jagged, irregular, or stellate may require complex repair. Layered closure is part of this wound repair.

To accurately code wound closures, the following questions must be answered:

- *What type of repair is being performed: simple, intermediate, or complex?*

- *What site or body part is involved, and what is the extent of the wound?* The operative report should be reviewed for mention of blood vessel, tendon, or nerve involvement. The wound repair codes include simple ligation of blood vessels and simple exploration of the nerves, vessels, or tendons, so they should not be reported separately. However, a separate code is warranted if the extent of the laceration requires repair of the nerves, vessels, or tendons.

- *What is the length of the repair (in centimeters)?*

When multiple wounds are repaired, the coder should add together the lengths of those in the same classification and from all anatomic sites that are grouped together into the same code descriptor. For example, add together the lengths of intermediate repairs to the trunk and extremities. Do not add lengths of repairs from different groupings of anatomic sites (for example, face and extremities). Also, do not add together the lengths of different classifications (for example, intermediate and complex repairs).

Example #1:   Simple wound repair of two lacerations of the arm measuring 2.5 cm and 1.5 cm. The sum of the two lacerations is 4.0 cm, and the code reported is 12002.

Example #2:   Emergency department physician documents a simple repair of the following lacerations: 2.0 cm of arm, 3.0 cm of leg, and 1.5 cm of cheek. In addition, the physician documented the following layered wound closures: 2.0 cm of foot, 1.5 cm of leg, and 3.0 cm of knee. Note the correct code assignment:

Simple Repairs	Intermediate Repairs
2.0 cm arm	2.0 cm foot
3.0 cm leg	1.5 cm leg
1.5 cm cheek	3.0 cm knee
Add 2.0 cm of arm and 3.0 of leg and assign CPT code 12002 (5.0-cm repair). An additional code of 12011 would be assigned for the repair of the cheek.	*Add 1.5 cm of leg and 3.0 cm of knee to assign CPT code 12032 (4.5-cm repair). An additional code of 12041 wound be assigned for the 2.0-cm repair of the foot.*

When more than one classification of wounds is repaired, the most complicated repair is listed first, followed by the less complicated repairs. Modifier 51 (for physician billing) also should be reported to identify the performance of more than one procedure. Debridement may be reported separately only when gross contamination requires prolonged cleansing, considerable amounts of devitalized or contaminated tissue are removed, or debridement is carried out separately without immediate primary closure.

To report excisional debridement, the coder must have the following information:

- Percentage of body surface debrided (11000–11001)

- Extent of skin debrided: full or partial thickness (11040–11041)

- Depth of the debridement: subcutaneous, muscle, or bone (11042–11044)

A note under the wound repair subheading refers the coder to codes 20100 through 20103 if the wound required any of the following:

- Enlargement

- Extension of dissection

- Debridement

- Removal of one or more foreign bodies

- Ligation or coagulation of minor subcutaneous and/or muscular blood vessel(s)

Superficial wound repairs requiring only Steri-Strips or bandages are reported with the appropriate E/M services code. Surgical codes are inappropriate because no surgical repair was performed. Repairs with tissue adhesive, such as 2-cyanoacrylate (Dermabond), are reported using the appropriate code from the repair category.

It is important to note that Medicare requires a Level II HCPCS code to identify a wound closed with tissue adhesives. Instead of assigning the CPT code for wound repair, the following code should be assigned: G0168, Wound closure utilizing tissue adhesive(s) only. (HCPCS Level II codes are discussed further in chapter 10.)

Exercise 4.4   Integumentary System

Assign appropriate CPT code(s) for the following procedures and indicate the index entries that were used to identify the codes. Assign only CPT surgical codes (no E/M codes) and append any applicable modifiers.

1. A child is seen in the physician's office for a superficial laceration of the right knee. The physician repairs the 3.0-cm laceration with simple suturing.

   Code(s): _____

   Index entries: _____

   _____

2. The patient is treated in the emergency department for a deep 3.5-cm wound of the right arm. A routine cleansing and layer closure was required.

   Code(s): _____

   Index entries: _____

   _____

3. A patient is treated for multiple wounds of the right forearm, hand, and knee. The physician sutured the following: simple repair, 2.5 cm forearm; intermediate repair, 1.5 cm hand; 2.0 cm simple repair, knee.

   Code(s): _____

   Index entries: _____

   _____

Exercise 4.5   Integumentary System

Emergency Department Record

Chief Complaint:	Laceration, left hand
History of Present Illness:	Patient is a 67-year-old female who tripped over a brick. As she tried to break her fall, she somehow cut her left hand. She has a laceration at the base of her fifth finger on the palm side, but no other injuries.
Past Medical History:	Unremarkable
Medications:	None
Allergies:	None
Physical Examination:	
General:	Alert female in no acute distress
Extremities:	Left upper extremity exam reveals a 2.5-cm full-skin-thickness laceration on the palm side of the left hand just at the base of the finger over the volar meta-carpal phalangeal joints. She has full active and passive range of motion.
Procedure:	Anesthesia local injection 2 cc 1% lidocaine plain; prepped and routine exploration revealed no foreign body. No neurovascular tendon injury noted. Repaired with six 5-0 nylon sutures. Polysporin ointment and dressing placed on the wound.
Diagnosis:	2.5-cm simple laceration, left hand
Disposition and Plan:	Wound care instructions given and advised to have sutures taken out in 10–12 days

Assign appropriate CPT code(s) for the preceding procedure and indicate the index entries that were used to identify the code(s). Assign only CPT surgical codes (no E/M codes) and append any applicable modifiers.

1. Code(s): _____

    Index entries: _____

    _____

Exercise 4.6   Integumentary System

Emergency Department Record

Chief Complaint:	Right arm laceration
History of Present Illness:	This 24-year-old male presents here after attempting to punch out a window in his garage door with his elbow in an attempt to enter his own house.
Medications:	None
Allergies:	Keflex
Last Known Tetanus:	Unknown
Review of Systems:	No shoulder pain, no wrist pain. Complains of multiple lacerations of the forearm.
Extremities:	Right elbow and right forearm reveal multiple lacerations in various lengths from proximal and working distally. Over the area of the olecranon, there is noted to be a 3-cm superficial laceration. There is also noted to be several simple lacerations distally: approximately four measuring 1 cm and three others measuring 2 cm each. There is noted to be a 5-cm laceration involving deeper layers of skin.
Procedure:	After adequate anesthesia was obtained with local infiltration of all lacerations with 1% lidocaine with epinephrine, the wounds were explored. No foreign bodies were appreciated. Each wound was vigorously irrigated and draped individually in a sterile fashion individually. Initially, the 3-cm laceration along the area of the olecranon was closed with two interrupted sutures of 4-0 Ethilon. The remaining smaller wounds were closed with simple sutures. The 5-cm laceration required closing with 3-0 Vicryl for the subcutaneous layer and 4-0 Vicryl to close the skin. Wound edges were painted with Benzoin and Steri-Strips applied. The patient tolerated the procedure well.

Assign appropriate CPT code(s) for the preceding procedure and indicate the index entries that were used to identify the code(s). Assign only CPT surgical codes (no E/M codes) and append any applicable modifiers.

1. Code(s): _____

    Index entries: _____

    _____

Exercise 4.7   Integumentary System

Emergency Department Operative Note

Chief Complaint: Head laceration

History of Present Illness: This 85-year-old male was found in his basement with a bleeding head laceration. Exam revealed a laceration on his scalp, which is at the superior occiput. The laceration was approximately 8 cm and required a complex repair. The wound was irrigated as well as possible with normal saline. Subsequently, using 4-0 Vicryl suturing, some of the deeper structures were reapproximated with some hemostasis. Approximately three Vicryl sutures were placed deep in these structures. Four-0 nylon interrupted suturing was used with multiple sutures placed, with eventual control of the hemostasis. Several other staples were placed as well for further cosmetic closure of the skin. The procedure did provide complete resolution of the symptoms. There was a very complex and deep wound with active hemorrhage. Subsequent to this, it was cleansed and Neosporin was placed. Please note that multiple areas of hair were trimmed with scissors prior to this procedure.

Assign appropriate CPT code(s) for the preceding procedure and indicate the index entries that were used to identify the code(s). Assign only CPT surgical codes (no E/M codes) and append any applicable modifiers.

1.   Code(s): _____

     Index entries: _____

     _____

Exercise 4.8   Integumentary System

Operative Report

Preoperative Diagnosis: Pigmented nevus, arm

Postoperative Diagnosis: Melanoma

Operation: Excision 1.5-cm nevus of arm

The patient was brought into the surgery center and prepped and draped in the usual manner. Local anesthesia was injected under the lesion. The lesion with 0.5-cm margins was excised taking full-thickness skin, transversely oblique. Hemostasis was obtained with cautery. The skin was closed in layers of 3-0 Vicryl in fascia, 5-0 Vicryl subcuticular, and 6-0 nylon in the skin. Dressing was applied.

Assign appropriate CPT code(s) for the preceding procedure and indicate the index entries that were used to identify the code(s). Assign only CPT surgical codes (no E/M codes) and append any applicable modifiers.

1.   Code(s): _____

     Index entries: _____

     _____

Skin Grafting

The first series of codes (14000–14350) includes both the lesion excision and the tissue transfer or rearrangement (also known as local skin flaps), such as Z-plasty, W-plasty, V-Y plasty, rotation, advancement, or double pedicle flap. These codes are categorized first by body part involved and then by size of defect in square centimeters. An additional code may be reported to describe any skin grafting required to close the secondary defect.

The following definitions are helpful when coding adjacent tissue transfer or arrangement procedures:

- *Advancement:* The sliding of a pedicle graft into its new position.

- *Pedicle graft:* Grafted tissue that remains connected to its vascular bed.

- *Z-plasty:* A tissue transfer that surgically releases tension in the skin caused by a laceration, contracted scar, or a wound along the flexion crease of joint. It is characterized by a Z-shaped incision that is above, through, and below the scar or defect.

- *W-plasty:* A tissue transfer performed to release tension along a straight scar. A W-shaped incision creates a series of triangular flaps of skin. The triangle flaps on both sides of the scar are removed, and the remaining skin triangles are moved together and sutured into place.

- *V-Y plasty:* A tissue transfer that begins with a V-shaped skin incision and with advancement and stretching of the skin and tissue. The defect is covered and forms a Y when sutured together.

- *Rotational flap:* These flaps are curved or semicircular and include the skin and subcutaneous tissues. A base is left, and the remaining portion of the flap is freed and rotated to cover the defect and then sutured into place.

The second series of codes (15000–15431) describes skin replacement surgery and skin substitute grafts that are completely separated from the donor site in a one-stage procedure. These codes are categorized by type of graft or skin substitute (for example, pinch graft, split-thickness graft, or full-thickness graft), body part involved, and size of defect in square centimeters (except for pinch grafts, which are measured in centimeters). The skin replacement/substitute procedures include simple debridement of granulations or recent avulsion. If the donor site requires skin grafting or local flaps, an additional code should be reported. CPT code 15040 is to be assigned for harvesting of skin for tissue-cultured skin autograft. (See Figure 4.3 for an illustration of a skin graft.)

The following definitions are helpful when coding free skin grafts:

- *Pinch graft:* This is a piece of skin graft about 0.25 inch in diameter that is obtained by elevating the skin with a needle and slicing it off with a knife.

- *Split-thickness graft:* This graft consists of only the superficial layers of the dermis.

- *Full-thickness graft:* This graft is composed of skin and subcutaneous tissues.

- *Allograft:* This graft is obtained from a genetically dissimilar individual of the same species (one individual to another). It is also known as allogenic graft and homograft.

- *Autograft:* A graft transferred from one part of the patient's body to another part.

- *Xenograft:* This graft is obtained from a species different from the recipient (for example, animal to human). It is also called xenogenic graft, heterograft, and hetero-transplant.

Removal of Skin Lesion with Skin Replacement/Substitute Graft

When an excision of a lesion requires a skin replacement/substitute graft for repair of the defect, the coder is directed to also assign a code to identify the excision of the lesion, using a code from the range 11400 through 11471 or 11600 through 11646.

Figure 4.3. Skin graft harvest

Preoperative Condition

Postoperative Condition

A full-thickness skin graft is taken from the thigh and sutured onto the right thumb.

Flaps (Skin and/or Deep Tissues)

This series of codes (15570–15738) includes procedures describing pedicle flaps, muscle, myocutaneous or fasciocutaneous flaps, and delayed flap transfers. The codes are categorized first by type of flap (for example, pedicle) and then by recipient body part.

Codes 15600 through 15630, which describe delayed transfer, identify the donor site, not the recipient site. An additional code should be reported when repair of the donor site requires skin grafting or local flaps.

The following definitions are helpful when coding flaps:

- *Pedicle flap:* This flap consists of detached skin and subcutaneous tissue in which the attached end or base contains an adequate blood supply. It is partially transferred to the recipient site with the base still attached to the donor site. After the recipient site has established a good blood supply, the base or pedicle is cut off and the graft completed.

- *Myocutaneous flap:* This flap involves the transfer of intact muscle, subcutaneous tissue, and skin as a single unit rotated on a relatively narrow blood supply of the muscle.

Exercise 4.9   Integumentary System

Assign appropriate CPT code(s) for the following procedure and indicate the index entries that were used to identify the code(s). Assign only CPT surgical codes (no E/M codes) and append any applicable modifiers.

1. Physician performs a wide resection of a 3.0-cm malignant skin lesion of the left leg. The defect required an adjacent tissue transfer measuring 15 cm^2.

    Code(s): _____

    Index entries: _____

    _____

Exercise 4.10   Integumentary System

Operative Report

Preoperative Diagnosis: Basal cell carcinoma of the forehead

Postoperative Diagnosis: Same

Procedure: Excision of basal cell carcinoma with split-thickness skin graft

The patient was given a local IV sedation and taken to the OR suite. The face and left thigh were prepped with Phisohex soap. The cancer was outlined for excision and measured 5 × 4 cm. The forehead was infiltrated with 1% Xylocaine with 1:100,000 epinephrine.

The cancer was excised and carried down to the frontalis muscle. A suture was placed at the 12 o'clock position. The specimen was sent to pathology for frozen section.

Attention was then turned to the skin graft. A pattern of the defect was transferred to the left anterior thigh using a new needle. A local infiltration was performed on the thigh. Using a freehand knife, a split-thickness skin graft was harvested. The thigh was treated with Tegaderm and a wraparound Kerliz and Ace wrap. The skin graft was applied and sutured to the forehead defect with running 5-0 plain catgut.

Xeroform with cotton soaked in glycerin was sutured with 4-0 silk. A sterile dressing was applied. The patient tolerated the procedure well, with no complications or blood loss.

Assign appropriate CPT code(s) for the preceding procedure and indicate the index entries that were used to identify the code(s). Assign only CPT surgical codes (no E/M codes) and append any applicable modifiers.

1. Code(s): _____

   Index entries: _____

   _____

Exercise 4.11   Integumentary System

Operative Report

Preoperative Diagnosis:	Open wound, left thigh, status post fasciotomy
Postoperative Diagnosis:	Same
Procedure:	Split-thickness skin graft, left thigh, donor site from left thigh. Graft was approximately 12 × 5 cm.

The patient is a status post trauma. He had a tree fall on him and sustained a significant injury to his thigh. He had compartment syndrome of his thigh requiring a fasciotomy. He presents today for a skin graft to the fasciotomy site.

The patient was brought to the operating room and placed supine on the operating table. Following the adequate induction of general anesthesia, his left thigh and fasciotomy site were prepped and draped in the standard surgical fashion. Attention was first directed to the patient's anterior thigh. The Betadine prep was gently removed with normal saline. We then applied mineral oil to the anterior thigh. We then used a dermatome to harvest an approximately 12 × 5-cm split-thickness skin graft in the depth of 0.015. Following removal of our donor site, an epinephrine-soaked sponge was applied to the donor site. We then went in to the back table and meshed our graft 1:1. Following this, we prepared our graft bed for graft placement. The excellent granulation tissue bed was roughed up using a gauze sponge, and the skin graft was applied and secured in place using surgical staples. The edge of the skin was then trimmed accordingly. Following adequate placement and securing our graft, we then fashioned the dressing. A Bacitracin-coated Adaptic was then applied over the graft and Reston foam was applied over that. Fine mesh gauze was then used to secure it in place, and the Reston and mesh gauze were secured also using surgical staples. There was an excellent compression against the graft. Following this, we turned our attention to the donor site. Epinephrine-soaked gauze was removed, and Calgiswab dressing was applied. There was excellent hemostasis from the donor site. Following this, a Kerlix roll was placed around the left thigh and secured with paper tape. The patient tolerated the procedure without complications. The patient was then taken to the PACU for recovery.

Assign appropriate CPT code(s) for the preceding procedure and indicate the index entries that were used to identify the code(s). Assign only CPT surgical codes (no E/M codes) and append any applicable modifiers.

1. Code(s): _____

    Index entries: _____

    _____

Surgical Procedures of the Breast

Codes 19000 through 19499 describe procedures performed on the breast, such as biopsy, mastectomy, and reconstruction. These codes are categorized first by general type of procedure (incision, excision, reconstruction/repair) and then by specific procedure.

The codes describing breast procedures refer to unilateral procedures, and modifiers LT or RT should be appended. If a bilateral procedure is performed, modifier 50 should be reported.

Breast Biopsy

In coding breast biopsies, the coder must determine the type of biopsy performed: percutaneous, excisional, or incisional:

- *Percutaneous biopsy:* A biopsy that involves the insertion of a hollow needle to remove a biopsy specimen of breast tissue. This procedure is reported with code 19100.

- *Excisional biopsy:* A biopsy that involves total removal of the lesion, whether malignant or benign, from the breast. To make this determination, the coder should review both the operative report and the pathology report. The operative report may indicate that the lesion was removed completely. In the case of malignant lesions, the pathology report may indicate that the margins of the specimen are negative for malignancy or free of tumor. If the excisional biopsy was performed with identification by preoperative placement of radiological marker, codes 19125 through 19126 should be reported. When appropriate, an additional code(s) to describe placement of the needle localization wire (19290–19291) or metallic localization clip (19295) should be reported.

- *Incisional biopsy:* A biopsy of the breast (19101) that typically involves removal of only a portion of the lesion for pathologic examination.

Mastectomy

Codes 19140 through 19240 describe the various types of mastectomy:

- Code 19160, Partial mastectomy, refers to the partial removal of part of the breast tissue, leaving the breast almost intact. This also may be referred to as a lobectomy or lumpectomy.

- Code 19180, Simple, complete mastectomy, is assigned for the excision of all the breast tissue, with the lymph nodes and muscle left intact.

- Code 19182, Subcutaneous mastectomy, is used for excision of breast tissue with the skin and nipple intact.

- Code 19200, Radical mastectomy, refers to the excision of breast tissue including the pectoral muscles and the axillary lymph nodes.

- Code 19220, also described as a radical mastectomy, is assigned for the excision of breast tissue including the pectoral muscles and axillary and internal mammary lymph nodes.

- Code 19240, Modified radical mastectomy, is used for the excision of breast tissue including the axillary lymph nodes. The pectoralis minor muscles may or may not be removed, but the pectoralis major muscles are left intact.

Insertion of breast prosthesis may be reported as an additional code when performed at the same time as the mastectomy (19340) or when performed at a later date (19342).

Exercise 4.12 Integumentary System

Physician Office Operative Note

This patient has come to see me for follow-up for a cyst present in the left breast area. I did a needle aspiration biopsy, and fluid was sent out for cytology. If the biopsy is negative, I can see him back in the office in four months, or earlier if there are any problems.

The right breast feels benign. There is no axillary adenopathy. No cervical adenopathy.

Hospital pathology of a sample from a left breast aspiration revealed only a few benign lipocytes.

Assign appropriate CPT code(s) for the preceding procedure and indicate the index entries that were used to identify the code(s). Assign only CPT surgical codes (no E/M codes) and append any applicable modifiers.

1. Code(s): _____

    Index entries: _____

    _____

Exercise 4.13 Integumentary System

Operative Report

Preoperative Diagnosis: Abnormal mammogram, left breast

Postoperative Diagnosis: Same

The patient is a 61-year-old G3, P3 female with a family history of positive carcinoma of the breast. She underwent a screening mammogram in the spring of this year that demonstrated a localized density in the subareolar tissue of the left breast. Physical exam demonstrated no palpable abnormality in the area.

The patient was brought to the OR after undergoing placement of a hook wire localizing needle in the mammography suite by the radiologist. She was placed on the OR table in a supine position. After ensuring an adequate level of conscious sedation, her left breast and chest wall were prepped and draped in a sterile fashion. A needle/wire complex was protruding from the left breast approximately 2 centimeters above the nipple. The skin surrounding the needle in the breast tissue in the subareolar area was infiltrated with 1% Xylocaine to achieve local anesthesia. A 5-centimeter incision was made around the localizing wire. Small superior and inferior skin flaps were elevated, exposing the underlying subcutaneous fat. Dissection with electrocautery was begun into the breast about the wire. The needle wire complex was grasped using Allis clamps and drawn into the operative wound. The breast tissue and subcutaneous fat surrounding the needle were excised in this fashion until all the tissue surrounding the needle/wire complex was excised. The specimen was then forwarded to the radiology suite for specimen mammography.

As the specimen mammogram was being obtained, the wound was examined for hemostasis, which was felt to be complete. The deeper breast tissues were closed using interrupted 3-0 Vicryl figure-of-eight sutures. Subcutaneous tissues were approximated in a similar fashion. The wound was irrigated and again examined for hemostasis, which was felt to be complete. The skin was closed using a running 5-0 Maxon subcuticular suture. The wound was washed and dried and sterile dressings applied. The operative field was not disturbed until a call was received from the radiology suite indicating that the specimen contained the area of interest identified on the patient's original mammogram. At this point, the patient was transferred to the recovery area in stable condition.

Assign appropriate CPT code(s) for the preceding procedure and indicate the index entries that were used to identify the code(s). Assign only CPT surgical codes (no E/M codes) and append any applicable modifiers.

1. Code(s): _____

    Index entries: _____

    _____

Exercise 4.14   Integumentary System

Operative Report

Preoperative Diagnosis: Probable carcinoma of the right breast

Postoperative Diagnosis: Carcinoma of the right breast

Operation: Excisional biopsy

The patient was brought to the OR. Under satisfactory general endotracheal anesthesia, the right breast was prepped and draped in the usual manner. Through an elliptical incision in the upper outer quadrant, a small nodule was excised. Bleeders were electrocoagulated. The deep layer was closed with interrupted 3-0 Vicryl. The skin was closed with clips. A dry sterile dressing was applied, and the patient returned to the recovery room in good condition.

Pathology Report

Clinical Diagnosis: Right breast mass

Specimen: Mass, right breast, frozen section

Pathological Diagnosis: Breast mass, right: infiltrating ductal carcinoma, Grade 2/3, 0.7 cm; resected margins negative for carcinoma

Assign appropriate CPT code(s) for the preceding procedure and indicate the index entries that were used to identify the code(s). Assign only CPT surgical codes (no E/M codes) and append any applicable modifiers.

1. Code(s): _____

    Index entries: _____

    _____

Exercise 4.15   Integumentary System Review

Assign appropriate CPT code(s) for the following procedures and indicate the index entries that were used to identify the code(s). Assign only CPT surgical codes (no E/M codes) and append any applicable modifiers.

1. Debridement and dressing of first-degree (partial-thickness) burn of the index finger

    Code(s): _____

    Index entries: _____

    _____

2. Wide excision of a malignant lesion of arm (3.0 × 2.0 cm) with adjacent skin graft

    Code(s): _____

    Index entries: _____

    _____

3. Layered closure of 2.0-cm laceration of right forearm and 2.5 cm of left elbow

    Code(s): _____

    Index entries: _____

    _____

(Continued on next page)

Exercise 4.15   (Continued)

4. With the use of imaging, the surgeon placed a metallic clip to identify the suspicious tissue in the left breast. A percutaneous needle core biopsy was performed.

   Code(s): _____

   Index entries: _____

   _____

5. Excision of malignant melanoma of left arm (3.0 × 1.5 cm, with 1.0-cm margins surrounding the lesion)

   Code(s): _____

   Index entries: _____

   _____

6. Excision of pilonidal cyst requiring single-layer suture

   Code(s): _____

   Index entries: _____

   _____

7. Complete excision of nail and matrix, left great toe

   Code(s): _____

   Index entries: _____

   _____

8. Dermabrasion of cheek for severe acne

   Code(s): _____

   Index entries: _____

   _____

9. Electrosurgical removal of 3.0-cm squamous cell carcinoma of the hand

   Code(s): _____

   Index entries: _____

   _____

10. Excision of sacral decubitus ulcer with primary suture

    Code(s): _____

    Index entries: _____

    _____

Musculoskeletal System

The musculoskeletal subsection is categorized first by body part and then by general type of procedure, with the individual codes describing the specific procedure performed. The first series of codes (20000–20999) describes general musculoskeletal procedures such as bone biopsy, application of fixation device, bone graft, replantation of body part, wound exploration, and arthrocentesis. A lengthy note at the beginning of this subsection defines terms related to the treatment of fractures.

The codes listed in this subsection include the application and removal of the first cast and/or traction device. Subsequent replacement of the cast and/or traction device may be reported with codes 29000 through 29799 and codes located at the beginning of the general subsection.

Fractures and Dislocations

To report the diagnosis and treatment of fractures and dislocations accurately, coders must answer the following questions:

- *What body site is involved?* The operative report and/or any diagnostic tests performed, such as x-rays or computed tomography (CT) scans, should be reviewed.

- *Was the fracture/dislocation treatment open or closed or with percutaneous skeletal fixation?* Closed treatment refers to treatment of the fracture/dislocation without a surgical incision into the site. Open treatment refers to the treatment of a fracture or dislocation that includes exposing the site via a surgical incision or when a fractured bone is opened remote from the fracture site in order to insert an intramedullary nail across the fracture site (fracture site is not opened and visualized). Percutaneous skeletal fixation involves treatment of a fracture by placing fixation devices such as pins across the fracture site, usually under x-ray imaging.

- *Was the fracture/dislocation manipulated?* Manipulation refers to the attempted reduction or restoration of a dislocated joint or fracture. CPT codes are available for reporting nondisplaced fractures treated without manipulation.

    Example: Code 27238 is used for reporting closed treatment of an intertrochanteric fracture, without manipulation.

- *Did the procedure include internal or external fixation?*

Application of Casts and Strapping

The series of codes (29000–29750) describing the application of casts and strapping can be reported in the following scenarios:

- To identify replacement of a cast or strapping during or after the period of normal follow-up care (global postoperative period)

- To identify an initial service performed without any restorative treatment or stabilization of the fracture, injury, or dislocation and/or to afford pain relief to the patient

- To identify an initial cast or strapping when the same physician does not perform, or is not expected to perform, any other treatment or procedure

- To identify an initial cast or strapping when another physician provided or will provide restorative treatment

CPT guidelines for hospital outpatient reporting of casting/strapping/splinting can be found in *CPT Assistant* (Vol. 12, Issue 4, April 2002).

Exercise 4.16 Musculoskeletal System

Assign appropriate CPT code(s) for the following procedures and indicate the index entries that were used to identify the codes. Assign only CPT surgical codes (no E/M codes) and append any applicable modifiers.

1. Diagnosis: Closed fracture of ulnar shaft, left
   Procedure: Open reduction of ulnar shaft fracture

   Code(s): _____

   Index entries: _____

   _____

2. Closed treatment of two uncomplicated rib fractures

   Code(s): _____

   Index entries: _____

   _____

3. Closed reduction of proximal humerus fracture, right

   Code(s): _____

   Index entries: _____

   _____

4. The orthopedic surgeon reduces a fracture of the right proximal tibia. After closed treatment and skeletal traction, the physician applies a short leg cast.

   Code(s): _____

   Index entries: _____

   _____

5. The patient was diagnosed with a dislocated right patella. Under anesthesia, the surgeon performed a closed reduction.

   Code(s): _____

   Index entries: _____

   _____

6. Open reduction with internal fixation, fracture of distal end (medial condyle) of left femur

   Code(s): _____

   Index entries: _____

   _____

7. Patient is diagnosed with right humeral shaft fracture. The orthopedic surgeon performs an open treatment of the fracture using an intramedullary implant and locking screws.

   Code(s): _____

   Index entries: _____

   _____

Exercise 4.17   Musculoskeletal System

Emergency Department Record

Chief Complaint: Right ankle injury

History of Present Illness: The patient is a 39-year-old female who injured her right ankle yesterday. While stepping around some puppies to avoid hitting them, she suffered an inversion injury to her ankle. She complains of lateral ankle and foot pain, and has pain on weight bearing.

Past Medical History: Status post hysterectomy

Medications: None

Allergies: Codeine, which causes nausea

Physical Examination: Alert female in no acute distress. Right lower extremity: proximal mid tibia-fibula are nontender. Ankle shows moderate diffuse swelling over the lateral ankle extending onto the dorsolateral foot with ecchymoses. Good distal neurovascular status. Decreased range of motion secondary to pain and swelling.

Emergency Department Course: X-ray of right foot and ankle shows an avulsion fragment off the distal fibula, otherwise soft tissue swelling.

Diagnosis: Acute right ankle sprain with avulsion fracture

Disposition and Plan: Short leg splint applied. Crutches. No weight bearing. Ice and elevate. Vicodin #30 1–2q 4–6 h. She tolerates it well. Orthopedic referral.

Assign appropriate CPT code(s) for the preceding procedure and indicate the index entries that were used to identify the code(s). Assign only CPT surgical codes (no E/M codes) and append any applicable modifiers.

1. Code(s): _____

   Index entries: _____

   _____

Exercise 4.18   Musculoskeletal System

Operative Report

Preoperative Diagnosis: Fracture of distal fibula, left

Postoperative Diagnosis: Same

Procedure: Closed reduction of fibular fracture

This 14-year-old gymnast feels pain in her left leg after vaulting at practice. She is unable to bear any weight on her foot.

Physical examination showed foot and ankle to be normal. The neurovascular status of the foot was normal. The ankle was nontender and not swollen. Findings were confined to the distal fibula, two inches proximal to the lateral malleolus. There was point tenderness in this area. An x-ray of the tibia and fibula shows a displaced fracture of the distal fibula.

The fracture was reduced and the patient placed in a short leg splint with extensive padding over the fracture site. She was given Tylenol #3 for pain and instructed to follow up with her physician in 10 days.

Assign appropriate CPT code(s) for the preceding procedure and indicate the index entries that were used to identify the code(s). Assign only CPT surgical codes (no E/M codes) and append any applicable modifiers.

1. Code(s): _____

   Index entries: _____

   _____

Arthroscopy

Procedures describing both diagnostic and therapeutic arthroscopy are reported with codes 29800 through 29909. These codes are categorized first by body part involved and then by type—surgical or diagnostic. The surgical arthroscopic codes are further divided to identify the specific procedure performed, such as synovectomy or debridement. A surgical arthroscopy always includes a diagnostic component that should not be reported separately. Figure 4.4 illustrates an arthroscopy of the knee.

Exercise 4.19   Musculoskeletal System

Assign appropriate CPT code(s) for the following procedures and indicate the index entries that were used to identify the codes. Assign only CPT surgical codes (no E/M codes) and append any applicable modifiers.

1. Arthroscopic synovectomy (limited) of the left knee

   Code(s): _____

   Index entries: _____

   _____

2. Arthroscopy of right shoulder with rotator cuff repair

   Code(s): _____

   Index entries: _____

   _____

3. Arthroscopy of the left wrist with repair of triangular fibrocartilage and joint debridement

   Code(s): _____

   Index entries: _____

   _____

4. Arthroscopy of the left elbow with limited debridement

   Code(s): _____

   Index entries: _____

   _____

Figure 4.4.   Knee surgery—injuries with arthroscopic repair

Grade II chondro-malacia

Radial tear

Horizontal tear

Medial

Lateral

Radial tear

Horizontal tear

Superior view of meniscii

Inflow and outflow cannula in superolateral portal

A. Entrance portals are created in the knee and the arthroscopic instruments are inserted.

Shaver in inferomedial portal

Arthroscope in inferolateral portal

B. The retropatellar chondromalacia is debrided with the shaver.

Postoperative Condition

C. Partial meniscectomies are performed on the medial meniscus and lateral meniscus.

Exercise 4.20 Musculoskeletal System

Operative Report

Preoperative Diagnosis: Tear of the right medial meniscus

Postoperative Diagnosis: Same

Operation: Meniscus repair

The patient was brought to the OR and anesthetized. An inflatable tourniquet was placed about the proximal thigh, and the operative area was prepped and draped in a sterile fashion with the leg placed in the instrument maker leg holder. Following this, incisions were made for insertion of the arthroscope inflow cannula and probe. Video arthroscopy was then carried out. He was found to have a tear of the posterior horn of the medial meniscus, and this was repaired. The anterior cruciate ligament was examined and found to be intact. The lateral meniscus also appeared to be intact. The patellofemoral joint was within normal limits. While the patient was asleep, the knee was examined and stressed. There was no opening of the medial collateral ligament region and no instability in that area. After completion of the arthroscopy, the instruments were withdrawn from the wound and the incisions closed. The incisions were injected marginally with local anesthetic for postoperative analgesia. After closure of the incisions, Betadine ointment and dressings were placed over the knee and the patient was returned to the recovery room in stable condition.

Assign appropriate CPT code(s) for the preceding procedure and indicate the index entries that were used to identify the code(s). Assign only CPT surgical codes (no E/M codes) and append any applicable modifiers.

1. Code(s): _____

   Index entries: _____

   _____

Exercise 4.21 Musculoskeletal System Review

Assign appropriate CPT code(s) for the following procedures and indicate the index entries that were used to identify the codes. Assign only CPT surgical codes (no E/M codes) and append any applicable modifiers.

1. Closed reduction of two metatarsal fractures of left foot

   Code(s): _____

   Index entries: _____

   _____

2. Repair of hammertoe, second digit of left foot

   Code(s): _____

   Index entries: _____

   _____

3. Open reduction of fracture of right medial malleolus with external fixation

   Code(s): _____

   Index entries: _____

   _____

Exercise 4.21   (Continued)

4. Surgical exploration of stab wound of chest with included coagulation of blood vessels and enlargement of the wound.

    Code(s): _____

    Index entries: _____

    _____

5. Incision and drainage of hematoma of shoulder

    Code(s): _____

    Index entries: _____

    _____

6. Repair of lateral collateral ligament of right elbow using local tissue

    Code(s): _____

    Index entries: _____

    _____

7. Midtarsal arthrodesis, left foot

    Code(s): _____

    Index entries: _____

    _____

8. Arthroscopy of the right wrist with partial synovectomy

    Code(s): _____

    Index entries: _____

    _____

9. Excision of bone cyst, toe (third digit of left foot)

    Code(s): _____

    Index entries: _____

    _____

10. Removal of sliver of metal from deep tissue in the right knee

    Code(s): _____

    Index entries: _____

    _____

Respiratory System

The respiratory subsection includes surgical procedures involving the nose and sinuses, larynx, trachea and bronchi, and lungs and pleura. Figures 4.5 and 4.6 illustrate the respiratory system.

Nasal Sinus Endoscopy

Codes 31231 through 31294 describe nasal sinus endoscopic procedures. These procedures allow the physician to visualize the interior of the nasal cavity, the middle and superior meatus,

Figure 4.5. The upper respiratory system

Figure 4.6.   The lower respiratory system

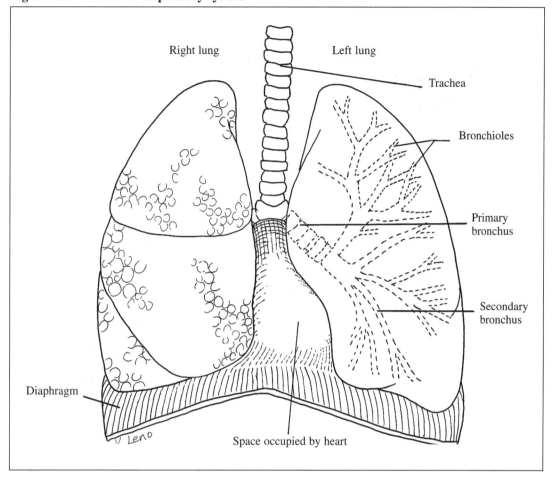

the turbinates, and the sphenoethmoid recess. The purpose of the procedures may be either diagnostic or surgical in nature. A surgical endoscopy may be performed to control a nosebleed or to perform a maxillary antrostomy or sphenoidotomy. The coder should always review the documentation carefully to clarify the extent of the procedure. A surgical endoscopy includes the diagnostic component. The diagnostic endoscopy should not be reported separately when performed during the same operative episode. Also, if performed, a sinusotomy is considered part of the endoscopic procedure and not reported separately.

Unless otherwise stated, codes in the 31231 through 31294 range are assumed to be unilateral. When the documentation indicates that a bilateral procedure was performed and the specific code does not state *bilateral,* modifier –50 may be assigned. Key points to remember include:

- Separate codes should not be assigned to identify a diagnostic nasal/sinus endoscopy when it is performed in conjunction with a surgical nasal/sinus endoscopy.

- A surgical endoscopy includes a sinusotomy. Only the code for the surgical endoscopy should be assigned when both are performed during the same operative episode.

- Modifier –50 should be assigned to identify a bilateral procedure only if the code does not specify bilateral.

Exercise 4.22   Respiratory System

Assign appropriate CPT code(s) for the following procedures and indicate the index entries that were used to identify the codes. Assign only CPT surgical codes (no E/M codes) and append any applicable modifiers.

1. Bilateral nasal endoscopy with total ethmoidectomy

    Code(s): _____

    Index entries: _____

    _____

2. Left nasal endoscopy for control of epistaxis

    Code(s): _____

    Index entries: _____

    _____

3. Diagnostic maxillary sinusoscopy, bilateral

    Code(s): _____

    Index entries: _____

    _____

Exercise 4.23 Respiratory System

Operative Report

Preoperative Diagnosis: Deviated nasal septum, chronic maxillary sinusitis, turbinate hypertrophy, nasal obstruction

Postoperative Diagnosis: Same

Procedure Performed:
1. Septoplasty
2. Nasal endoscopy, with bilateral maxillary antroscopy, removal of maxillary polyp
3. Submucous resection of the inferior turbinates, bilaterally

This twenty-six-year-old female was seen by ENT Service for complaints of chronic sinusitis and difficulty breathing through the nose. She was noted to have a severely deviated septum toward the right with turbinate hypertrophy, nasal obstruction (CT scans confirmed this), as well as obstruction of the ostiomeatal complexes with mucosal thickening. A decision for the above-stated procedure was then made after she had failed conservative care.

The patient was brought to the operative suite, given general anesthetic, and properly prepped and draped. 5% cocaine pledgets were placed in each nasal chamber. 1% lidocaine with 1:100,000 epinephrine were injected into the caudal columnar region into the septum, as well as the middle uncinate middle turbinate region. Then, with the #1 scalp blade, an incision was made along the left caudal columnar region in the septum, down to the mucoperichondrium. The mucoperichondrium was carefully elevated off the nasal septum cartilage, exposing a portion of the deviation. The contralateral portion was also freed up. With a Seiler knife, a portion of the deviation was removed. A large septal spur, touching the lateral wall, was carefully freed up and removed.

After the patient exhibited a much improved nasal septum, a piece of cartilage was morselized and inserted between the septal mucosa layers and the submucosa was closed with 4-0 plain suture in interrupted form. Attention was then brought to the middle turbinates, which were found to be lateralized. A decision to medialize them was made by placing 4-0 Vicryl to the left middle turbinate, sent through the right middle turbinate, back to the septum, and tied off on the left side.

Next, with the scope, the left nasal chamber was examined. The natural os was located. With the frontal probe, it was further enlarged with microbiter straight shot and back-biters. There was a moderate amount of mucosal thickening around this opening, just on the inside. After it was widely patent and cleaned out, attention was brought to the right side. The right os was located in a similar fashion and widely enlarged with the microbiter straight shot and back-biters. Again, a moderate amount of mucosal thickening was noted around this opening. When this was completed, attention was brought to the inferior turbinates.

The inferior turbinates were infractured and clamped with a Carmel clamp for five minutes, then submucosal resection was performed in the usual fashion. The rods of the turbinates were then cauterized with suction cautery. This was repeated in a similar fashion bilaterally. Silastic splints were sewn into place along the septum with 3-0 Ethilon, and tampons coated in Bactroban were inserted into both nasal chambers. The oral cavity was suctioned of all serosanguineous debris, and the patient exhibited good hemostasis. She was taken out of her anesthetic and transferred to the recovery room in stable condition.

Assign appropriate CPT code(s) for the preceding procedure and indicate the index entries that were used to identify the code(s). Assign only CPT surgical codes (no E/M codes) and append any applicable modifiers.

1. Code(s) to be submitted for the *hospital* services: _____

    _____

    Index entries: _____

    _____

Laryngoscopy

A laryngoscopy is an endoscopic procedure that allows the physician to visualize the larynx, or voice box. This examination may be diagnostic only or may be performed for surgical purposes such as for a biopsy or removal of a lesion. Codes 31505–31579 describe these diagnostic and surgical endoscopic procedures.

Codes 31505 through 31513 refer to an indirect laryngoscopy. An indirect laryngoscopy is the simplest way to examine the larynx. One technique involves the use of a small mirror placed in the back of the throat. With the aid of a light source, the image of the larynx can be visualized in the mirror. The physician may view the image of the oropharynx, posterior third of the tongue, lateral laryngeal walls, posterior pharyngeal wall, epiglottis, valleculae, and piriform sinuses. He or she also may be able to view the aryepiglottic folds, posterior epiglottis, and vocal cords. Although an indirect laryngoscopy is the simplest and least expensive way to examine the larynx, it does require a great deal of skill on the part of the physician. Moreover, this technique may be impossible to perform on a patient who has a strong gag reflex and cannot be used on small children.

Codes 31515 through 31571 are used to identify a direct laryngoscopy. This range of codes identifies the performance of procedures such as biopsy, removal of a lesion, arytenoidectomy, and removal of a foreign body. Laryngoscopes that are commonly used include Kleinsasser, Jako, Dedo, Jackson, Lindholm, Nagashima, Holinger, and Benjamin. During this complex procedure, the physician looks directly at the larynx. The patient is usually placed under general anesthesia to avoid the difficulties associated with the gag reflex. A microscope also may be used during the procedure to magnify the image of the larynx. Because the code assignment will be affected, the coder should review the operative report carefully for any mention of a microscope or for terms such as "microlaryngoscopy." It is inappropriate to use code 69990, Use of operating microscope, in addition to any laryngoscopy code identified as being done with an operating microscope.

Codes 31575 through 31578 are used for a laryngoscopy performed with flexible fiberoptic equipment. After administration of a topical anesthesia and vasoconstrictor, the instrument is passed through the nasal cavity. This type of laryngoscope provides a more comfortable approach to visualizing the larynx, the pharynx, and the nasal cavity.

Code 31579 identifies a laryngoscopy with stroboscopy. A strobe light provides a very bright light in short flashes. Because of the flashing produced by the stroboscopy, the physician is better able to examine moving vocal cords.

The following questions should be answered before assigning codes for laryngoscopies:

- *What was the purpose of the laryngoscopy?*

- *Which type of laryngoscope was used: direct, indirect, or flexible fiberoptic?*

- *Was a stroboscopy used?*

In cases during which an operating microscope was used, the combination code should be assigned and not code 69990.

Exercise 4.24   Respiratory System

Assign appropriate CPT code(s) for the following procedures and indicate the index entries that were used to identify the codes. Assign only CPT surgical codes (no E/M codes) and append any applicable modifiers.

1. Direct laryngoscopy with stripping of vocal cords

    Code(s): _____

    Index entries: _____

    _____

2. Flexible fiberoptic laryngoscopy performed for removal of a dime lodged in the patient's larynx

    Code(s): _____

    Index entries: _____

    _____

3. Indirect laryngoscopy with biopsy

    Code(s): _____

    Index entries: _____

    _____

4. Using an operating microscope, the surgeon performs a laryngoscopy with excision of a polyp

    Code(s): _____

    Index entries: _____

    _____

Exercise 4.25   Respiratory System

Operative Report

Preoperative Diagnosis: Laryngeal lesion

Postoperative Diagnosis: Same

Operation: Direct laryngoscopy and biopsy of vocal cord lesion using an operating microscope

The patient was placed on the OR table in the supine position, induced under general anesthesia, and intubated. The Dedo laryngoscope was introduced into the oral cavity, slipped under the tip of the epiglottis, and suspended from the Lewy suspension apparatus. The lesion involved the entire left vocal cord and extended through the ventricle to the false vocal cord and into the anterior commissure area. It also slightly involved the anterior portion of the right vocal cord. In addition, some subglottic extension was present. A biopsy was taken and sent out for frozen section. The laryngoscope was then removed and the procedure terminated. The patient tolerated the procedure well and left the room in good condition.

Assign appropriate CPT code(s) for the preceding procedure and indicate the index entries that were used to identify the code(s). Assign only CPT surgical codes (no E/M codes) and append any applicable modifiers.

1. Code(s): _____

    Index entries: _____

    _____

Bronchoscopy

A bronchoscope is an instrument that can be inserted into either the nose or the mouth and passed through the trachea, past the larynx, and into the bronchial tubes. Indications for this procedure include hemoptysis, a persistent cough that is unresponsive to medication, shortness of breath, an acute upper airway obstruction, or an abnormal chest x-ray or infection.

A physician may elect to use a flexible or rigid bronchoscope. The rigid scope, also referred to as an open-tube bronchoscope, is inserted through the mouth and most often is used to remove foreign objects or to secure a larger-than-normal biopsy sample. The more commonly performed flexible bronchoscopy consists of a flexible tube with many small glass fibers that allow the transmission of light. Codes in the 31622 through 31656 range are used to identify a variety of procedures using either type of bronchoscope.

The note at the beginning of this section advises coders that a surgical bronchoscopy includes a diagnostic bronchoscopy. It is important to note that codes 31622–31646 include fluoroscopic guidance. Fluoroscopic equipment serves as an image intensifier and is frequently used during bronchoscopies. It is incorrect to use an additional code to identify fluoroscopy.

Frequently, the purpose of the bronchoscopy is to obtain tissue to allow the physician to make an accurate diagnosis. Specimens may be collected in several ways. Cell washings may be obtained by introducing saline solution into the airways, which then is removed and sent to the lab for cytological examination. Code 31622 identifies a bronchoscopy *with* or *without* cell washings.

Brushings of tissue is another method of specimen collection. One advantage to this method is that brushings allow the diagnosis to be made on the basis of tissue that could not be obtained normally with biopsy forceps. Either a fixed brush or a protected specimen brush (PSB) may be introduced through the bronchoscope. A PSB is a brush contained in a double catheter. A wax plug at the top prevents contamination of the specimen by upper airway flora. Code 31623 is assigned when a bronchoscopy is performed to collect specimen(s) with either a fixed brush or a PSB.

Code 31624 identifies a bronchoscopy with bronchial alveolar lavage (BAL). This procedure is performed to collect cells from peripheral lung tissue. During a BAL, sterile saline is instilled into the airway in aliquots of 20 ml up to 50 ml. The saline is suctioned out and sent for cytological examination. Code 32997 is assigned for total lung lavage (unilateral).

When a lesion can be visualized with the bronchoscope, the physician may elect to use forceps to obtain a sample of tissue. This procedure allows a more precise piece of tissue to be obtained for pathological diagnosis. Code 31625 is used to identify a bronchoscopy with bronchial or endobronchial biopsy, single or multiple sites.

When the diagnosis of a lung disease requires a sample of lung tissue, a transbronchial lung biopsy may be performed. During the bronchoscopy, forceps are used to puncture the bronchus and take samples of the lung tissue. This procedure is less invasive than an open-lung biopsy and thus carries less risk of morbidity. Code 31628 is assigned to identify a bronchoscopy with a transbronchial lung biopsy of a single lobe. To report transbronchial lung biopsies performed in additional lobes, assign add-on code 31632.

The following questions should be answered before assigning a code for a bronchoscopy:

- *Why was the bronchoscopy performed?*

- *Was a diagnostic bronchoscopy performed in conjunction with a surgical bronchoscopy?* If so, only the code for the surgical procedure should be assigned.

- *Was the procedure one of the bronchoscopies described by a code from the series 31622 through 31646?* If so, a separate code to identify fluoroscopy should not be assigned because fluoroscopic guidance is considered part of the procedures identified by that series of codes.

Exercise 4.26   Respiratory System

Assign appropriate CPT code(s) for the following procedures and indicate the index entries that were used to identify the codes. Assign only CPT surgical codes (no E/M codes) and append any applicable modifiers.

1.   Bronchoscopy with transbronchial biopsy of lung

   Code(s): _____

   Index entries: _____

   _____

2.   Bronchoscopy with laser destruction of a lesion of the bronchus

   Code(s): _____

   Index entries: _____

   _____

3.   Flexible bronchoscopy with cell washings, brushings, and biopsy

   Code(s): _____

   Index entries: _____

   _____

Exercise 4.27   Respiratory System

Operative Report

Preoperative Diagnosis:	Persistent cough, dyspnea
Postoperative Diagnosis:	Probable bronchitis
Procedure:	Bronchoscopy
Medications:	Versed 13 mg given just prior to and during the procedure; topical aerosolized lidocaine and atropine 0.4 mg IM and aerosolized albuterol 2.5 mg

The left nares was cannulated. The posterior nasopharynx was normal. The vocal cords, although with exogenous tissue consistent with obesity, were normal and normally apposed. The main carina was normal as was the trachea itself. The left lower lobe anatomy was a variant of normal with two main subsegments, each having three sub-subsegments in the left upper lobe. Very slight erythema is seen in the medial aspect of the left upper lobe subsegment. Brushings were obtained from this area.

The right inside anatomy was entirely normal. No endobronchial lesions were seen throughout.

Pathology

Gross Description:	Received are two prepared slides
Microscopic Description:	The bronchial brushing slides demonstrate benign bronchial epithelial cells and macrophages. The background contains mucus with minimal inflammation. There is no atypia or malignancy.
Diagnosis:	Lung, left upper lobe, bronchial brushings. Negative for malignant cells.

Assign appropriate CPT code(s) for the preceding procedure and indicate the index entries that were used to identify the code(s). Assign only CPT surgical codes (no E/M codes) and append any applicable modifiers.

1.   Code(s): _____

   Index entries: _____

   _____

Exercise 4.28   Respiratory System Review

Assign appropriate CPT code(s) for the following procedures and indicate the index entries that were used to identify the codes. Assign only CPT surgical codes (no E/M codes) and append any applicable modifiers.

1. Thoracoscopy with wedge resection of lung

   Code(s): _____

   Index entries: _____

   _____

2. Scalpel excision of polyp from inside the nose performed in the physician's office

   Code(s): _____

   Index entries: _____

   _____

3. Flexible bronchoscopy with bronchial biopsies

   Code(s): _____

   Index entries: _____

   _____

4. Removal of pebble from child's nasal passage performed in the physician's office

   Code(s): _____

   Index entries: _____

   _____

5. Nasal endoscopy with polypectomy

   Code(s): _____

   Index entries: _____

   _____

6. Patient treated in the emergency department for severe epistaxis; physician performs extensive anterior packing, bilateral

   Code(s): _____

   Index entries: _____

   _____

7. Direct laryngoscopy for removal of lesion

   Code(s): _____

   Index entries: _____

   _____

Exercise 4.28 (Continued)

8. Puncture aspiration of lung

   Code(s): _____

   Index entries: _____

   _____

9. Flexible fiberoptic laryngoscopy with biopsy of tissue

   Code(s): _____

   Index entries: _____

   _____

10. Partial excision of inferior turbinate

    Code(s): _____

    Index entries: _____

    _____

Cardiovascular System

The cardiovascular subsection includes surgical procedures involving the heart and pericardium, arteries, and veins. (Figure 4.7 illustrates the heart, veins, and arteries.) The codes are categorized first by body part involved and then by procedure performed, such as insertion of pacemaker, coronary artery bypass, embolectomy, and venipuncture. Assignment of codes for many of the cardiac procedures requires advanced knowledge and skill. The reference section of this book provides a list of recommended resources for coding cardiac procedures.

Vascular Injection Procedures

Careful review of the note at the beginning of this subsection will help the coder select the appropriate codes.

Intra-Arterial/Intra-Aortic Injections
Selective arterial catheterizations require that the catheter be removed, manipulated, or guided into a part of the arterial system other than the aorta or the vessel punctured. Nonselective arterial catheterizations involve placement of a catheter or needle directly into an artery, or a needle is negotiated only into the thoracic or abdominal aorta from any approach.

Intravenous Injections
Selective venous catheterizations include catheter placement in those veins that rise directly from the vena cava or the vein punctured directly (primary branches) and any subsequent (secondary) branches of the primary venous branches. Nonselective venous catheterizations involve direct puncture of peripheral veins and the vena cavae or placement of the catheter in the inferior or superior vena cava by any route.

Figure 4.7. The heart and the veins and arteries that branch from it

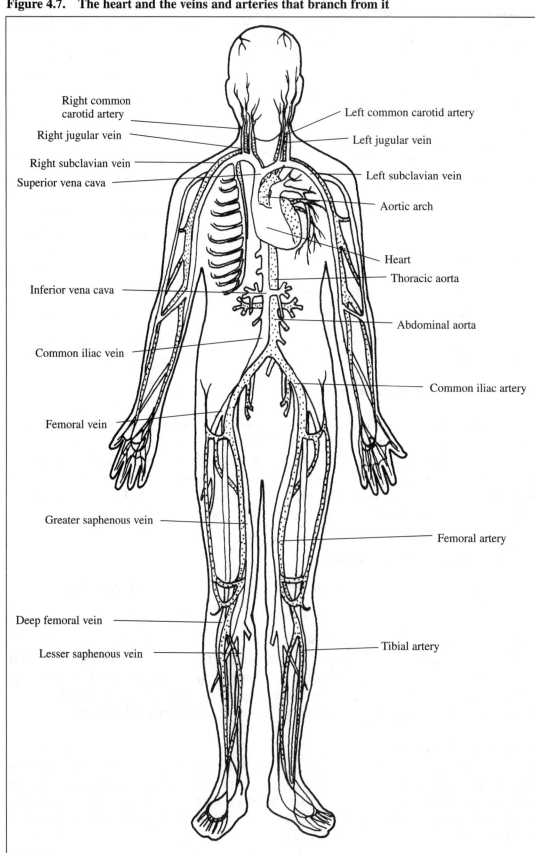

Right common carotid artery
Right jugular vein
Right subclavian vein
Superior vena cava
Left common carotid artery
Left jugular vein
Left subclavian vein
Aortic arch
Heart
Thoracic aorta
Inferior vena cava
Abdominal aorta
Common iliac vein
Common iliac artery
Femoral vein
Greater saphenous vein
Femoral artery
Deep femoral vein
Tibial artery
Lesser saphenous vein

Coronary Artery Bypass Grafting

Codes 33510 through 33545 describe procedures related to coronary artery bypass grafting (CABG). The first series of codes (33510–33516) is reported when the CABG uses only venous grafts, such as those obtained from the saphenous vein. To code this procedure accurately, the coder must review the operative report to determine the number of coronary venous grafts that were performed.

> **Example:** CABG of two coronary arteries using saphenous vein grafts. The code reported is 33511.

The second series of codes (33517–33530) describes a CABG that uses both arterial and venous grafts. As already mentioned, the saphenous vein usually provides the venous grafts and the arterial graft is usually created from the internal mammary artery. To fully code arterial-venous bypass grafting, two codes must be assigned: one from the 33517 through 33523 series to identify the number of venous grafts performed, and one from the 33533 through 33545 series to identify the number of arterial grafts. Careful review of the operative report is required to determine the type and number of grafts performed.

Cardioverter–Defibrillator Insertion/Removal

Pacemakers, pacing cardioverters, and defibrillator systems are classified with codes from the series 33200 through 33249. Guidelines in this section should be reviewed for descriptions of what comprises the various kinds of pacemaker and defibrillator systems. Figure 4.8 illustrates a pacemaker insertion.

Figure 4.8. Pacemaker insertion

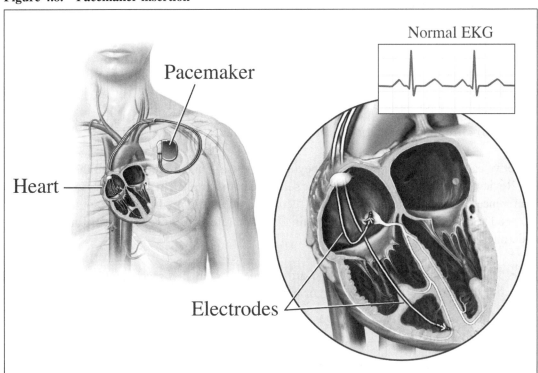

Interventional Radiology Procedures for Cardiovascular Conditions

Coding interventional radiology procedures for cardiovascular conditions requires a thorough understanding of coding guidelines and anatomy. Coders often refer to anatomic diagrams of the vascular families to assist with accurate coding assignment. Appendix L of the CPT book provides a reference list for the vascular families. The Society of Interventional Radiology publishes a book titled *Interventional Radiology Coding Users' Guide,* and AHIMA has offered several audio seminars that concentrate on CPT coding in this area. The purpose of this lesson is to provide an overview of coding guidelines. In order to be proficient at interventional radiology coding, more advanced study and practice are necessary.

Angiography

Most interventional angiography procedures have two components: a surgical component (involving, for example, injection of contrast solutions, implantation of devices, and removal of strictures with angioplasty balloons), and an imaging (radiology) component, which includes supervision and interpretation (S&I) of images.

Codes for diagnostic radiology are in the 70000 series of the CPT codebook. Most interventional radiology procedures require at least two codes. Hospitals generally bill for both of the above-mentioned components, and radiologists bill for both components (provided they performed both components).

Coding guidelines state that codes must be assigned for both the catheter placement (surgical component) and the imaging procedure (S&I component). There is not always a one-to-one correlation between the number of surgical codes and the number of S&I codes. Several anatomic areas may be imaged from the same catheter placement; therefore, the number of S&I codes may exceed the number of surgical component codes.

CPT coding decisions for angiography are based on whether the physician performed a selective or nonselective catheter placement. Nonselective catheter placement is one in which the vascular catheter is left in the vessel it punctured and not advanced any further or it is advanced into the aorta and not beyond. Examples of nonselective catheter placement CPT codes are as follows:

- 36200 Introduction of needle or intracatheter; retrograde brachial artery

- 36140 Introduction of needle or intracatheter, extremity artery

- 36145 Introduction of needle or intracatheter, arteriovenous shunt

Selective catheter placement is moved beyond the vessel punctured or beyond the aorta.

Review of the coding descriptions for selective catheter placement (36215–36248) reveals a reference to "order," such as first order, second order, and so on. It is important to emphasize the need to review anatomic diagrams/definitions and reference materials before attempting to code interventional radiology cases.

- CPT codes 36215 through 36217 are assigned for catheter placement in first-, second-, or third-order arteries (thoracic or brachiocephalic).

- CPT codes 36245 through 36247 are used for first-, second-, and third-order placement in abdominal, pelvic, and lower extremity arteries.

- Only two codes represent catheter placement on the venous side: 36011 and 36012.

The vascular family is divided into two parts:

- *Arterial vascular family:* A group of arteries fed by a primary branch of the aorta or a primary branch of the vessel punctured (that is, left common iliac artery, innominate artery, right renal artery)

- *Venous vascular family:* A group of veins that flows into a primary branch of the vena cava or a primary branch of the vessel punctured (that is, left iliac vein, right renal vein, left brachiocephalic vein)

Coding guidelines instruct coders to assign a code to the highest-order catheter placement within a vascular family. Each vascular family that is catheterized is coded separately. A code for nonselective catheter placement should not be assigned in addition to a selective catheter placement code unless there are multiple accesses (punctures).

> **Example:** A catheter is inserted in the femoral artery and passed into the aorta, into the brachiocephalic artery, and then further into the right common carotid artery.

The brachiocephalic is a first-order vessel and the right common carotid artery is a second-order vessel within the same vascular family. A code (36216) would be assigned for the second order only.

Supervision and interpretation (S&I) codes are used to describe the imaging component of the procedure. S&I codes are assigned based upon the vessels that are imaged, not the vessels that are catheterized.

> **Example:** A catheter is inserted into the femoral artery and advanced into the right common carotid (second order) and contrast injected, with imaging of the cervical and cerebral portions of the carotid circulation.

The correct coding assignment for this case would be 36216 for catheter placement and 75665 (cerebral) and 75676 (cervical) imaging.

Arteriovenous Fistulas and Grafts

Creating an arteriovenous (AV) fistula is the most desirable method for hemodialysis access because AV fistulas are less likely to clot or become infected than other methods and last longer. This procedure requires the surgeon to connect the artery to the vein. This abnormal connection between these two vessels causes more blood to flow from the artery directly to the vein under high arterial pressure. Eventually, the vein grows stronger and becomes thick-walled. This thick-walled vein becomes an ideal target to place the dialysis needles.

The CPT coding decision is based on whether the fistula was created by vein transposition or direct anastomosis. Codes for vein transposition are assigned according to the vein used:

- 36818 Upper arm (cephalic or brachiocephalic)
- 36819 Upper arm basilic vein
- 36820 Forearm vein (radio-cephalic)

The direct anastomosis method (36821) involves attaching an artery and a vein directly.

If an AV fistula is not possible because the patient's veins are too small or too far apart or there is not enough time to perform the procedure, the surgeon may elect to perform an arteriovenous (AV) graft (36825-36830) that connects the artery to the vein. AV fistulas require weeks or months to mature, but AV grafts require less time. A major disadvantage of AV grafts is that they often clot or become infected.

Complications of AV Fistulas and Grafts

Common complications of AV fistulas and grafts include clotting, obstruction, and narrowing of the access. Several CPT codes are provided for the procedures necessary to correct these complications.

There are several methods of treatment for stenoses, including angioplasty, stent placement, and thrombectomy. Thrombectomies can be performed with or without a revision of the graft, and CPT provides several codes to describe the various procedures:

- Thrombectomy, open, without revision (36831)

- Revision, open, without thrombectomy (36832)

- Revision, open, with thrombectomy (36833)

Percutaneous thrombectomy of a graft is coded with 36870, which includes all the work required to restore flow to the access. For this procedure, the thrombus may be removed pharmaceutically (that is, urokinase) or mechanically (AngioJet, small Fogarty-type balloons).

In addition to code 36870, additional procedures may be reported to identify the punctures of the graft. Two punctures are usually performed (both arterial and venous), each would be reported with CPT code 36145. Modifier –59 should be appended to the second code to indicate that a distinct, separate procedure was performed.

Because the venous anastomotic stenosis is a common problem among hemodialysis patients, balloon angioplasties are often performed to restore patency and flow. CPT code 35476 (Transluminal balloon angioplasty, percutaneous; venous) is provided for this procedure.

Central Venous Access Procedures

Many therapies can be administered via various types of catheters and ports. CPT coding for catheterization procedures depends on the type and use of the catheter. In general, CPT codes are assigned only to catheters inserted by physicians and not to catheters inserted by nursing personnel.

Central venous access devices (CVADs) are small, flexible tubes placed in large veins for patients who require frequent access to their bloodstream. CVADs are commonly used for the following purposes:

- Administration of medications (for example, antibiotics, chemotherapy)

- Administration of fluids and nutritional compounds (for example, hyperalimentation)

- Transfusion of blood products

- Multiple blood draws for diagnostic testing

Before assigning codes in this section, coders should read the note that precedes code 36555. First, CPT classifies venous access procedures into five distinct categories:

- Insertion

- Repair

- Partial replacement
- Complete replacement
- Removal

The definitions for each of these categories are provided in CPT. Additional information must be abstracted from the health record to determine the correct code. As an example, refer to the decision tree in Figure 4.9 for insertion of a central venous access device. From this decision tree, documentation is needed to determine the following:

- Catheter inserted centrally or peripherally
- Tunneled or nontunneled
- Pump or port
- Age of patient

A centrally inserted catheter is placed in the jugular, subclavian, femoral vein, or inferior vena cava. The peripherally inserted catheters are typically placed in the arm and advanced forward into the larger subclavian vein. The documentation may state that the catheter was inserted into the basilic or cephalic vein. For the centrally inserted catheter, the coder must check the documentation to determine whether the catheter was tunneled. Tunneled catheters have an entrance site at a distance from where they enter the vascular system. These are "tunneled" through the skin and subcutaneous tissue to a great vein. Typically, these catheters are for long-term use. The code descriptions also differentiate between the use of subcutaneous ports or pumps. Implanted ports are placed below the skin, and blood is drawn or medication is delivered by placing a tiny needle through the overlying skin into the port or reservoir. Pumps use a computerized mechanism for infusion.

Unlike centrally inserted central catheters, peripherally inserted central catheter (PICC) lines are not inserted into the central vein.

CPT provides codes for the removal of CVADs (36589–36590) but instructs the coder not to assign the codes for nontunneled central venous catheters. Removal of some catheters does not warrant a separate code when no surgical procedure is required and the catheter is simply pulled out.

Exercise 4.29 Cardiovascular System

Operative Report

Preoperative Diagnosis: Heart block ⟶ Peripherally

Postoperative Diagnosis: Same

Procedure: Insertion of permanent pacemaker

The patient was premedicated before arriving at the OR. The patient was prepped and draped in the usual manner. A pocket was created for the pacemaker. The bipolar electrode was introduced, taken to the pulmonary artery, and brought out slowly to the apex of the right ventricle. Measurements were taken, and the position was excellent. The electrode was anchored to the fascia over the sleeve and connected to the pacemaker battery. The wound was closed. Patient tolerated the procedure well and returned to the outpatient recovery area.

Assign appropriate CPT code(s) for the preceding procedure and indicate the index entries that were used to identify the code(s). Assign only CPT surgical codes (no E/M codes) and append any applicable modifiers.

1. Code(s): _____

   Index entries: _____

   _____

Figure 4.9. Central venous access procedures coding decision tree

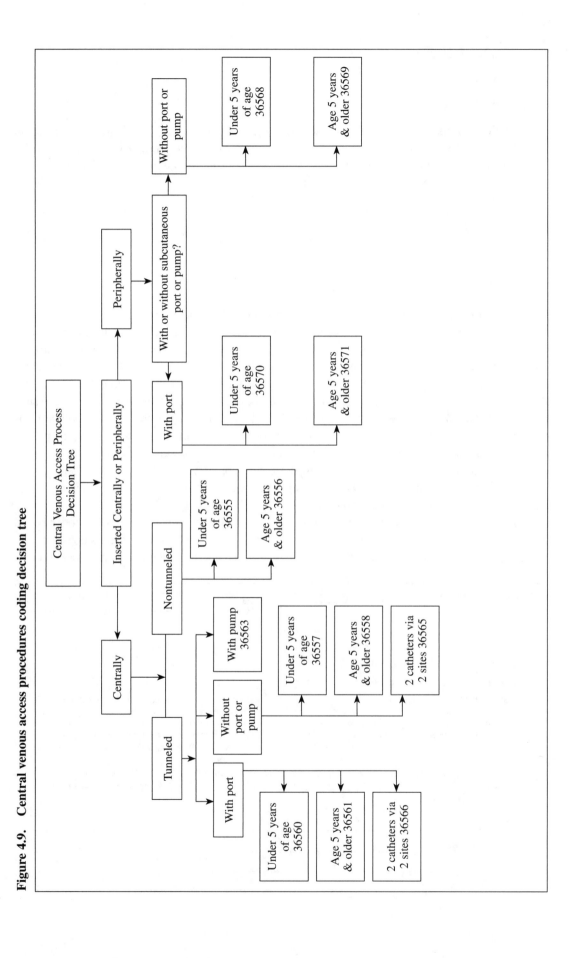

Exercise 4.30   Cardiovascular System

Operative Report

Preoperative Diagnosis: Breast carcinoma

Postoperative Diagnosis: Same

Operation: Removal of venous access port

The patient is a 44-year-old woman who had a left, modified radical mastectomy in 2002. In August, she had a Port-a-Cath placed in the right side. However, it has caused an extreme amount of discomfort so she has requested that it be removed.

The patient was taken to the OR and placed in a supine position on the table. She was then prepped and draped in the usual sterile fashion. The area was anesthetized with 1% Carbocaine. An incision was made over the venous access device and carried down to the place of the device. After freeing it up and cutting the retention sutures, the venous access device was removed. Hemostasis was obtained with cautery and pressure. The wound was then closed in layers and a dressing applied. The patient tolerated the procedure well and was returned to the surgicenter in stable condition.

Assign appropriate CPT code(s) for the preceding procedure and indicate the index entries that were used to identify the code(s). Assign only CPT surgical codes (no E/M codes) and append any applicable modifiers.

1.   Code(s): _____

     Index entries: _____

     _____

Exercise 4.31   Cardiovascular System

Operative Report

Preoperative Diagnosis: Renal failure

Postoperative Diagnosis: Same

Operation: Insertion of subclavian venous catheter

With this elderly patient in the head-down position, the entire left upper chest was prepared with Betadine scrub and painting, and draped in the usual sterile fashion. Then, 1% Xylocaine was used for local anesthetic. A percutaneously subclavian venous catheter was inserted without difficulty and secured at the skin level with 3-0 Nylon, and a sterile dressing was applied. The catheter also was irrigated with Heparin solution. Patient tolerated the procedure well. Will follow with a chest x-ray.

Assign appropriate CPT code(s) for the preceding procedure and indicate the index entries that were used to identify the code(s). Assign only CPT surgical codes (no E/M codes) and append any applicable modifiers.

1.   Code(s): _____

     Index entries: _____

     _____

Exercise 4.32 Cardiovascular System Review

Assign appropriate CPT code(s) for the following procedures and indicate the index entries that were used to identify the codes. Assign only CPT surgical codes (no E/M codes) and append any applicable modifiers.

1. Relocation of pacemaker pocket

    Code(s): _____

    Index entries: _____

    _____

2. Open revision of AV fistula with thrombectomy, patient receiving hemodialysis

    Code(s): _____

    Index entries: _____

    _____

3. Repair of patent ductus arteriosus by division (18-year-old patient)

    Code(s): _____

    Index entries: _____

    _____

4. Catheter placement into the brachiocephalic artery (first order)

    Code(s): _____

    Index entries: _____

    _____

5. Complete replacement of tunneled centrally inserted central venous catheter with subcutaneous port; replacement performed through original access site (45-year-old patient)

    Code(s): _____

    Index entries: _____

    _____

6. Percutaneous thrombectomy of AV graft

    Code(s): _____

    Index entries: _____

    _____

7. Percutaneous transluminal femoral-popliteal atherectomy

    Code(s): _____

    Index entries: _____

    _____

Exercise 4.32   (Continued)

8.   Valvuloplasty of tricuspid valve with ring insertion

     Code(s): _____

     Index entries: _____

     _____

9.   Insertion of epicardial dual-chamber pacing cardioverter-defibrillator system (pulse generator
     and electrodes) by thoracotomy

     Code(s): _____

     Index entries: _____

     _____

10. Long saphenous vein stripping from saphenofemoral junction to below knee of left and
     right legs

     Code(s): _____

     Index entries: _____

     _____

Digestive System

The digestive subsection includes surgical procedures involving the lips, mouth and tongue, palate and uvula, salivary glands and ducts, pharynx, adenoids and tonsils, esophagus, stomach, intestines, appendix, rectum, biliary tract, abdomen, peritoneum, and omentum. The codes are categorized first by body part involved and then by procedure, such as herniorrhaphy, esophagotomy, ileostomy, cholecystectomy, and hemorrhoidectomy. Figure 4.10 shows the digestive system.

Endoscopies

In general, gastrointestinal endoscopies are categorized by body part involved, type or purpose of endoscopy (diagnostic or surgical), and specific procedure performed, such as biopsy, ablation of tumor or polyp, and removal of foreign body. The endoscopy should always be coded as far as the scope was passed.

An esophagoscopy allows the physician to visualize the esophagus. Codes in the range 43200 through 43232 are used to report esophagoscopies.

An upper gastrointestinal endoscopy, also known as an esophagogastroduodenoscopy, or EGD, or upper endoscopy, involves the visual examination of the esophagus, stomach and upper duodenum, and/or jejunum. Indications for these procedures include gastrointestinal (GI) bleeding, ulceration, or inflammation; abdominal pain; narrowing of the esophagus; and suspected tumors or polyps. EGDs are reported with codes in the range 43234 through 43259. The code ranges can be located in the alphabetic index under Endoscopy, Gastrointestinal, Upper. See Figure 4.11 for illustration.

Figure 4.10.   The digestive system

Figure 4.11. Upper GI endoscopy

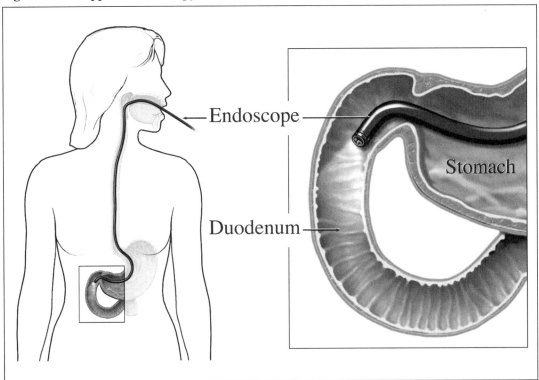

Lower GI endoscopies can be classified by the area of the intestine examined, as follows:

- *Proctosigmoidoscopy:* An examination limited to the rectum and sigmoid colon (45300–45327).

- *Sigmoidoscopy:* An examination of the entire rectum and sigmoid colon that may also include a portion of the descending colon (45330–45345).

- *Colonoscopy:* An examination of the entire colon, from the rectum to the cecum, that may include the terminal ileum (45355–45392). Figure 4.12 illustrates the anatomy of the colon with colonoscopy procedure.

Indications for performing lower GI procedures include an abnormal barium enema, lower gastrointestinal bleeding, iron deficiency anemia of unknown etiology, and diarrhea. They may also be performed for follow-up examination after removal of a neoplastic growth.

When coding a colonoscopy, the coder must review the operative report to determine the approach: through an existing colostomy (44388–44397), a colotomy (45355), or the rectum (45378–45392).

The following questions should be answered before a code is assigned for an endoscopy:

- *Was the diagnostic endoscopy performed as part of a surgical endoscopy?* If so, only the surgical endoscopy should be coded.

- *What was the purpose of the endoscopy?*

- *What approach was used to insert the endoscope?*

Figure 4.12.   Anatomy of colon with colonoscopy procedure

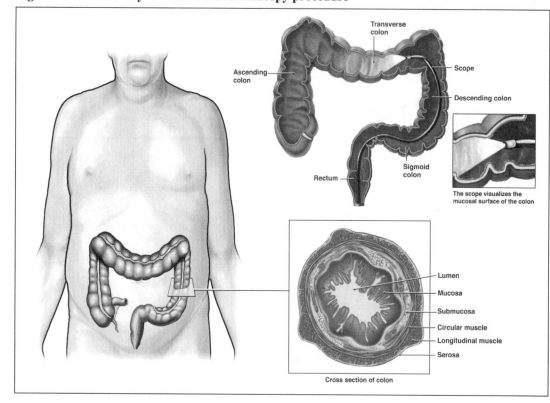

Cross section of colon

Removal of Tumors or Polyps

Because the endoscopic removal of a tumor or polyp can be accomplished with several tech-niques, the coder should review the documentation carefully before selecting a code. It is also possible for a physician to use different techniques to remove polyps during the same operative episode. In this case, an appropriate CPT code would be assigned to identify each technique.

One technique uses hot biopsy forceps or bipolar cautery. Hot biopsy forceps resemble tweezers connected to an electrosurgical unit. Grasping the polyp, the physician pulls the growth away from the wall of the structure. A portion of the neoplasm may be removed for pathological analysis. The remaining portion is destroyed with the electrocoagulation current. Bipolar cautery also uses electrical current to remove the polyp.

The snare technique uses a wire loop that is slipped over the polyp or tumor. The stalk is then cauterized and the growth removed.

Finally, the physician may elect to use a neodymium yttrium aluminum garnet (Nd:YAG) laser to remove the lesion. When a laser is used during the endoscopy, the coder should assign the code for the endoscopy that states "with ablation of tumor(s), polyp(s), or other lesion(s) not amenable to removal by hot biopsy forceps, bipolar cautery or snare technique."

Incomplete Colonoscopies

There are several guidelines for coding discontinued procedures for physicians and hospitals. (See chapter 3 of this book and appendix A of the CPT codebook for descriptions of modifiers –52, –53, –73, and –74.) In the case of a colonoscopy, the procedure may be attempted, but circumstances may prevent the entire colon from being visualized (for instance, poor prep). In this case, CPT guidelines instruct the coder to assign the colonoscopy code with modifier –52 for reduced services (for physician services).

It should be noted that some Medicare carriers have different guidelines for reporting incomplete colonoscopies. According to Program Memorandum AB-03-114 issued August 1, 2003, Medicare covers colorectal cancer screening test/procedures for the early detection of colorectal cancer when coverage conditions are met. Among the screening procedures covered are screening colonoscopies:

- G0105   Colorectal cancer screening; colonoscopy on individual at high risk

- G0121   Colorectal screening; colonoscopy on individual not meeting criteria for high risk

Coverage of these services is subject to certain frequency limitations. The memorandum further explains that when a covered colonoscopy is attempted but cannot be completed, the professional provider should add modifier –53 to the colonoscopy code to indicate that the procedure was interrupted. When submitting a facility claim for the interrupted colonoscopy, providers are to suffix the colonoscopy codes with modifier –73 or –74, as appropriate.

Biopsies and Lesion Removal

When performing a GI endoscopy, the physician may encounter one or many lesions. Biopsies of some or all lesions may be taken. Lesion removal may be performed after a biopsy or without a biopsy. Therefore, the following guidelines should be applied:

- When a biopsy of a lesion is taken and the remaining portion of the *same* lesion is excised during the same operative episode, assign a code for the excision only (*CPT Assistant,* February 1999).

- When one lesion is biopsied and a *different* lesion is excised, assign a code for the biopsy and a code for the excision. This rule is applicable unless the excision code narrative includes the phrase "with or without biopsy." In this case, only the excision code is assigned. It would be appropriate to append the biopsy code with modifier –59, Distinct Procedural Service.

- Biopsy codes use the terminology "with biopsy, single or multiple." These codes are to be used only once, regardless of the number of biopsies taken.

Exercise 4.33   Digestive System

Assign appropriate CPT code(s) for the following procedures and indicate the index entries that were used to identify the codes. Assign only CPT surgical codes (no E/M codes) and append any applicable modifiers.

1. Esophagoscopy with biopsy of a small lesion in the esophagus and a snare removal of a polyp from another area of the esophagus

    Code(s): _____

    Index entries: _____

    _____

2. Proctosigmoidoscopy with biopsy of four separate lesions

    Code(s): _____

    Index entries: _____

    _____

3. EGD with laser removal of duodenal polyp

    Code(s): _____

    Index entries: _____

    _____

4. Endoscopic biopsy of a lesion of the transverse colon

    Code(s): _____

    Index entries: _____

    _____

5. ERCP with removal of bile duct stones

    Code(s): _____

    Index entries: _____

    _____

Exercise 4.34   Digestive System

Operative Note

Procedure: EGD with foreign body removal

Clinical Note: This patient is a 47-year-old male who experienced acute odynophagia after eating a meal consisting of fish. The patient felt a foreign body-like sensation in his proximal esophagus. He was evaluated with lateral, C-spine films, and soft tissue films without any evidence of perforation.

Findings: After obtaining informed consent, the patient was endoscoped. He was premedicated without any complication. Under direct visualization, an Olympus Q20 was introduced orally and the esophagus was intubated without any difficulty. The hypopharynx was carefully reviewed, and no abnormalities were noted. There were no foreign bodies and no lacerations to the hypopharynx. The proximal esophagus was normal. No active bleeding was noted. The endoscope was advanced farther into the esophagus, where careful review of the mucosa revealed no foreign bodies and no obstructions. However, the gastroesophageal junction did show a very small fish bone, which was removed without any complications. The endoscope was advanced into the stomach, where partially digested food was noted. The duodenum was normal. The endoscope was then removed. The patient tolerated the procedure well, and his postprocedural vital signs are stable.

Assign appropriate CPT code(s) for the preceding procedure and indicate the index entries that were used to identify the code(s). Assign only CPT surgical codes (no E/M codes) and append any applicable modifiers.

1. Code(s): _____

    Index entries: _____

    _____

Exercise 4.35   Digestive System

Operative Report

Procedure: Colonoscopy

Instrument Used: Olympus CF100L

Indications: The patient has a family history of carcinoma of the colon and colonic polyps.

The digital and anal exams were normal. The colonoscope was inserted to the cecum. The prep was good. Eight to ten very sessile and diminutive polyps were identified, all but one located in the rectum. The other polyp was located in the proximal transverse colon. All were coagulated and removed with the hot biopsy forceps. No other mucosal lesions were identified.

Pathology Report

Results of Gross Examination:

1. The specimen labeled biopsy of polyp, transverse colon, consists of a pale tan, slightly firm tissue measuring 0.2 cm in greatest diameter; completely submitted.

2. The specimen labeled biopsy of polyp, rectum, consists of six pieces of slightly firm pinkish-tan tissue ranging from 0.2 to 0.3 cm in greatest diameter; completely submitted.

Results of Microscopic Examination:

No high-grade dysplasia or malignant change is seen in the colorectal polyps.

Pathological Diagnosis:

1. Biopsy of polyp, transverse colon: Hyperplastic polyp

2. Biopsy of polyp, rectum: Hyperplastic polyp

Assign appropriate CPT code(s) for the preceding procedure and indicate the index entries that were used to identify the code(s). Assign only CPT surgical codes (no E/M codes) and append any applicable modifiers.

1.   Code(s): _____

     Index entries: _____

     _____

Exercise 4.36   Digestive System

Operative Report

Preoperative Diagnosis: Residual inflammatory changes

Postoperative Diagnosis: See below

Operation: Flexible fiberoptic sigmoidoscopy

The sigmoidoscope was inserted into the rectum and eventually advanced up to a level 60 cm from the anus. The mucosa throughout the colon and rectum were examined and appeared completely normal with no inflammation, ulceration, or exudate. There was no bleeding. I did not see any narrowed areas, polyps, or masses. I did see a few sigmoid diverticula.

With the exception of a few sigmoid diverticula, the examination up to a level of 60 cm from the anus was noted to be normal. The previous inflammatory changes have completely subsided.

Assign appropriate CPT code(s) for the preceding procedure and indicate the index entries that were used to identify the code(s). Assign only CPT surgical codes (no E/M codes) and append any applicable modifiers.

1.   Code(s): _____

     Index entries: _____

     _____

Hernia Repairs

An abdominal hernia occurs when internal organs, such as the intestines, break through a hole or tear in the musculature of the abdominal wall. This protrusion produces a bulge that can be seen or felt. Symptoms include burning and pain with activity.

Codes 49491 through 49659 describe procedures related to hernia repair. To assign these codes accurately, the coder must be able to specify the type and/or site of the hernia, the history of the hernia, the age of the patient, and the clinical presentation of the hernia.

The following terms are used to describe the type and/or location of different hernias:

- *Inguinal hernia:* A common herniation of the inguinal canal in the groin area

- *Lumbar hernia:* A rare herniation in the lumbar region of the torso

- *Incisional hernia:* A herniation at the site of a previous surgical incision

- *Femoral hernia:* A common herniation in the femoral canal in the groin area

- *Epigastric hernia:* A herniation above the navel

- *Umbilical hernia:* A herniation at the navel

- *Spigelian hernia:* A herniation usually above the inferior epigastric vessel along the outer border of the rectus muscle

Some codes provide historical information specifying whether the hernia is an *initial* repair (first surgical repair of the hernia) or a *recurrent* repair (hernia has been surgically repaired previously). Other codes differentiate patients by age: any age, under six months, six months to under five years, or five years or over. Finally, a number of terms are used to describe the clinical presentation of hernias. These include:

- *Reducible:* The protruding organs can be returned to normal position by surgical (not medical) manipulation.

- *Sliding:* The colon or cecum is part of the hernia sac. (In some cases, the urinary bladder also may be involved.)

- *Incarcerated:* The hernia cannot be reduced without surgical intervention.

- *Strangulated:* The hernia is an incarcerated hernia in which the blood supply to the contained organ is reduced. A strangulated hernia presents a medical emergency.

The following example illustrates how the different variables describing hernias can be represented in a specific code assignment:

> **Example:** 49550 Repair initial femoral hernia, any age; reducible
> 49553 incarcerated or strangulated

More than 600,000 hernia repairs (herniorrhaphies) are performed each year. A physician may perform one of three common types of repairs. The first type is the traditional or conventional repair. Under general anesthesia, the physician pushes the bulging tissue back into the abdominal cavity. The defect is closed by pulling together and stitching the surrounding muscles and ligaments. A recovery period of four to six weeks is usually needed.

The second type of herniorrhaphy uses mesh rather than stitches to repair the abdominal defect. Because stitches are not used, the patient experiences less postoperative pain. Commonly used meshes are Marlex and Prolene. When coding a mesh repair of an incisional or ventral hernia, code 49568, Implantation of mesh or other prosthesis for incisional or ventral hernia repair, must be assigned in addition to the repair code. The use of mesh with other hernia repairs is not coded.

The third type of hernia repair is performed by a laparoscope. A laparoscopic repair is commonly performed to repair bilateral and recurrent hernias. Less discomfort and faster recovery are the main advantages of this approach. As with other endoscopies, a surgical laparoscopy includes a diagnostic laparoscopy. See Figure 4.13 for a laparoscopic ventral hernia repair.

It is important to note that diaphragmatic and hiatal hernias are not assigned to the digestive system. To identify these hernias, the coder should use codes from the 39502–39541 range in the diaphragm subsection of the CPT codebook.

Exercise 4.37   Digestive System

Assign appropriate CPT code(s) for the following procedures and indicate the index entries that were used to identify the codes. Assign only CPT surgical codes (no E/M codes) and append any applicable modifiers.

1. Initial herniorrhaphy for repair of an inguinal hernia and a unilateral hydrocelectomy of the spermatic cord (4-year-old patient)

   Code(s): _____

   Index entries: _____

   _____

2. Right incarcerated initial incisional hernia repair with mesh (49-year-old patient)

   Code(s): _____

   Index entries: _____

   _____

3. Diagnosis: recurrent inguinal hernia; procedure: laparoscopic hernia repair

   Code(s): _____

   Index entries: _____

   _____

4. Recurrent incarcerated inguinal hernia repair with implantation of mesh (56-year-old patient)

   Code(s): _____

   Index entries: _____

   _____

5. Umbilical herniorrhaphy (35-year-old patient)

   Code(s): _____

   Index entries: _____

   _____

Figure 4.13. Laparoscopic ventral hernia repair

Preoperative View

Small bowel adherent to the anterior abdominal wall and bulging through the previous incision site

Sagittal view

Trocar Placement in the Abdomen

A. Trocars are placed in the inflated abdomen.

Grasping forceps

Previous incision site

Scope

Anterior view

Dissection of the Adhesions

B. Grasping cautery forceps are used to dissect the adhesions.

Grasping forceps

Scope

Placement of the GORE-TEX Mesh

C. GORE-TEX mesh is inserted and sutured onto the anterior abdominal wall.

GORE-TEX mesh

Exercise 4.38   Digestive System

Operative Report

Preoperative Diagnosis: Left inguinal hernia

Postoperative Diagnosis: Same

Procedure: Left initial inguinal hernia repair with mesh

Anesthesia: General

The patient is a 23-year-old male who presented with several weeks' history of pain in his left groin associated with a bulge. Examination revealed that his left groin did indeed have a bulge and his right groin was normal. We discussed the procedure as well as the choice of anesthesia.

After preoperative evaluation and clearance, the patient was brought into the operating suite and placed in a comfortable supine position on the OR table. Monitoring equipment was attached, and general anesthesia was induced. His left groin was sterilely prepped and draped, and an inguinal incision made. This was carried down through the subcutaneous tissues until the external oblique fascia was reached. This was split in a direction parallel with its fibers, and the medial aspect of the opening included the external ring. The ileo inguinal nerve was identified, and care was taken to retract this inferiorly out of the way. The cord structures were encircled and the cremasteric muscle fibers divided. At this point, we examined the floor of the inguinal canal, and the patient did appear to have a weakness here. We then explored the cord. There was no evidence of an indirect hernia. A piece of 3×5 mesh was obtained and trimmed to fit. It was placed down in the inguinal canal and tacked to the pubic tubercle. It was then run inferiorly along the pelvic shelving edge until lateral to the internal ring and tacked down superiorly using interrupted sutures of 0-Prolene. A single stitch was placed lateral to the cord to recreate the internal ring. Details of the mesh were tucked underneath the external oblique fascia. The cord and the nerve were allowed to drop back into the wound, and the wound was infiltrated with 30 cc of half percent Marcaine. The external oblique fascia was then closed with a running suture of 0-Vicryl. Subcutaneous tissues were approximated with interrupted sutures of 3-0 Vicryl. The skin was closed with a running subcuticular suture of 4-0 Vicryl. Benzoin and Steri-Strips and a dry sterile dressing were applied. All sponge, needle, and instrument counts were correct at the end of the procedure. The patient tolerated the procedure well and was taken to the recovery room in stable condition.

Assign appropriate CPT code(s) for the preceding procedure and indicate the index entries that were used to identify the code(s). Assign only CPT surgical codes (no E/M codes) and append any applicable modifiers.

1.   Code(s): _____

     Index entries: _____

     _____

Exercise 4.39   Digestive System Review

Assign appropriate CPT code(s) for the following procedures and indicate the index entries that were used to identify the codes. Assign only CPT surgical codes (no E/M codes) and append any applicable modifiers.

1.   Laser removal of external hemorrhoids

     Code(s): _____

     Index entries: _____

     _____

2.   Laparoscopic gastric bypass and Roux-en-Y gastroenterostomy performed for obesity

     Code(s): _____

     Index entries: _____

     _____

Exercise 4.39   (Continued)

3.   EGD with suturing of esophagogastric junction

   Code(s): _____

   Index entries: _____

   _____

4.   Palatoplasty for cleft palate, soft

   Code(s): _____

   Index entries: _____

   _____

5.   Colonoscopy with laser removal of lesions

   Code(s): _____

   Index entries: _____

   _____

6.   Laparoscopic cholecystectomy with exploration of common duct

   Code(s): _____

   Index entries: _____

   _____

7.   Repair of recurrent, incarcerated inguinal hernia (34-year-old patient)

   Code(s): _____

   Index entries: _____

   _____

8.   Laparoscopic aspiration of ovarian cyst

   Code(s): _____

   Index entries: _____

   _____

9.   Anoscopy with removal of polyp via hot biopsy forceps

   Code(s): _____

   Index entries: _____

   _____

10.   Removal of a chicken bone from pharynx

   Code(s): _____

   Index entries: _____

   _____

Urinary System

The urinary subsection includes surgical procedures involving the kidney, ureter, bladder, and urethra. These codes are categorized first by body part involved and then by procedure performed, such as cystourethroscopy, percutaneous renal biopsy, transurethral resection of the prostate, and urethroplasty. Figure 4.14 provides an illustration of the urinary system.

Urodynamics

Codes 51725 through 51798 describe urodynamic procedures that may be reported separately or in combination when more than one procedure is performed. Modifier –51 should be reported when multiple procedures are performed (modifier –51 is for physician use only). These procedures are performed either by the physician or under his or her direction. The following services/supplies are considered part of the procedure and should not be reported separately: instruments, equipment, fluids, gases, probes, catheters, technicians' fees, medications, gloves, trays, tubing, and other sterile supplies.

Figure 4.14.   The urinary system

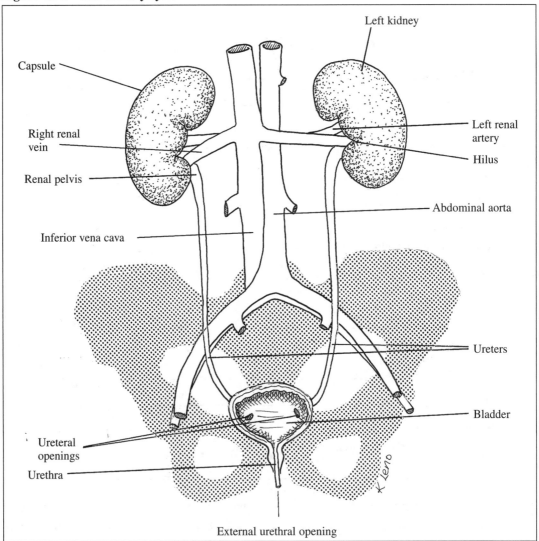

If the physician is providing only the professional component (that is, the supervision and interpretation), modifier −26 also should be reported for physician services.

The following definitions (Rogers 2004) describing the various urodynamic procedures will help the coder assign the appropriate CPT code:

- *Cystometrogram:* An examination performed to determine the capacity of the urinary bladder. A simple cystometrogram is the measurement of the bladder's capacity, sensation of filling, and intravesical pressure. A complex cystometrogram involves the measurement of the bladder's capacity, sensation of filling, and intravesical pressure using a rectal probe to distinguish between intra-abdominal pressure and bladder pressure.

- *Uroflowmetry:* An examination performed to determine the functional capacity of the urinary bladder. Simple uroflowmetry is the measurement of voiding time and peak flow. Complex uroflowmetry involves the measurement and recording of mean and peak flow and the time taken to reach peak flow during continuous urination.

- *Urethral pressure profile (UPP):* An examination that involves the recording of pressures along the urethra as a special catheter is slowly withdrawn.

- *Electromyography:* Studies performed to record muscle activity during voiding and to simultaneous recording urine flow rate.

Genitourinary Endoscopies

In general, genitourinary endoscopies are categorized by body part involved—urethra, prostate, or ureter—and specific procedure performed, such as cystourethroscopy with biopsy of the bladder or urethra, transurethral incision of prostate, cystourethroscopy with ureteral meatotomy, and cystourethroscopy with insertion of indwelling ureteral stent. The endoscopic procedures described in codes 52000 through 52700 are listed so that the main procedure can be identified without having to list all the minor related functions performed at the same time.

Example: Code 52647 describes laser coagulation of the prostate, including control of postoperative bleeding. The description indicates a complete procedure that includes vasectomy, meatotomy, cystourethroscopy, urethral calibration and/or dilatation, and internal urethrotomy. Minor procedures such as meatotomy, calibration, and so on are part of code 52647 and should not be reported separately.

Figure 4.15 illustrates a ureteral calculus with attempted ureteroscopy.

Figure 4.15. Ureteral calculus with attempted ureteroscopy

ANTERIOR VIEW

GUIDE WIRE INSERTION

LEFT KIDNEY

TIP OF GUIDE WIRE COILED WITHIN THE RENAL PELVIS

LEFT URETER

GUIDE WIRE

LEFT MID-URETERAL CALCULUS

DILATING BALLOON INSERTION

GUIDE WIRE

DEFLATED DILATING BALLOON ADVANCED OVER GUIDE WIRE

DILATING BALLOON INFLATION

GUIDE WIRE

BALLOON DILATED TO 13mm

ATTEMPTED URETEROSCOPE INSERTION

GUIDE WIRE

URETEROSCOPE BLOCKED AT SITE OF NARROWING OF LEFT URETER

NARROWING OF LEFT URETER

ILIAC VESSELS

ENLARGEMENT OF LEFT URETER

Exercise 4.40   Urinary System

Assign appropriate CPT code(s) for the following procedures and indicate the index entries that were used to identify the codes. Assign only CPT surgical codes (no E/M codes) and append any applicable modifiers.

1. Cystoscopy for insertion of double-J ureteral stent

    Code(s): _____

    Index entries: _____

    _____

2. Cystoscopy with fulguration of 1.0-cm lesion of bladder

    Code(s): _____

    Index entries: _____

    _____

3. Cystoscopy, left ureteroscopy with laser lithotripsy

    Code(s): _____

    Index entries: _____

    _____

4. Cystoscopy with insertion of urethral stent

    Code(s): _____

    Index entries: _____

    _____

Exercise 4.41   Urinary System

Operative Report

Preoperative Diagnosis: Right ureteral stone

Postoperative Diagnosis: Same

Procedure: Right ureteroscopy, stone extraction, stent

The patient was taken to the operating suite and placed in the dorsal lithotomy position, and then sterilely prepped and draped in the usual fashion. Cystoscope was then inserted into the urethra; it was normal. The prostate was nonobstructed, and the bladder was free of neoplasm, infection, or calculus. There was some edema of the right intramural ureter. A guide wire was introduced into the right ureteral orifice, advanced to the right renal-collecting system without difficulty. A balloon was used to dilate the ureter, and a scope was introduced. The gravel was noted from the stone being fragmented from the balloon. This was washing out. The remainder of the ureter was examined and found to be free of neoplasm, perforation, or calculus. The stent was inserted. A string was kept attached. The patient was transferred to the recovery room in satisfactory condition.

Assign appropriate CPT code(s) for the preceding procedure and indicate the index entries that were used to identify the codes. Assign only CPT surgical codes (no E/M codes) and append any applicable modifiers.

1. Code(s): _____

    Index entries: _____

    _____

Exercise 4.42   Urinary System

Operative Report

Preoperative Diagnosis:	Recurrent bladder cancer
Postoperative Diagnosis:	Recurrent bladder cancer
Procedure:	Cystoscopy with bladder biopsies and fulguration
Anesthesia:	General

The patient has prior transitional cell carcinoma of the bladder and also carcinoma in situ. He has received MVAC therapy and BCG. Surveillance cystoscopy demonstrated erythema of the bladder wall. He is being admitted for cystoscopy, bladder biopsy, and fulguration now. Procedure, reasons, risks, and complications were reviewed and consent was granted.

He was brought to the Operating Room under general anesthesia, placed in the dorsolithotomy position, and prepped and draped in a sterile manner. A #21 French cystoscope was inserted, urethra was normal, veru-montanum intact. Prostate revealed evidence of prior transurethral resection and moderate outlet obstruction. There were erythematous areas throughout the bladder, and a 0.5-cm lesion was fulgurated. Both ureteric orifices were normal size, shape, and caliber with clear efflux. The erythematous areas were then biopsied with flexible biopsy forceps. After obtaining biopsies, the area was then fulgurated with Bugbee electrode. Reinspection was carried out; no gross bleeding was noted. The bladder was drained, cystoscope was with-drawn, and the patient was transferred to the Recovery Room in satisfactory condition with all vital signs stable.

Pathology Report

Final Diagnosis: 1.   Urothelial carcinoma in situ, focal

2.   Chronic nonspecific cystitis

Assign appropriate CPT code(s) for the preceding procedure and indicate the index entries that were used to identify the codes. Assign only CPT surgical codes (no E/M codes) and append any applicable modifiers.

1.   Code(s): _____

Index entries: _____

_____

Exercise 4.43   Urinary System Review

Assign appropriate CPT code(s) for the following procedures and indicate the index entries that were used to identify the codes. Assign only CPT surgical codes (no E/M codes) and append any applicable modifiers.

1.   Laparoscopic sling procedure for stress incontinence

Code(s): _____

Index entries: _____

_____

2.   Excision of urethral polyp

Code(s): _____

Index entries: _____

_____

Exercise 4.43   (Continued)

3. Cystoscopy with fulguration of 2.0-cm benign tumor

   Code(s): _____

   Index entries: _____

   _____

4. Cystotomy with excision of bladder diverticulum

   Code(s): _____

   Index entries: _____

   _____

5. Needle renal biopsy

   Code(s): _____

   Index entries: _____

   _____

6. Cystoscopy with ureteroscopy

   Code(s): _____

   Index entries: _____

   _____

7. Cystourethroscopy with bilateral ureteral meatotomy

   Code(s): _____

   Index entries: _____

   _____

8. Needle EMG studies of urethral sphincter

   Code(s): _____

   Index entries: _____

   _____

9. Insertion of straight catheter

   Code(s): _____

   Index entries: _____

   _____

10. Closure of ureterocutaneous fistula

    Code(s): _____

    Index entries: _____

    _____

Male Genital System

The codes in the male genital system subsection are used to report procedures on the penis, testis, epididymis, tunica vaginalis, scrotum, vas deferens, spermatic cord, seminal vesicles, and prostate. Figure 4.16 illustrates these structures.

Removal of lesions (for example, condyloma, papilloma, molluscum contagiosum, herpetic vesicle) of the penis is not located in the integumentary system subsection but, rather, in the male genital system (54050–54065) subsection. The code selection is determined by the method of removal. For destruction or excision of other lesions, reference the integumentary system subsection of the surgery section.

Prostatectomy

The prostate gland lies under the bladder and surrounds the first part of the urethra that carries urine to the penis. When the prostate becomes enlarged, it tends to obstruct the urethral and makes urination difficult. There are three common methods of prostatectomy, each involving a different approach: transurethral (most common), retropubic, and perineal. Transurethral resection of the prostate (52601–52640 and 53850–53852) uses a scope inserted through the urethra to remove the prostate tissue piece by piece. A perineal prostatectomy (55801–55815)

Figure 4.16. The male genital system

requires an incision between the back of the scrotum and the anus. A retropubic prostatectomy (55821–55845) requires the surgeon to make an incision in the front wall of the abdomen, just above the pubic bone, to directly reach the prostate. CPT also provides a code for laparoscopic retropubic prostatectomy (55866).

Exercise 4.44   Male Genital System

Assign appropriate CPT code(s) for the following procedures and indicate the index entries that were used to identify the codes. Assign only CPT surgical codes (no E/M codes) and append any applicable modifiers.

1. Laser destruction of four condylomas of the penis

    Code(s):_____

    Index entries: _____

    _____

2. Incision and drainage of subcutaneous abscess of the penis

    Code(s):_____

    Index entries: _____

    _____

3. Radical retropubic prostatectomy with excision of lymph nodes

    Code(s):_____

    Index entries: _____

    _____

4. Bilateral epididymectomy

    Code(s):_____

    Index entries: _____

    _____

5. Clamp circumcision, newborn

    Code(s):_____

    Index entries: _____

    _____

Exercise 4.45   Male Genital System

Operative Report

Preoperative Diagnosis:	Adenocarcinoma of the prostate
Postoperative Diagnosis:	Same
Procedure:	Transrectal ultrasound
	Transperineal implant of I–125 seeds into the prostate
Anesthesia:	General

The patient was brought to the cysto suite and placed in the lithotomy position at a 90° angle. General anesthesia was induced, and a Foley catheter was placed. The ultrasound probe was positioned in the rectum, and the appropriate reference points were identified and compared to his previous volumetric studies.

Under fluoroscopic and ultrasound guidance, 19 needles were inserted into the prostate based on a pre-measured template. Approximately 70 seeds were placed.

A cystoscopic examination was performed at the end of the case, and no seeds were identified within the urinary bladder.

A Foley catheter was replaced into the bladder and will be removed later today. The appropriate postimplantation radiation and postoperative instructions were given. He tolerated the procedure well and was taken to the recovery room in satisfactory condition.

Assign appropriate CPT code(s) for the preceding procedure and indicate the index entries that were used to identify the codes. Assign only CPT surgical codes (no E/M codes) and append any applicable modifiers.

1. Code(s): _____

    Index entries: _____

    _____

Exercise 4.46   Male Genital System

Operative Report

Preoperative Diagnosis: Chronic left orchialgia
Chronic epididymitis

Procedure: Left inguinal orchiectomy

Anesthesia: Local standby; 0.25% Marcaine, 1%, Xylocaine, 1/1 dilution. Total 25 cc used as inguinal block

Estimated Blood Loss: Minimal

This is an 82-year-old male with chronic left gonadal pain due to chronic granulomatous epididymitis. This has failed to respond to conservative measures and has caused him marked discomfort in the left groin. As a result, we recommended that he consider outpatient orchiectomy. The risks and potential complications were discussed and informed consent obtained.

The patient was given Ancef IV as well as IV sedation and placed on the operating table in the supine position. The lower groin and abdomen were shaved, prepped, and draped in the standard fashion. The external inguinal ring was identified, and an area just distal to the external inguinal ring was anesthetized with the local anesthetic, and a small transverse incision was made down to the spermatic cord. The testis was then brought out through the inguinal incision after the spermatic cord blockade with local anesthetic. The testis was separated from the scrotum by incision in the gubernaculum with needle tip Bovie. The spermatic cord was identified, dissected back to the external inguinal ring, and bisected with a curved Kelly clamp and then clamped and transected with Metzenbaum scissors. The spermatic cord was closed with suture ligature of 0 Vicryl and a free tie of 0 Vicryl proximal to this on each side of the spermatic cord. The incision was inspected for hemostasis. No further bleeding was noted, and the testis was delivered for pathologic evaluation. The Scarpa's fascia was closed with interrupted 2-0 Vicryl, and the skin was closed with a running 4-0 Vicryl subcuticular closure. Steri-Strips and four by fours were applied as a dressing. He was returned to the recovery room in stable condition. Estimated blood loss was minimal.

Assign appropriate CPT code(s) for the preceding procedure and indicate the index entries that were used to identify the codes. Assign only CPT surgical codes (no E/M codes) and append any applicable modifiers.

1. Code(s): _____

    Index entries: _____

Exercise 4.47 Male Genital System Review

Assign appropriate CPT code(s) for the following procedures and indicate the index entries that were used to identify the codes. Assign only CPT surgical codes (no E/M codes) and append any applicable modifiers.

1. Excision of spermatocele with epididymectomy

   Code(s): _____

   Index entries: _____

   _____

2. Removal of inflatable penial prosthesis (no replacement)

   Code(s): _____

   Index entries: _____

   _____

3. Laparoscopic orchiectomy

   Code(s): _____

   Index entries: _____

   _____

4. One-stage distal hypospadia repair with simple meatal advancement

   Code(s): _____

   Index entries: _____

   _____

5. Biopsy and exploration of epididymis

   Code(s): _____

   Index entries: _____

   _____

6. Incision into abscess of scrotal wall to drain pus

   Code(s): _____

   Index entries: _____

   _____

7. Plethysmography of penis

   Code(s): _____

   Index entries: _____

   _____

8. Excision of condylomas of the penis

   Code(s): _____

   Index entries: _____

   _____

Exercise 4.47 (Continued)

9. Bilateral orchiopexy, inguinal approach with hernia repair

   Code(s): _____

   Index entries: _____

   _____

10. Laparoscopic retropubic radical prostatectomy

   Code(s): _____

   Index entries: _____

   _____

Female Genital System

The female genital system subsection of the CPT surgery chapter includes codes for various surgical repairs, dilatation and curettage, and hysterectomies and hysteroscopies. This section also contains codes for maternity care and delivery. Figure 4.17 provides an illustration of the female genital system.

Hysteroscopy

A hysteroscope is a thin, telescopelike instrument that allows the physician to look inside the uterus. After insufflation of the uterine cavity with CO_2, the hysteroscope is inserted through

Figure 4.17.   The female genital system

the cervical canal and into the uterus. This direct visualization improves the accuracy of diagnosis and treatment. Accessory instruments that may be used with a hysteroscope procedure include scissors, forceps, lasers, and various electrodes. A dilatation and curettage (D&C) is commonly performed with a hysteroscopic biopsy or polypectomy. Therefore, no additional code is assigned to identify the D&C. Codes for hysteroscopies are included in the range 58555 through 58579.

Hysterectomy

CPT bases the hysterectomies codes on the surgical approach. Codes for the laparoscopic removal of the uterus (58550–58554) differentiate between procedures that include the removal of the uterus only and those that include the removal of the fallopian tubes and ovaries in addition to the uterus. The excisional operation can be performed through the vagina (58260–58294) or through a conventional incision in the front wall of the abdomen (58150–58240).

Maternity Care and Delivery Subsection (Guidelines for Physician Services)

Along with codes for surgery and other procedures involving the female reproductive organs, the female genital system subsection includes CPT codes for maternity care and delivery services. Antepartum care includes initial and subsequent history, physical examination, recording of clinical information, and monthly visits up to 28-week gestation, biweekly visits to 36-week gestation, and weekly visits until the time of delivery. According to the CPT codebook, any additional visits are to be coded separately using E/M codes. Health plans may have specific rules about the reporting of services beyond those included in the global service package that often accompanies maternity coverage. This may affect the reporting of services, particularly if more than one physician is required to care for the patient, as may occur with unexpected Cesarean delivery.

Postpartum care codes include both hospital and office visit codes following either vaginal or Cesarean delivery.

Some CPT codes address global care, and some are used to report only a portion of care.

Example: CPT code 59425 is for antepartum care only, four to six visits. It may be used by a family practice physician who refers a patient in the second trimester of pregnancy to an obstetrician due to a high risk of complications.

Code 59510 would be reported by a physician providing global care for a Cesarean delivery from start to finish.

Patients who attempt vaginal delivery after previous Cesarean delivery or who successfully deliver vaginally after previous Cesarean delivery have specific CPT codes assigned from the 59610 through 59622 range. These codes should always be used when they apply.

Exercise 4.48 Female Genital System

Assign appropriate CPT code(s) for the following procedures and indicate the index entries that were used to identify the codes. Assign only CPT surgical codes (no E/M codes) and append any applicable modifiers.

1. Laparoscopic fulguration of fallopian tubes

    Code(s): _____

    Index entries: _____

    _____

2. D&C performed for a patient with dysfunctional bleeding

    Code(s): _____

    Index entries: _____

    _____

3. D&C performed for patient with diagnosis of incomplete abortion (8 weeks pregnant)

    Code(s): _____

    Index entries: _____

    _____

4. Laparoscopy with aspiration of ovarian cyst

    Code(s): _____

    Index entries: _____

    _____

5. Laparoscopic removal of two fibroids (total weight 150 gm)

    Code(s): _____

    Index entries: _____

    _____

6. Vaginal hysterectomy with salpingo-oophorectomy (uterus weight 250 gm)

    Code(s): _____

    Index entries: _____

    _____

Exercise 4.49   Female Genital System

Operative Report

Preoperative Diagnosis: Moderate dysplasia of the cervix

Postoperative Diagnosis: Same

Procedure: LEEP

Anesthesia: General inhalation anesthesia per mask

The patient was brought to the OR with IV fluids infusing and placed on the table in the supine position. General inhalation anesthesia per mask was administered after acquisition of an adequate anesthetic level, and the patient was placed in the lithotomy position. The perineum was draped. A laser speculum was placed in the vaginal vault. The cervix was rinsed with a solution of acetic acid, and colposcopic examination of the cervix showed areas of wide epithelium across the anterior lip of the cervix, consistent with the previous biopsy showing moderate dysplasia. Using the 2-cm electrosurgical loop excision, the endocervical canal was cauterized with bipolar cautery. Then the procedure was completed. The speculum was removed. The patient was taken out of the lithotomy position. Her anesthesia was reversed. She was awakened and taken to the recovery room in stable condition. Sponge, instrument, and needle counts were correct times three. Estimated blood loss was less than 25 cc.

Assign appropriate CPT code(s) for the preceding procedure and indicate the index entries that were used to identify the codes. Assign only CPT surgical codes (no E/M codes) and append any applicable modifiers.

1. Code(s): _____

    Index entries: _____

    _____

Exercise 4.50   Female Genital System

Operative Report

Preoperative Diagnosis: Dysfunctional uterine bleeding, failed hormonal therapy

Postoperative Diagnosis: Same

Procedure Performed: Diagnostic hysteroscopy

                               Fractional dilatation and curettage

The patient is a 35-year-old Gravida V Para IV AB I female from the Towne Health Center. She has been bleeding the majority of each month over the past four months. She has been tried on Ortho-Novum 7/7 to control the bleeding, but this has been of no help. The patient is here for the above procedure.

Description of Procedure: With the patient under satisfactory general anesthesia in the dorsal lithotomy position, a pelvic exam revealed a cervix that came down to the introitus, constituting a second-degree uterine prolapse. The patient had many hymenal tags on both the right and left side. A large speculum was placed inside the vagina. The anterior lip of the cervix was grasped with a single-toothed tenaculum. The cervix was sounded to 8.5 cm. The endocervical canal was now serially dilated. Using the hysteroscope and Ringer's Lactate as a distending solution, the hysteroscope was passed through the internal os into the uterine cavity. Inspection of the uterine contents revealed both right and left ostia identified. Some lining was on the floor of the uterus and some on the roof. The fundus was devoid of any lining. There were no submucosal fibroids and no submucosal septa. The hysteroscope was removed, and the next procedure was fractional dilatation and curettage. Using a Kevorkian—Younge curet, the endocervical canal was curetted and the cervical canal was further dilated using a medium-size curet. The endometrial cavity was curetted with moderate curettings obtained. These were sent for pathological diagnosis. The patient tolerated the procedure fairly well and was escorted to the recovery room in satisfactory condition.

Assign appropriate CPT code(s) for the preceding procedure and indicate the index entries that were used to identify the codes. Assign only CPT surgical codes (no E/M codes) and append any applicable modifiers.

1. Code(s): _____

    Index entries: _____

    _____

Exercise 4.51   Female Genital System Review

Assign appropriate CPT code(s) for the following procedures and indicate the index entries that were used to identify the codes. Assign only CPT surgical codes (no E/M codes) and append any applicable modifiers.

1. Colposcopy with biopsy of cervix

   Code(s): _____

   Index entries: _____

   _____

2. Vulvectomy, partial removal of skin and superficial subcutaneous tissues

   Code(s): _____

   Index entries: _____

   _____

3. Laparoscopy with fulguration of peritoneal lesions

   Code(s): _____

   Index entries: _____

   _____

4. Total abdominal hysterectomy with bilateral salpingo-oophorectomy

   Code(s): _____

   Index entries: _____

   _____

5. Incision and drainage of vaginal hematoma, posttrauma

   Code(s): _____

   Index entries: _____

   _____

6. Biopsy of two lesions, one from labia minora and another from the vaginal orifice

   Code(s): _____

   Index entries: _____

   _____

7. Laparoscopic vaginal hysterectomy with bilateral salpingo-oophorectomy (uterus weighing 280 gm)

   Code(s): _____

   Index entries: _____

   _____

8. Hysteroscopy with removal of fibroids

   Code(s): _____

   Index entries: _____

   _____

(Continued on next page)

Exercise 4.51   (Continued)

9. Vaginal hysterectomy (uterus weighing 260 gm)

    Code(s): _____

    Index entries: _____

    _____

10. Endometrial cryoablation with ultrasonic guidance

    Code(s): _____

    Index entries: _____

    _____

Endocrine System

No specific coding guidelines apply to the subsection that provides codes for the endocrine system.

Exercise 4.52   Endocrine System Review

Assign appropriate CPT code(s) for the following procedures and indicate the index entries that were used to identify the codes. Assign only CPT surgical codes (no E/M codes) and append any applicable modifiers.

1. Excision of thyroglossal duct cyst

    Code(s): _____

    Index entries: _____

    _____

2. Laparoscopic adrenalectomy, complete

    Code(s): _____

    Index entries: _____

    _____

3. Patient had a previous surgery for removal of part of thyroid, now has a bilateral thyroidectomy for remaining tissue

    Code(s): _____

    Index entries: _____

    _____

4. Fine needle aspiration of thyroid cyst (with imaging)

    Code(s) (surgical procedure only): _____

    Index entries: _____

    _____

5. Parathyroidectomy

    Code(s): _____

    Index entries: _____

    _____

Nervous System

The nervous system subsection of the CPT surgery chapter includes the procedures that involve the brain, spinal cord, and peripheral nerves. The CPT codes for procedures performed to manage pain such as nerve blocks and epidural procedures also are part of this subsection. Examples of procedures in this subsection include major brain operations such as craniectomies and craniotomies as well as relatively minor spinal injections and catheter insertions into the nerves and the spinal cord.

Laminotomy and Laminectomy

Laminotomy and laminectomy procedures involve the nerves that occupy the space inside the vertebrae that make up the spinal column. (Figure 4.18 illustrates the sections of the spine.) The CPT codes for surgical procedures involving the spine are based on the surgical approach, the anatomic location of the precipitating condition, and the specific procedures performed.

Laminotomy (hemilaminectomy) codes are based on the anatomic location of the specific interspace involved. When surgery is performed on more than one interspace, the coder should locate the appropriate code(s) in that section of CPT for each additional interspace.

Spinal Injections

Spinal injections are coded according to the site of the injection and the substance injected. Spinal injections (or infusions) involve injecting medications through a needle placed into a structure or space in the spine in order for the physician to be able to diagnose the source of pain or to reduce it. Typical medications used include local anesthetics and corticosteroids. Local anesthetics numb the nerves and corticosteroids help reduce inflammation.

To accurately assign codes for these procedures, coders must abstract documentation from the operative report to determine the injection site (cervical, lumbar) and the substance injected (neurolytic). For example, a single steroid injection into the lumbar spine would be assigned CPT code 62311.

Figure 4.18.   Anatomy of the nervous system

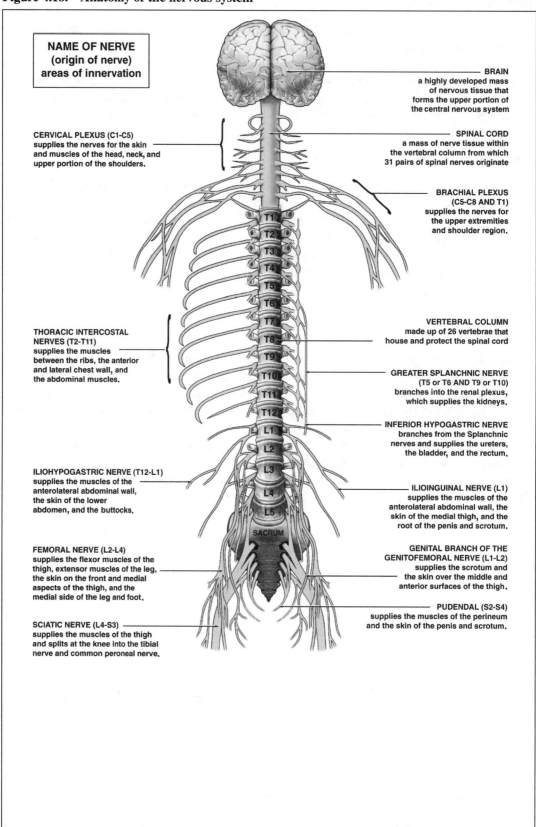

Exercise 4.53   Nervous System

Assign appropriate CPT code(s) for the following procedures and indicate the index entries that were used to identify the codes. Assign only CPT surgical codes (no E/M codes) and append any applicable modifiers.

1. Patient with chronic pain receives a nerve block; anesthetic agent into the branch of sciatic nerve

    Code(s): _____

    Index entries: _____

    _____

2. Using an operating microscope, the physician performs a neuroplasty of the right ring finger

    Code(s): _____

    Index entries: _____

    _____

3. Cervical epidural spinal injection of phenol

    Code(s): _____

    Index entries: _____

    _____

4. Neurorrhaphy of digital nerves of right thumb and ring finger

    Code(s): _____

    Index entries: _____

    _____

Exercise 4.54   Nervous System

Operative Report

Preoperative Diagnosis:	C5–C6 disc herniation
Postoperative Diagnosis:	Same
Procedure:	Anterior cervical discectomy

This 45-year-old gentleman presents with a six-month history of neck pain, right shoulder pain, right intra-scapular pain, and pain radiating on the outer aspect of the right arm. He was found to have wasting of the supra and infra-spinatus muscles and EMG confirmed an C-6 radiculopathy.

Magnetic resonance imaging scan showed a lateral disc herniation at the level of C5–C6. The patient tried initial conservative measures, which did not help him; hence recommendation of surgery was made. The risks and benefits included infection, hemorrhage, injury to the nerve roots, paralysis, injury to the spinal cord with paralysis, failure to improve, or even death. The patient fully understands and agrees to go ahead with the procedure.

The patient was anesthetized and positioned supine with a shoulder support, and the neck was prepared and draped in the usual manner. Mid-cervical crease incision was marked, both four cm. Incisions were placed transversely and the skin was sharply cut, and then the platysma was cut in the line of incision. The cervical fascia was dissected. Then we entered the plane between the trachea and the carotid sheath by blunt dissection reaching the prevertebral space. The prevertebral fascia was incised longitudinally. The disc bulge at 5–6 was easily identified, and a spinal needle placed confirmed the position to be at 5–6. The anterior osteophytes were prominent. They were removed and then we entered the disc space. The disc space itself had collapsed, and there was only desiccated disc material. We curetted out the disc and the cartilage plate, and the vertebral spreader was put in. More disc was removed from the lateral parts of the disc extending toward the uncus on both sides. As we moved posteriorly toward the ligament, there was subligamentous disc herniation to the right side. It was removed, and the ligament was reached. The ligament was lifted with a blunt hook and opened with micro-punches. Using a Midas Rex drill, the posterior parts of the bone in this region were drilled doing a right foraminotomy on the right, and the nerve root was decompressed. A no-free fragment was identified inside the canal, and the entire ligamentum disc was removed over the nerve root. The bone was punched in those corners to give adequate space. The ligament was cut across the width of the space, and on the left side also foraminotomy was done removing the osteophytes in the corner and decompressing the nerve root. After we were satisfied with the decompression, the space was irrigated with antibiotic solution and hemostasis was achieved with some Gelfoam powder, and the wound was thoroughly irrigated. Hemostasis was achieved in the muscle plane, and closure was done with 3-0 Vicryl for the platysma and subcutaneous layer, and the skin was closed with 4-0 subcuticular Vicryl. Dressings were applied in the usual manner with Steri-Strips, Telfa gauze, and Tegaderm. The patient was reversed from anesthesia and had an uneventful recovery. He was moving all the limbs well and was transferred in a stable condition to the Recovery Room.

Assign appropriate CPT code(s) for the preceding procedure and indicate the index entries that were used to identify the codes. Assign only CPT surgical codes (no E/M codes) and append any applicable modifiers.

1. Code(s): _____

    Index entries: _____

    _____

Exercise 4.55   Nervous System Review

Assign appropriate CPT code(s) for the following procedures and indicate the index entries that were used to identify the codes. Assign only CPT surgical codes (no E/M codes) and append any applicable modifiers.

1. Cable nerve grafts, 2.0 cm right leg and left 4.0 cm right arm

    Code(s): _____

    Index entries: _____

    _____

Exercise 4.55   (Continued)

2. Sciatic neuroplasty, left leg

    Code(s): _____

    Index entries: _____

    _____

3. Excision of neuroma of peripheral nerve of left foot

    Code(s): _____

    Index entries: _____

    _____

4. Suture repair of posterior tibial nerve

    Code(s): _____

    Index entries: _____

    _____

5. Laminectomy and excision of intradural lumbar lesion

    Code(s): _____

    Index entries: _____

    _____

6. Lumbar epidural steroid injection, L5–S1 interspace

    Code(s): _____

    Index entries: _____

    _____

7. Removal of implanted spinal neurostimulator pulse generator

    Code(s): _____

    Index entries: _____

    _____

8. Repair of 6-cm myelomeningocele

    Code(s): _____

    Index entries: _____

    _____

9. Vagus nerve block injection

    Code(s): _____

    Index entries: _____

    _____

10. Craniotomy for evacuation of subdural hematoma

    Code(s): _____

    Index entries: _____

    _____

Eye and Ocular Adnexa

The eye and ocular adnexa subsection includes procedures involving the eyeball, anterior and posterior segment, ocular adnexa, and conjunctiva. (Figure 4.19 shows the structure of the eye.) The codes are categorized first by body part involved and then by type of procedure, such as retinal and choroid repair, conjunctivoplasty, cataract removal, and removal of foreign body. Many of the refractive procedures performed for vision correction (such as LASIK procedures) are categorized in the unlisted category for the anterior segment, CPT code 66999, rather than having specific CPT codes.

Cataract Extraction

The note at the beginning of the cataract extraction subsection (66830–66986) identifies the following procedures as part of the extraction: lateral canthotomy, iridectomy, iridotomy, anterior capsulotomy, posterior capsulotomy, use of viscoelastic agents, enzymatic zonulysis, use of other pharmacologic agents, and subconjunctival or sub-Tenon injections. When performed as part of the cataract extraction, these procedures should not be coded separately because they are incorporated into the bigger procedure of the cataract removal.

The two types of cataract extraction are extracapsular and intracapsular. Extracapsular extraction, which includes removal of the lens material without removing the posterior capsule, is reported with codes 66840 through 66852, 66940, 66982, and 66984. Intracapsular extraction, which involves removal of the entire lens including the capsule, is reported with codes 66920, 66930, and 66983.

Figure 4.19.   Structure of the eye

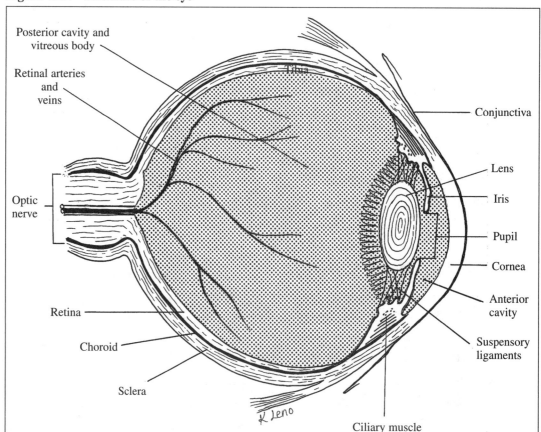

Codes 66982, 66983, and 66984 describe cataract extraction with insertion of intraocular lens (IOL) prosthesis during the same operative episode. Insertion of IOL prosthesis performed during a subsequent encounter is reported with code 66985.

Exercise 4.56   Eye and Ocular Adnexa

Operative Report

Preoperative Diagnosis: Cataract of the left eye

Postoperative Diagnosis: Cataract of the left eye

Operative Procedure: Phacoemulsification of cataract of the left eye with lens implantation

Complications: None

The patient is a 77-year-old female with a history of decreasing vision to a level of 20/100 in her left eye. Slit lamp examination showed a nuclear sclerotic cataract. Fundus examination view appeared to be normal. The patient requested removal of the cataract for improvement in her vision.

Procedure: The patient was brought to the OR and placed on the operating table in the supine position. A small amount of Brevital was given intravenously for relaxation, and then a local anesthetic using 0.75% Marcaine in a peribulbar manner and a modified Van Lint manner was administered. After obtaining proper anesthetic effect, the eye was prepped and draped in the usual manner. A blepharostat was placed between the lids of the eye, and a bridle suture using 4-0 silk was placed through the superior rectus tendon. A peritomy was performed from the 2 to 10 o'clock position superiorly with cautery used to obtain hemostasis. A 3.5-mm grooved incision was placed tangent to the limbus approximately 2 mm posterior to the surgical limbus, and a scleral tunnel was formed anteriorly toward clear cornea. A stab incision was made at the 2 o'clock position in the limbus with a #75 Beaver blade forming an irrigating peritomy site, and the anterior chamber was entered at the base of the scleral tunnel, using a #55 Keratome blade. Healon was instilled in the anterior chamber, and then an irrigating cystotome blade was used to perform a smooth capsulorrhexis opening of the anterior capsule. A balanced salt solution was used to perform hydrodissection, and the phacoemulsification tip was used to break up and remove the nucleus of the lens. The remaining cortical material was removed from the eye using the irrigation-aspiration tip. The posterior capsule of the lens was polished using a Kratz scratcher. The wound was extended very slightly, and then a 6-mm folding posterior chamber lens was placed in the eye with the lens within the capsular bag. Excess Healon was removed from the eye using the irrigation-aspiration tip.

The corneosclera was tested and found to be watertight and free of any iris incarceration. The conjunctiva was repositioned to its original site and tacked down using bipolar cautery. A collagen shield, which had been soaked in a suspension of Tobradex eyedrops, was then placed over the cornea and one drop of Timoptic was instilled on the conjunctiva. The blepharostat and the bridle suture were removed from the eye, and a dry dressing and Fox shield were placed over the eye. The patient tolerated the procedure well and left the OR in good condition. She was instructed to leave the eye dressing intact for the remainder of the day and to return to the office the following day for follow-up care and instructions.

Assign appropriate CPT code(s) for the preceding procedure and indicate the index entries that were used to identify the codes. Assign only CPT surgical codes (no E/M codes) and append any applicable modifiers.

1. Code(s): _____

    Index entries: _____

    _____

Strabismus Surgery

Strabismus is a condition in which there is abnormal deviation of one eye in relation to the other. Surgical correction is performed on the muscles that regulate the movement of the eyeball. CPT codes from the series 67311 through 67318 require documentation of the number and types of muscles involved in the procedure. The procedure descriptions are considered to be unilateral. Note the following definitions:

- *Extraocular muscles:* Six extraocular muscles are attached to each eye, two horizontal and four vertical.

- *Horizontal muscles:* Two horizontal extraocular muscles—lateral rectus and medial rectus—move the eye from side to side.

- *Vertical muscles:* Four vertical extraocular muscles—inferior rectus, superior rectus, inferior oblique, and superior oblique—move the eye up and down.

Exercise 4.57   Eye and Ocular Adnexa Review

Assign appropriate CPT code(s) for the following procedures and indicate the index entries that were used to identify the codes. Assign only CPT surgical codes (no E/M codes) and append any applicable modifiers.

1. With the use of a slit lamp, the physician removes a piece of metal from the patient's cornea.

   Code(s): _____

   Index entries: _____

2. Biopsy of left upper eyelid

   Code(s): _____

   Index entries: _____

3. Excision of 0.5-cm lesion of conjunctiva

   Code(s): _____

   Index entries: _____

4. Excision of a chalazion, right upper eyelid

   Code(s): _____

   Index entries: _____

5. Strabismus correction involving the lateral rectus muscle

   Code(s): _____

   Index entries: _____

6. Incision into upper right eyelid to drain abscess

   Code(s): _____

   Index entries: _____

Exercise 4.57 (Continued)

7. Repair of left blepharoptosis using superior rectus technique with fascial sling

    Code(s): _____

    Index entries: _____

    _____

8. Excisional transverse blepharotomy with one-quarter lid margin rotation graft

    Code(s): _____

    Index entries: _____

    _____

9. Ectropion repair using absorbable sutures

    Code(s): _____

    Index entries: _____

    _____

10. Orbitotomy of right eye to remove a piece of glass

    Code(s): _____

    Index entries: _____

    _____

Auditory System

The auditory system subsection includes codes for procedures performed on the inner, outer, and middle ear. (Figure 4.20 depicts the structure of the ear.) Diagnostic services such as audiometry and vestibular testing, however, are found in the medicine section of CPT. Surgical procedures are found in the code range from 69000 through 69979 and have no specific coding guidelines designated that impact code assignment.

One of the most commonly performed auditory surgical procedures is the tympanostomy for insertion of ventilating tubes for children with chronic ear infections. Under direct visualization with a microscope, the physician makes an incision in the eardrum (tympanum). The physician also may remove fluid from the middle ear. A ventilating tube is inserted through the opening in the tympanum. Coders may be confused by the terminology when the physicians state that they performed a "myringotomy for insertion of ventilating tubes." For coding purposes, this describes a tympanostomy (code 69433 or 69436).

Figure 4.20. Structure of the ear

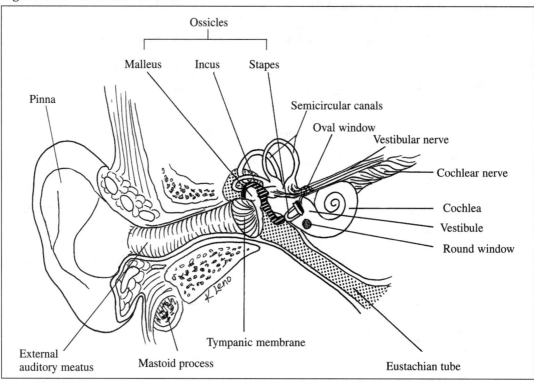

Exercise 4.58   Auditory System

Operative Report

Preoperative Diagnosis: Bilateral otitis media

Postoperative Diagnosis: Same

Procedure: Bilateral myringotomy with tubes

The patient was brought to the operating room, placed in a supine position, and given a general anesthesia. Myringotomies were performed bilaterally in the anterior-superior quadrant of each tympanic membrane. The left middle ear cavity contained a mucopurulent material; the right middle ear cavity contained a thick mucoid material. Tympanostomy tubes were placed bilaterally without difficulty. The patient tolerated the procedure well and was discharged to the recovery area.

Assign appropriate CPT code(s) for the preceding procedure and indicate the index entries that were used to identify the codes. Assign only CPT surgical codes (no E/M codes) and append any applicable modifiers.

1. Code(s): _____

    Index entries: _____

    _____

Exercise 4.59   Auditory System Review

Assign appropriate CPT code(s) for the following procedures and indicate the index entries that were used to identify the codes. Assign only CPT surgical codes (no E/M codes) and append any applicable modifiers.

1. Labyrinthectomy with mastoidectomy

    Code(s): _____

    Index entries: _____

    _____

2. Under general anesthesia, a surgeon removes a pebble from the left external auditory canal of a 1-year-old child.

    Code(s): _____

    Index entries: _____

    _____

3. Tympanoplasty with mastoidotomy and ossicular chain reconstruction

    Code(s): _____

    Index entries: _____

    _____

4. Drainage of external left ear hematoma requiring an extensive amount of time

    Code(s): _____

    Index entries: _____

    _____

5. Physician inflates blocked eustachian tube by increasing air pressure in nasopharynx.

    Code(s): _____

    Index entries: _____

    _____

Exercise 4.60   Chapter 4 Review

Assume that the following procedures were performed in either the outpatient department or the emergency department of Central Hospital. Assign the appropriate CPT code(s) and modifiers that the *hospital* would submit to payers for reimbursement. Also indicate the index entries you used to find the codes.

1. Incision and drainage of complicated parotid gland abscess

   Code(s): _____

   Index entries: _____

   _____

2. Bilateral tympanostomy with insertion of ventilating tube performed under general anesthesia

   Code(s): _____

   Index entries: _____

   _____

3. Colposcopy of cervix (upper vagina) with biopsy of the cervix

   Code(s): _____

   Index entries: _____

   _____

4. Cystourethroscopy with fulguration of bladder tumor (1.0 cm)

   Code(s): _____

   Index entries: _____

   _____

5. Open incisional biopsy of left breast (Medicare patient)

   Code(s): _____

   Index entries: _____

   _____

6. Intermediate wound repair of a 2-cm laceration of the face

   Code(s): _____

   Index entries: _____

   _____

7. Closed treatment of distal phalangeal fracture of right thumb without manipulation (Medicare patient)

   Code(s): _____

   Index entries: _____

   _____

8. Direct laryngoscopy with biopsy and use of operating microscope

   Code(s): _____

   Index entries: _____

   _____

Exercise 4.60 (Continued)

9. Placement of central venous catheter via basilic vein in 50-year-old patient for hemodialysis

   Code(s): _____

   Index entries: _____

   _____

10. Flexible sigmoidoscopy with removal of polyp by hot biopsy forceps

    Code(s): _____

    Index entries: _____

    _____

11. Repair of bilateral, initial inguinal hernia with strangulation in a 10-year-old

    Code(s): _____

    Index entries: _____

    _____

12. Arthroscopy of the left elbow with removal of loose body

    Code(s): _____

    Index entries: _____

    _____

13. Drainage of abscess of left thumb and second finger

    Code(s): _____

    Index entries: _____

    _____

Exercise 4.61   Chapter 4 Review

Assume that the following procedures were performed by physicians in the surgery department of a hospital. Assign the appropriate CPT codes and modifiers for the *physician services only.* Also indicate which index entries you used to find the codes.

1. Craniectomy for excision of cerebellopontine angle tumor, a complex procedure that required the services of two neurosurgeons

   Code(s) for physician #1: _____

   Code(s) for physician #2: _____

   Index entries: _____

   _____

2. Induced abortion by dilatation and curettage

   Code(s): _____

   Index entries: _____

   _____

(Continued on next page)

Exercise 4.61   (Continued)

3. Diagnostic and surgical arthroscopy of the right shoulder with complete synovectomy

   Code(s): _____

   Index entries: _____

   _____

4. Insertion of permanent cardiac pacemaker and atrial and ventricular transvenous electrodes; physician #1 provided the postoperative management for this patient; physician #2 provided the preoperative management and performed the procedure at a university hospital

   Code(s): _____

   Index entries: _____

   _____

5. Endoscopic retrograde cholangiopancreatography (ERCP) with endoscopic retrograde insertion of tube into pancreatic duct

   Code(s): _____

   Index entries: _____

   _____

6. Laparoscopy with removal of tubes and ovaries; the operative report indicates that the procedure was extremely difficult to perform and took two hours longer to complete than usual

   Code(s): _____

   Index entries: _____

   _____

7. Bilateral probing of lower nasolacrimal ducts with irrigation under general anesthesia

   Code(s): _____

   Index entries: _____

   _____

8. Bilateral sinus endoscopy with maxillary antrostomy and removal of maxillary sinus tissue

   Code(s): _____

   Index entries: _____

   _____

9. Total abdominal colectomy with continent ileostomy

   Code(s): _____

   Index entries: _____

   _____

10. Closed treatment of distal fibular fracture without manipulation; the patient was in the postoperative period for an arthroscopy of the shoulder performed two weeks ago; the same physician performed both surgeries

    Code(s): _____

    Index entries: _____

    _____

11. Microdermabrasion of the epidermis to remove tattoo of arm

    Code(s): _____

    Index entries: _____

    _____

Chapter 4 Test

Write the appropriate answers.

1. Excision of solar keratosis, face, .5 cm in diameter, with no significant margins

   Code(s): _____

2. Repair of 3.4-cm laceration of the left forearm, single-layer closure with 4-0 Dexon, repair of 2.0-cm laceration of the left upper arm, single-layer closure

   Code(s): _____

3. Open reduction of knee dislocation with repair of the anterior cruciate ligament by Anchor suture

   Code(s): _____

4. Putti-Platt procedure, left shoulder

   Code(s): _____

5. Nasal sinus endoscopy with anterior ethmoidectomy

   Code(s): _____

6. Bronchoscopy with tracheal dilation and stenting

   Code(s): _____

7. Insertion of permanent pacemaker with atrial and ventricular transvenous leads

   Code(s): _____

8. Insertion of intra-aortic balloon pump, percutaneous

   Code(s): _____

9. Ligation and stripping of long and short saphenous veins

   Code(s): _____

10. Percutaneous transluminal iliac angioplasty

    Code(s): _____

11. Needle biopsy of inguinal lymph nodes

    Code(s): _____

12. ERCP with manipulation and removal of stone from the common bile duct

    Code(s): _____

13. Uvulopalatopharyngoplasty for sleep apnea

    Code(s): _____

14. Laparoscopic Nissen fundoplication

    Code(s): _____

(Continued on next page)

Chapter 4 Test   (Continued)

15. Small bowel endoscopy with control of hemorrhagic site in ileum using bipolar cautery

    Code(s): _____

16. Colonoscopy with removal of five colonic polyps using hot biopsy forceps

    Code(s): _____

17. Cystourethroscopy with fulguration of three bladder tumors ranging in size from 0.4 to 1.6 cm

    Code(s): _____

18. Cystourethroscopy with biopsy of bladder wall

    Code(s): _____

19. Insertion of semirigid penile prosthesis

    Code(s): _____

20. Vaginal hysterectomy (weight of uterus 230 grams) with enterocele repair

    Code(s): _____

21. Excision of adenoma of thyroid

    Code(s): _____

22. Diagnostic lumbar spinal tap

    Code(s): _____

23. Injection of bupivacaine and Depo-Medrol, L4 facet

    Code(s): _____

24. Strabismus surgery, recession of superior oblique muscle

    Code(s): _____

25. Repair of tympanic membrane perforation using synthetic patch

    Code(s): _____

Chapter 5

Radiology

The radiology section of CPT includes the following subsections:

Subsection	Code Range
Diagnostic Radiology (Diagnostic Imaging)	70010–76499
Diagnostic Ultrasound	76506–76999
Radiation Oncology	77261–77799
Nuclear Medicine	78000–79999

It is important to understand the differences between the subsections and not to assign codes based on the area of the body being treated or studied. Some of the subsections contain instructions that are unique to them, and notes are included throughout each subsection to explain important instructions, such as the definitions of A-mode, M-mode, or B-scan ultrasounds.

Many of the conventions and guidelines discussed in earlier chapters of *Basic CPT/HCPCS Coding* also apply to this chapter. Specific conventions pertinent to the radiology section are included in this chapter.

Links to the Society of Interventional Radiology and MedLearn that are pertinent to the discussion in this chapter are located in the Web resources at the back of this book.

Hospital Billing and Radiology Code Reporting

When reporting radiological procedures, many hospitals use a computer program called a chargemaster. The chargemaster contains all the codes, abbreviated definition descriptions, charges, and sometimes other information used by any given hospital, physician office, or clinic. (See Table 5.1 for an example excerpt from a radiology chargemaster.) Thus, whenever a radiological procedure is ordered and performed, the computer automatically assigns the code and applies the charge from the requisition form the physician used to order the service. The chargemaster is known by several other names, including charge description master, standard charge file, service item master, or charge compendium. In most cases, each ancillary department is responsible for maintaining its codes in the chargemaster. Requests for input, however, often are made to health information management (HIM) departments.

Periodic review of these systems is mandatory for correct reimbursement and data quality control. The wrong code attached to a procedure can result in significant revenue loss or overpayment for a hospital or large clinic. Inappropriate unbundling of codes can result in

Table 5.1. Example excerpt from radiology chargemaster

Charge Seq Number	Revenue Center*		Description	CPT Code
	DEPT 721	RADIOLOGY—DIAGNOSTIC		
1700004 999	320	X RAY	NO CHARGE	
1701101 999	320	X RAY	MANDIBLE	70110
1701309 999	320	X RAY	MASTOIDS STENVERS LAWS	70130
1701341 999	320	X RAY	INT AUD CANAL	70134
1701341 999	320	X RAY	FACIAL BONES	70150
1701606 999	320	X RAY	NASAL BONES	70160
1701903 999	320	X RAY	OPTIC FORAMINA	70190
1702000 999	320	X RAY	ORBITS	70200
1702208 999	320	X RAY	SINUSES	70220
1702406 999	320	X RAY	SELLA TURCICA	70240
1702604 910	320	X RAY	SKULL	70260
1703305 999	320	X RAY	TEMPMAND JT BI	70330
1703552 999	320	X RAY	DENTAL PANOREX	70355
1703602 999	320	X RAY	NECK FOR SOFT TISSUE	70360
1703800 999	320	X RAY	SALIVARY GLAND	70380
1710102 910	324	X RAY	CHEST PA	71010

*73010320 = MDLAB, 910 = ER, 920 = OUTP, 921 = OUTP, 999 = INP

fraudulent charges to insurance companies, so the accuracy of any automated coding via a chargemaster program is an important data quality concern.

Physician Billing

When a radiology service is performed in a physician's office or a freestanding center owned by the radiologist, the Medicare Part B carrier will pay the radiologist for both the professional component (PC) and the technical component (TC). Payment for the technical component covers the cost for personnel, equipment, and supplies involved in the nonphysician portion of the services. Because many physicians do not have radiological equipment in their offices, they usually refer patients who need radiological procedures to the local hospital or a freestanding radiological center. In such cases, coders and billers for referring physicians do not assign radiology codes unless the physicians or facilities provide supervision and interpretation. Usually, radiological procedures are reported by radiologists associated with a hospital, clinic, or freestanding radiology center. Individuals providing billing services for radiologists and/or radiation oncologists must have a thorough understanding of radiological procedures, ultrasound procedures, nuclear medicine procedures, and radiation therapy.

In some cases, hospitals employ radiologists and report both technical and professional components of procedures or, when available, CPT codes representing complete procedures or CPT codes without modifiers. Revisions have been made to CPT that have created fewer complete procedures and more procedures where the professional and technical components are reported using separate codes. The Medicare Physician Fee Schedule database contains a list of codes that have been approved for splitting.

Radiological Supervision and Interpretation

Many codes in the radiology section of CPT include the term *radiological supervision and interpretation* in their description. These codes are used to describe the radiological portion of a procedure that two physicians often perform. In situations where one physician performs the procedure and also provides the supervision and interpretation, two codes are reported: a radiological code and a code from another section of the CPT codebook, such as surgery. This is often referred to as a complete procedure.

Example: Unilateral lymphangiography of the extremity—complete procedure. The physician submits codes 75801 and 38790. Code 75801 identifies the radiological procedure, including interpretation of the results, and code 38790 identifies the injection provided for the lymphangiography.

It should be noted that the radiological supervision and interpretation codes do not apply to the radiation oncology subsection.

Modifiers in the Radiology Section

A complete listing of modifiers is in appendix A of the CPT codebook. Some of the common modifiers used with the radiology section follow:

22 **Unusual Procedural Services:** This modifier is intended for physician use only when the service provided is greater than that usually required for the listed procedure. The CPT codebook states that modifier –22 may be reported with computerized tomography codes when additional slices are required or when a more detailed examination is necessary.

26 **Professional Component:** In circumstances where a radiological procedure includes both a physician (professional) component and a technical component, modifier –26 may be reported to identify the physician (professional) component. The professional component includes supervising the procedure, reading and interpreting the results, and documenting the interpretation in a report. This service can be provided by the physician who ordered the procedure or by the radiologist on staff at the hospital or freestanding radiology clinic. The technical component includes performance of the actual procedure and expenses for supplies and equipment. Usually, this service is provided by a radiologic technician at a hospital or a freestanding radiology clinic. The physician reports the professional component by attaching modifier –26 to the appropriate radiologic procedure. The freestanding radiology clinic reports the technical component by attaching modifier –TC (technical component) to the same procedure. Modifier –TC is a Level II HCPCS modifier that may not be recognized by all payers.

Example: Code 74220, Radiologic examination of the esophagus. The physician should report 74220–26, and the clinic should report 74220–TC.

When reporting a code that includes "radiologic supervision and interpretation" in the description, modifier –26 should not be appended to the procedure code. Because the radiologic supervision and interpretation code already describes the professional component, the modifier is unnecessary.

Example: Cervical myelography with the physician providing only the supervision and interpretation of this procedure. The physician should report as follows: 72240, Myelography, cervical, radiological supervision and interpretation.

In this example, modifier –26 is inappropriate because the descriptor for code 72240 already indicates that the physician provided only supervision and interpretation of the procedure.

51 **Multiple Procedures:** Modifier –51 (for physician use only) may be reported to identify that multiple radiological procedures were performed on the same day or during the same radiological episode. The first procedure listed should identify the major procedure or the one that is most resource intensive.

52 **Reduced Services:** Modifier –52 may be reported by hospitals or physicians to indicate that a radiological procedure has been partially reduced or eliminated at the discretion of the physician.

The CPT codebook states that modifier –52 may be reported with computerized tomography codes for a limited study or a follow-up study.

53 **Discontinued Procedure:** Modifier –53 is appropriate in circumstances where the physician elected to terminate or discontinue a diagnostic procedure, usually because of risk to the patient's well-being. Modifier –73 or –74 would be used for hospital reporting.

> **Example:** A patient planned to have urography with KUB, which would be reported with code 74400. Because the patient fainted during the procedure, it was discontinued before completion. The physician should report 74400–53.

59 **Distinct Procedural Services:** Modifier –59 may be used by both hospitals and physicians to identify that a procedure or service was distinct or independent from other services provided on the same day. Modifier –59 is appropriate for procedures that have been performed together because of specific circumstances, although they usually are not integral to one another or not performed together.

RT/LT Modifiers: Modifiers –RT and –LT are Level II HCPCS modifiers that should be reported when bilateral radiological procedures are performed. To report these modifiers to reflect a bilateral radiological procedure, the procedure code should be assigned twice and –RT attached to one code and –LT to the other.

> **Example:** 73650–RT and 73650–LT, Radiologic examination of the calcaneus with a minimum of two views, bilateral

Both modifiers apply to Medicare claims, and their use varies according to the reporting requirements of Medicaid programs and other third-party payers. The CMS guidelines for hospitals state that –RT and –LT are not to be used to report bilateral surgical procedures. Instead, modifier –50 is to be used because of the effect on payment.

Diagnostic Radiology (Diagnostic Imaging)

Codes 70010 through 76499 describe diagnostic radiology services and are subdivided first by anatomic site and then by specific type of procedure performed: x-ray, computed tomography (CT) scan, magnetic resonance imaging (MRI) scan, and magnetic resonance angiography (MRA) scan. These radiology procedures may be found in the alphabetic index of the CPT codebook by referencing the following main entries: X-ray, CT scan, Magnetic Resonance Imaging, and Magnetic Resonance Angiography. They also may be referenced under the specific site with a subterm identifying the specific procedure.

The CPT codebook differentiates between radiological procedures with and without contrast material. Contrast material consists of radiopaque substances that obstruct the passage of x-rays and cause the areas containing the material to appear white on the x-ray film, thus outlining the contour of body structures and permitting the identification of abnormal growths. Contrast material may be administered orally or intravenously. Examples of contrast agents include barium or Gastrografin, iohexol, iopamidol, ioxaglate, Hypaque, and Renografin. Commonly performed radiologic examinations using contrast material include barium enema, angiography, cystogram, endoscopic retrograde cholangiopancreatogram, fistulogram, intravenous pyelogram, excretory urogram, lymphangiography, oral cholecystogram, retrograde pyelogram, and voiding cystourethrogram.

CT scans also may be performed with or without contrast material. Although this radiological procedure can scan any body part, it is most helpful in evaluating the brain, lung, mediastinum, retroperitoneum, and liver.

When coverage requirements are met, reimbursement for the supply of contrast media may be obtained by reporting the appropriate HCPCS code.

MRI scans are almost equal to CT scans, although they are considered superior for scanning the brain, spinal cord, soft tissues, and adrenal and renal masses. This radiological procedure is contraindicated for patients who have metallic objects in their bodies, such as pacemakers, shrapnel, cochlear implants, metallic eye fragments, and vascular clips in the central nervous system. Contrast material also can be used when performing MRI scans. Gadolinium (gadopentetate dimeglumine) is the contrast agent most often used.

Exercise 5.1   Diagnostic Radiology

Assign the appropriate codes for the following procedure(s). Append modifiers if applicable.

1. MRI of abdomen with contrast

    _____

2. CT scan of lumbar spine without contrast

    _____

3. X-ray of pelvis, AP

    _____

4. Upper GI series with KUB

    _____

5. Cystography, three views, supervision and interpretation only

    _____

Interventional Radiology

Interventional radiology is the branch of medicine that diagnoses and/or treats diseases using percutaneous or minimally invasive techniques with the use of imaging guidance. Assigning codes for interventional radiology requires advanced study and thorough knowledge of anatomy and physiology. Suggested references are provided in this book.

Diagnostic Ultrasound

The subsection of diagnostic ultrasound includes codes 76506 through 76999, which are subdivided by anatomic site. The diagnostic ultrasound codes can be found in the alphabetic index of the CPT codebook by referencing the main entries of Ultrasound or Echography. Diagnostic ultrasound involves the use of ultrasonic waves, or high-frequency sound waves, to visualize internal structures of the body. Ultrasounds are commonly performed for evaluation of the abdomen, the pelvis (for both gynecologic and obstetric diagnoses), and the heart.

Four types of diagnostic ultrasounds are recognized:

*   An A-mode ultrasound is a one-dimensional ultrasonic measurement procedure.

*   An M-mode ultrasound is a one-dimensional ultrasonic measurement procedure with movement of the trace to record amplitude and velocity of moving echo-producing structures.

- A B-scan ultrasound is a two-dimensional ultrasonic scanning procedure with a two-dimensional display.

- A real-time scan is a two-dimensional ultrasonic scanning procedure with display of both two-dimensional structure and motion with time.

The medicine section of the CPT codebook includes ultrasounds involving the following areas:

- Cerebrovascular arterial studies (93875–93893)

- Arterial studies of the extremities (93922–93931)

- Venous studies of the extremities (93965–93971)

- Visceral and penile vascular studies (93975–93981)

- Ultrasounds of the heart (echocardiography) (93303–93350)

Exercise 5.2 Diagnostic Ultrasound

Assign the appropriate codes for the following procedure(s). Append modifiers if applicable.

1. Saline infusion hysterosonography with color flow Doppler

_____

2. Limited ultrasound of pregnant uterus to determine fetal position

_____

3. Bilateral ultrasound of breasts

_____

Radiation Oncology

The radiation oncology codes (77261–77799) describe the therapeutic use of radiation to treat diseases, especially neoplastic tumors. Radiation therapy may be used as primary therapy to treat certain types of malignancies, such as early stages of Hodgkin's disease. It also may be used:

- As adjuvant treatment in small-cell lung cancer and head and neck cancers

- As palliative treatment to alleviate pain caused by metastasis to bone

- To control bleeding caused by gynecologic malignancies

- To relieve obstruction and compression from advanced lung cancer, brain lesions, and spinal cord lesions

The most common type of radiation used in the treatment is electromagnetic radiation with x-rays and gamma rays. X-rays are photons generated inside a machine; gamma rays are photons emitted from a radioactive source. Radiation is measured in units known as the radiation-absorbed dose (rad) or the gray (Gy). The Gy is equal to 100 rad.

The delivery of radiation therapy may be external or internal. *External* radiation therapy involves delivery of a beam of ionizing radiation from an external source through the patient's skin toward the tumor region. *Internal* radiation therapy, also known as brachytherapy, involves applying a radioactive material inside the patient or in close proximity. This material may be contained in various types of devices, including tubes, needles, wires, seeds, and other small containers. Common radioactive materials used in brachytherapy include radium-226, cobalt-60, cesium-137, and iodine-125. Three types of brachytherapy are recognized in the CPT codebook:

- Interstitial brachytherapy involves placing a radiation source directly into tissues.

- Intracavitary brachytherapy utilizes radiation source(s) placed in special devices and then implanted in body cavities.

- Surface application brachytherapy uses radioactive material that is contained on the surface of a plaque or mold and applied directly or close to the surface of the patient.

Radiation Consultation, Treatment Management, and Treatment Delivery

Radiation oncologists often provide consultative services before a treatment plan is developed for the patient. Such treatment planning consultations should be reported with the appropriate E/M, medicine, or surgery code.

The actual management of radiation treatment services is reported in units of five fractions or treatment sessions, regardless of the actual time period in which the services are furnished. The services need not be furnished on consecutive days. Multiple fractions representing two or more treatment sessions furnished on the same day may be counted as long as there has been a distinct break in therapy sessions and the fractions are of the character usually furnished on different days.

Codes 77401 through 77421 describe the technical component of delivering the radiation treatment, as well as the various energy levels administered. To assign the appropriate code, the following information is needed:

- Number of treatment areas involved

- Number of ports involved

- Number of shielding blocks used

- Total million electron volts (MeV) administered

Hyperthermia Treatment

Hyperthermia involves the use of heat to raise the temperature of a specific area of the body to increase cell metabolism and destroy cancer cells. Usually, it is performed as an adjunct to radiation therapy or chemotherapy. The hyperthermia codes (77600–77615) in the CPT codebook include external, interstitial, and intracavitary treatment. If administered at the same time, radiation therapy should be reported separately.

Codes 77600 through 77615 include management during the hyperthermia treatment and follow-up care for three months after completion.

Clinical Brachytherapy

Clinical brachytherapy uses natural or manufactured radioactive elements that are applied in or around a particular treatment field. A therapeutic radiologist supervises the use of radioactive elements and interprets appropriate dosage. When the services of a surgeon are needed, modifier 66 or 62 may be reported to ensure that both physicians are reimbursed.

Codes 77750 through 77799 include admission to the hospital and daily visits by the physician. The codes differentiate between interstitial and intracavitary brachytherapy, and are subdivided further to identify the number of sources/ribbons applied: simple, intermediate, or complex. The CPT codebook includes definitions for each of these levels. (In the context of clinical brachytherapy, the term *sources* refers to intracavitary or permanent interstitial placement of radioactive material and the term *ribbons* refers to temporary interstitial placement of radioactive material.)

Nuclear Medicine

Nuclear medicine involves the administration of radioisotopes, which are radioactive elements that diagnose diseases. The radioactive isotope deteriorates spontaneously and emits gamma rays from inside the body that enable the physician to view internal abnormalities. Some radioisotopes are selectively absorbed by tumors or specific organs in the body, making them visible on the scan.

Nuclear medicine procedures are organized in codes 78000 through 79999 according to body systems, such as the cardiovascular system. The provision of radium or other radioelements is not included in the services listed in this section. These procedures may be found in the alphabetic index of the CPT codebook by referencing "Nuclear Imaging" or "Nuclear Medicine."

Some of the more common diagnostic nuclear medicine scans include the following:

- Bone scans are performed as part of metastatic workups to identify infections such as osteomyelitis, to evaluate hip prosthesis, to distinguish pathologic fractures from traumatic fractures, and to evaluate delayed union of fractures.

- Cardiac scans are performed for diagnosis of myocardial infarction, stress testing, ejection fractures, measurement of cardiac output, and diagnosis of ventricular aneurysms.

  —The thallium 201 scan examines myocardial perfusion, with normal myocardium appearing as "hot" and ischemic or infarcted areas appearing as "cold."

  —The technetium 99m pyrophosphate scan identifies recently damaged myocardial tissue and is most sensitive 24 to 72 hours after an acute myocardial infarction.

  —The technetium 99m ventriculogram scan identifies abnormal wall motion, cardiac shunts, size and function of heart chambers, cardiac output, and ejection fraction. The multigated acquisition (MUGA) scan is another form of this type of study.

When the following tests are performed during exercise and/or pharmacologic stress, the appropriate stress-testing code from the 93015 through 93018 range should be reported in addition to the appropriate code from the nuclear medicine subsection:

- Hepatobiliary scans (HIDA scans) are performed for diagnosis of biliary obstruction, acute cholecystitis, or biliary atresia.

- Lung scans (ventilation-perfusion [V/Q] scans) can reveal pulmonary disease, chronic obstructive pulmonary disease, and emphysema. When performed along with chest x-rays, these scans are important tools in evaluating pulmonary emboli.

- Renal scans are performed to evaluate the overall function of the kidneys.

- Thyroid scans are most commonly performed with technetium 99m pertechnetate and are useful in detecting nodules.

Exercise 5.3 Chapter 5 Review

Assign the appropriate codes for the following procedure(s). Include CPT modifiers and HCPCS Level II modifiers when applicable.

1. Radiological examination (x-ray) of the forearm, anteroposterior (A/P) and lateral views. What code(s) should be submitted on the claim form if the physician provided only the supervision and interpretation (professional component) for this procedure?

   _____

2. MRI of the cervical spine with contrast material. What code(s) should be submitted on the claim form for the radiologist to receive payment?

   _____

3. Physician performed the radiological supervision and interpretation for cystography (minimum of three views). What code(s) should be submitted?

   _____

4. Myocardial perfusion imaging (nuclear medicine) single study performed at rest; myocardial perfusion study with ejection fraction. What code(s) should be submitted?

   _____

5. Bilateral screening mammogram. What code(s) should be submitted?

   _____

6. Radiologic supervision and interpretation for transluminal atherectomy of renal artery. What code(s) should be submitted?

   _____

7. CT scan of the head with contrast material. What code(s) and modifier should the radiology clinic report on the claim it submits?

   _____

8. Pelvic ultrasound, pregnant uterus. Real-time with image documentation, transvaginal. What code(s) should be submitted?

   _____

9. Radiologist provided radiological supervision and interpretation for ultrasonic guidance needle biopsy. What code(s) should be submitted?

   _____

10. Whole-body bone scan (nuclear medicine). What code(s) should be submitted?

   _____

11. Barium enema with KUB. What code(s) should be submitted?

   _____

12. SPECT liver imaging. What code(s) should be submitted?

   _____

(Continued on next page)

Exercise 5.3   (Continued)

13. Delivery of radiation therapy to single area with single port and simple blocks–13 MeV. What code(s) should be submitted?

_____

14. Renal scan with vascular flow and function study (nuclear medicine) without pharmacological intervention. What code(s) should be submitted?

_____

15. Chest x-ray, two views. What code(s) should be submitted?

_____

16. Intracavitary placement of four radioelement sources. What code(s) should be submitted?

_____

17. Cervical myelogram (S&I). What code(s) should be submitted?

_____

18. Retroperitoneal ultrasound, limited study. What code(s) should be submitted?

_____

19. X-ray of the hips and pelvis in a five-year-old, with minimum of two views. What code(s) should be submitted?

_____

20. Gastroesophageal reflux study. What code(s) should be submitted?

_____

Assign the appropriate CPT codes to the following reports. Assume that you are billing for the professional and technical component.

21. RENAL ULTRASOUND

   History: Pyelonephritis

   Findings: The right kidney measures 11.1 cm and left measures 11.5 Both kidneys are normal in echo texture and smooth in contour. There is no mass, calcification, or evidence of hydronephrosis. There is no perinephric fluid collection or abscess. There is no evidence of focal nephronia.

   There is a cyst in the upper pole of the right kidney. This measures just under 2 cm. It has typical ultrasound characteristics of a benign renal cyst.

_____

22. AP PELVIS AND LEFT HIP

   There is generalized demineralization of the bone.

   There is an intertrochanteric fracture of the left hip with moderate angulation and displacement present. There is a free fracture fragment of the lesser trochanter.

Exercise 5.3   (Continued)

23.   PA AND LATERAL CHEST

Coronary artery bypass graft changes are noted. The heart is mildly enlarged in size. The lung fields are clear, without infiltrate or effusion. Moderate spondylitic changes are noted in the thoracic spine.

24.   KUB, UPPER GI SERIES

A preliminary KUB study reveals a large amount of fecal matter present in the colon. Staples are seen in the right upper quadrant.

A barium meal reveals a normal filling of the esophagus. The stomach is high and transverse in type. There is a small sliding hiatal hernia and there is small gastroesophageal reflux. The duodenal bulb fills without ulceration. The stomach empties well.

Opinion: Small sliding hiatal hernia with intermittent gastroesophageal reflux

25.   CT SCAN OF THE HEAD WITHOUT INTRAVENOUS CONTRAST

Reveals a diffuse, moderately large area of localized atrophy involving the superior-most portion of the left parietal region. This is seen on images #14, 15, and 16. There is no extra-axial fluid collection, acute intracranial bleeding, midline shift, mass effect, or other significant abnormality.

IMPRESSION: Localized atrophy involving the superior-most portion of the left parietal lobe as described above. This could be old or recent. Short-term interval follow-up CT scan is suggested for further evaluation.

Chapter 5 Test

Write in the appropriate answers.

1. X-ray of mandible, five views

   _____

2. X-ray of soft tissues of the neck for foreign body

   _____

3. MRI of chest with contrast

   _____

4. Cervical myelogram, radiological supervision and interpretation

   _____

5. X-ray of fractured hip in the operating room to confirm reduction

   _____

6. Barium enema with KUB

   _____

7. Percutaneous transhepatic cholangiography, radiological supervision and interpretation

   _____

8. Ultrasound, pregnant uterus, first trimester

   _____

9. SPECT bone scan

   _____

10. Retroperitoneal ultrasound

    _____

Chapter 6

Pathology and Laboratory Services

The pathology and laboratory section of the CPT codebook includes services provided by physicians, including pathologists and technologists under the supervision of a pathologist or other physician. It includes codes for services and procedures such as organ or disease panel tests, automated multichannel tests, urinalysis, hematologic and immunologic studies, and surgical and anatomic pathologic examinations. This chapter discusses specific subsections of the pathology and laboratory section.

Subsection	Code Range
Organ or Disease Oriented Panels	80048–80076
Drug Testing	80100–80103
Therapeutic Drug Assays	80150–80299
Evocative/Suppression Testing	80400–80440
Consultations (Clinical Pathology)	80500–80502
Urinalysis	81000–81099
Chemistry	82000–84999
Hematology and Coagulation	85002–85999
Immunology	86000–86849
Transfusion Medicine	86850–86999
Microbiology	87001–87999
Anatomic Pathology	88000–88099
Cytopathology	88104–88199
Cytogenetic Studies	88230–88299
Surgical Pathology	88300–88399
Transcutaneous Procedures	88400
Other Procedures	89050–89356

Alphabetic Index

Laboratory and pathology procedures/services are listed in the alphabetic index of the CPT codebook under the following main terms:

- Specific name of the test, such as urinalysis, evocative/suppression test, and fertility test

- Specific substance/specimen/sample, such as glucose, CPK, cyanide, enterovirus, bone marrow, and nasal smear

- Specific method used, such as culture, fine needle aspiration, and microbiology

Hospital Billing for Laboratory and Pathology Procedures

In the hospital setting, the chargemaster is used to automate the billing of laboratory and pathology services. (See table 6.1 for an example excerpt from a laboratory chargemaster.) As mentioned in chapter 5, the chargemaster is a computer program containing codes, abbreviated definition descriptions, charges, and possibly other information used by a given hospital. Therefore, when patients visit the outpatient department with a requisition from their physician for laboratory work, the computer automatically assigns the appropriate code and charge for that particular service. Although coders are not really involved in the actual coding of these services, the health information management (HIM) department may be asked to help the laboratory and pathology department update its portion of the chargemaster.

Physician Billing

When reporting laboratory services provided by a physician, the coder must determine whether the physician performed the complete procedure or only a component of it. Some physician offices and physician-owned clinics have sophisticated laboratory equipment on the premises that enables the physicians to provide complete laboratory testing. A complete test would involve ordering the test, obtaining the sample (for example, blood or urine), handling the specimen, performing the actual test or procedure, and analyzing and interpreting the results. However, most physicians typically send the sample to a freestanding or hospital-based laboratory for testing and analysis. In this instance, the physician may report only the collection and handling of the blood sample or specimen.

Physicians also may send the patient for laboratory testing to a local hospital, where the sample or specimen is taken, the test or procedure is performed, and the results are analyzed and interpreted. The physician may seek reimbursement for these tests from some insurance plans when the tests are purchased from a reference laboratory or a hospital acting as a reference lab. Medicare, however, does not allow any provider who does not perform the test to bill for it. The reporting of laboratory tests depends on the organizations involved and the health plan guidelines applicable to the patient.

> **Example:** Dr. Reynolds performed a bone marrow needle biopsy in an oncology clinic and sent the specimen to a pathologist for review and interpretation. Dr. Reynolds reports 38221 for the actual biopsy of the bone marrow, and the pathologist reports 88305 for the review and interpretation of the specimen. If Dr. Reynolds pays the pathologist for the interpretation, he may report both codes, depending on the guidelines of the health plan involved.

Quantitative and Qualitative Studies

Throughout the laboratory and pathology section of the CPT codebook, code descriptions state whether the test performed is quantitative or qualitative in nature. *Qualitative* screening refers to tests that detect the presence of a particular analyte, constituent, or condition. Typically, qualitative studies are performed to determine whether a particular substance is present in the sample being evaluated. In contrast, *quantitative* studies provide results expressing specific numerical amounts of an analyte in a specimen. Usually, these tests are performed after a qualitative study to identify the specific amount of a particular substance in the sample.

Table 6.1. Excerpt from a laboratory chargemaster in numeric order by department

Charge Seq Number	Revenue Center*	Description	CPT Code
		DEPT 703 CHEMISTRY	
2120053 320	301	HEPATITIS B CORE HBc AbO	86704
2120053 910	301	HEPATITIS B CORE IgM antibody	86705
2120103 320	301	ELECTROLYTES PROFILE I	80051
2120111 999	301	BASIC METABOLIC 4	80048
2120129 320	301	GLUCOSE FASTING	82947
2120137 320	301	ACETONE SERUM	82009
2120145 320	301	GLUCOSE 1HR PP	82950
2120152 999	301	HDL CHOLESTEROL	83718
2120160 320	301	GLUCOSE 2HR PP	82950
2120186 999	301	UREA NITROGEN	84540
*320 = MDLAB, 999 = INP			

Modifiers in the Laboratory Section

Because most of the commonly used modifiers in the pathology and laboratory section have been discussed in earlier chapters, only a brief summary of each is offered here.

22   **Unusual Procedural Services:** This modifier is intended for use by physicians when the service provided is greater than the one usually required for the listed procedure.

26   **Professional Component:** In circumstances where a laboratory or pathology procedure includes both a physician (professional) component and a technical component, modifier –26 can be reported to identify the physician component.

32   **Mandated Services:** Modifier –32 may be reported when a group such as a third-party payer or a PRO mandates a service.

52   **Reduced Services:** Modifier –52 may be reported by both hospitals and physicians to indicate that a laboratory or pathology procedure was partially reduced or eliminated at the discretion of the physician.

53   **Discontinued Procedure:** Modifier –53 may be reported by physicians only to indicate that the physician elected to terminate a procedure due to circumstances that put the patient's well-being at risk.

59   **Distinct Procedural Service:** Modifier –59 may be used by both hospitals and physicians to identify that a procedure or service was distinct or independent from other services provided on the same day. This modifier may be used when procedures are performed together because of specific circumstances, even though they usually are not.

90   **Reference (Outside) Laboratory:** Modifier –90 may be reported by physicians to indicate performance of the test by a party other than the treating or reporting physician.

91   **Repeat Clinical Diagnostic Laboratory Test:** Modifier –91 shows the need to repeat the same laboratory test on the same day to obtain multiple test results. It may be used by both hospitals and physicians. It is not to be used to confirm initial results due to testing problems with specimens or equipment or for any reason when a normal one-time reportable result is all that is required. In addition, it is inappropriate for tests where codes describe a series of test results, such as with glucose tolerance or evocative suppression testing.

Example: Dr. Reynolds performed a venipuncture to obtain a blood sample for a lipid panel. He prepared the sample for transport and had it sent to an outside laboratory for testing, analysis, and interpretation. Dr. Reynolds should report 80061–90 to describe the laboratory test with the interpretation and analysis being performed at an off-site laboratory, along with code 36415 for the venipuncture. If this were a Medicare patient, HCPCS code G0001 would be used to report the venipuncture and the off-site laboratory would report code 80061 for the lipid panel.

Organ- or Disease-Oriented Panels

The organ- or disease-oriented panels describe the laboratory procedures performed most commonly for specific diseases, such as hepatitis and arthritis, or for specific organs, such as thyroid and hepatic function. All the tests listed in a panel must be performed for that code to be reported. When additional tests are performed that are not part of that particular panel, the codes describing those tests also must be reported. When some, but not all, of the tests in the panel are performed, the individual CPT codes should be reported, rather than the panel code. In the index, reference the main term Organ for a list of the panels.

Example: Code 80051 describes an electrolyte panel and includes the following tests: carbon dioxide, chloride, potassium, and sodium. For code 80051 to be reported, all four tests must be performed. If the carbon dioxide test is omitted, separate codes must be assigned for the remaining tests: chloride (82435), potassium (84132), and sodium (84295). Code 80051 should not be reported.

If a glucose test is performed in addition to the electrolyte panel, a separate code is reported for the glucose test (82947), along with the electrolyte panel (80051).

Evocative/Suppression Testing

The codes used for evocative/suppression testing (80400–80440) allow the physician to determine a baseline and the effects on the body after evocative or suppressive agents are administered. In reviewing the codes in this series, it should be noted that the description for each panel identifies the type of test(s) included in that panel and the number of times a specific test must be performed.

Example: Code 80420, Dexamethasone suppression panel, 48-hour. This panel must include:
Free cortisol, urine (82530 × 2)
Cortisol (82533 × 2)
Volume measurement for timed collection (81050 × 2)

Physician attendance and monitoring during the test should be reported with the appropriate E/M services code, as well as the prolonged physician care codes, if they apply.

Chemistry

This series of codes (82000–84999) is used to report individual chemistry tests that are not performed as part of the automated organ- or disease-oriented panels (80048–80076). Unless otherwise noted in the code description, these tests are quantitative in nature.

Example: Patient was seen in the laboratory department and the calcium level test was performed. Results: total calcium: 82310

Hematology and Coagulation

The codes in the hematology and coagulation subsection (85002–85999) are used to report hematological procedures, such as complete blood count (CBC), and coagulation procedures, such as clotting factor and prothrombin time.

To assign the appropriate code, careful attention must be paid to the specific type of procedure performed. Collaboration with the medical laboratory director or technician is helpful in ensuring that CPT codes are correct and consistent with the equipment available and the actual test performed.

Surgical Pathology

In surgical pathology coding (88300–88399), the unit of service is known as the specimen. The CPT codebook defines a specimen as tissue or tissues submitted for individual and separate attention, requiring individual examination and pathologic diagnosis. Codes are differentiated by six levels. Level I (88300) identifies the gross examination of tissue only. Levels II through VI (88302–88309) refer to the gross and microscopic examination of tissue. Selection of a level between II and VI is made based on the type of specimen submitted. When two or more specimens are obtained from one patient, separate codes identifying the appropriate level for each should be reported.

Example #1: Gross examination of a gallstone. The pathologist reports code 88300.

Example #2: Gross and microscopic examination of a pituitary adenoma. The pathologist reports code 88305.

Example #3: Gross and microscopic examination of two separate colon polyps. The pathologist reports codes 88305 and 88305 to identify examination of two separate specimens.

It should be noted that codes 88300 through 88309 include the accession or acquisition, examination, and reporting of a specimen.

Exercise 6.1   Chapter 6 Review

Assign the appropriate codes for the following pathology and laboratory procedures.

1. Gross and pathologic examination of transurethral resection of the prostate

   _____

2. Natriuretic peptide

   _____

3. ACTH stimulation panel for 21-hydroxylase deficiency

   _____

4. Automated urinalysis (dip stick), without microscopy

   _____

5. Reticulated platelet assay

   _____

6. Gross and microscopic examination of left mastectomy with regional lymph nodes

   _____

7. Candida skin test

   _____

8. Confirmatory test for HTLV-1 antibody

   _____

9. The following tests were performed as a group from one blood sample: (lipid panel) total serum cholesterol, HDL and triglycerides; (electrolyte panel) carbon dioxide, chloride, potassium, and sodium

   _____

10. Quantitative testing (therapeutic drug assay) of theophylline level

    _____

11. Evaluation of blood gases—pH, pCO_2, pO_2, CO_2, and HCO_3

    _____

12. Hepatitis B surface antibody (HBsAb)

    _____

13. Partial thromboplastin time of whole blood (PTT) and prothrombin time (PT)

    _____

14. Gross and microscopic autopsy, including brain and spinal cord

    _____

15. Pathology consultation provided during surgery with frozen section of single specimen

    _____

Chapter 6 Test

Write the appropriate answer.

1. Iron-binding capacity

    _____

2. Screen for mercury

    _____

3. Spinal fluid pH

    _____

4. Protein, by refractometry

    _____

5. Urine sodium

    _____

6. Automated CBC with automated differential

    _____

7. Lee-White clotting time

    _____

8. Surgical pathology, examination (gross and microscopic) of breast and regional lymph nodes

    _____

9. Lyme disease antibody

    _____

10. Protoporphyrin screen

    _____

Chapter 7

Evaluation and Management Services

The section dedicated to evaluation and management (E/M) services was added to the CPT codebook in 1992. The E/M codes are designed to classify the cognitive services provided by physicians during skilled nursing facility (SNF) visits, consultations, and hospital and office visits. The various levels of the E/M codes describe the wide variety of skills and the amount of effort, time, responsibility, and medical knowledge that physicians dedicate to the prevention, diagnosis, and treatment of illnesses and injuries as well as the promotion of optimal health. Healthcare facilities such as hospitals also report E/M codes to designate encounters or visits for outpatient services.

In claims processing for physicians, E/M codes are reported to document the professional services provided to patients. The level of medical decision making is a key factor in the selection of appropriate E/M codes, but the level of decision making is sometimes difficult to quantify in documentation. Generally, it is preferable that physicians select E/M codes. Coding professionals can then validate and verify the physicians' code selections according to the documentation guidelines developed jointly by the American Medical Association (AMA) and the Centers for Medicare and Medicaid Services (CMS).

Assignment of an E/M code for hospital services is required in most of the prospective payment systems developed by third-party payers, such as ambulatory payment group (APG) or ambulatory payment classification (APC) systems. E/M code assignment helps distinguish medical services from surgical services when assigning patients to a particular payment group. It also facilitates data collection by counting patients rather than services for outpatient reporting because one patient may have a number of outpatient services during a single visit. Under the prospective payment system, CMS instructed hospitals to develop their own method for assignment of the facility E/M codes.

CMS and the American Academy of Family Physicians Web sites provide additional information pertinent to E/M coding. (See appendix A of this workbook for a list of relevant Web sites.)

Classification of the Evaluation and Management Services

The E/M services section of CPT is divided into broad subsections that are further divided into subcategories. The subsections and subcategories include the following:

Office or Other Outpatient Services
New Patient   99201–99205
Established Patient   99211–99215

Hospital Observation Services
    Observation Care Discharge Services   99217
    Initial Observation Care   99218–99220

Hospital Inpatient Services
    Initial Hospital Care   99221–99223
    Subsequent Hospital Care   99231–99233
    Hospital Observation or Inpatient Care Services
        (Including Admission and Discharge Services)   99234–99236
    Hospital Discharge Services   99238–99239

Consultations
    Office or Other Outpatient Consultations   99241–99245
    Initial Inpatient Consultations   99251–99255

Emergency Department Services
    New or Established Patient   99281–99285
    Other Emergency Services   99288

Pediatric Critical Care Patient Transport   99289–99290

Critical Care Services   99291–99292
    Inpatient Pediatric Critical Care   99293–99294
    Inpatient Neonatal Critical care   99295–99296
    Continuing Intensive Care Services   99289–99300

Nursing Facility Services
    Initial Nursing Facility Care   99304–99306
    Subsequent Nursing Facility Care   99307–99310
    Nursing Facility Discharge Services   99315–99316
    Other Nursing Facility Services   99318

Domiciliary, Rest Home, or Custodial Care Services
    New Patient   99324–99328
    Established Patient   99334–99337
    Home Care Plan Oversight Services   99339–99340

Home Services
    New Patient   99341–99345
    Established Patient   99347–99350

Prolonged Services
    With Direct Patient Contact   99354–99357
    Without Direct Patient Contact   99358–99359
    Standby Services   99360

Case Management Services
    Team Conferences   99361–99362
    Telephone Calls   99371–99373

Care Plan Oversight Services   99374–99380

Preventive Medicine Services

New Patient	99381–99387
Established Patient	99391–99397
Individual Counseling	99401–99404
Group Counseling	99411–99412
Other Preventive Medicine Services	99420–99429

Newborn Care	99431–99440

Special Evaluation and Management Services

Basic Life/Disability Evaluation Services	99450
Work-Related or Medical Disability Evaluation Services	99455–99456

Other Evaluation and Management Services	99499

Many of the E/M categories and subcategories include three to five levels of service codes.

Format of Evaluation and Management Codes

The basic format of the E/M service codes followed in most of the categories in the section consists of five elements:

1. A unique code number beginning with 99

2. The place or type of service (for example, physician office or other outpatient service or initial or subsequent hospital care)

3. The extent or level of service (for example, detailed history and detailed examination)

4. The nature of the presenting problem (for example, moderate severity)

5. The amount of time typically required to provide a service

Documentation Guidelines for Evaluation and Management Services

Documentation is the basis for all coding, including E/M services. In the fall of 1994, the AMA and CMS developed documentation guidelines for E/M reporting in an effort to clarify code assignment for both physicians and claims reviewers. These guidelines were implemented in 1995.

In 1997, CMS and the AMA collaborated again on a revised edition of the guidelines that includes specific elements that should be performed and documented for general multisystem and selected single-specialty examinations. However, the 1997 revised version did not replace the 1995 documentation guidelines. Physicians may use either set of guidelines, whichever is more advantageous to the individual physician. (See appendix B of this workbook, which includes an excerpt from the 1997 documentation guidelines for E/M. A complete set of the 1995 and 1997 documentation guidelines is available on the CMS Web site: cms.hhs.gov/ medlearn/emdoc.asp.)

Code Assignment for Evaluation and Management Services

Before an E/M service code can be assigned, the coder should review the documentation and answer three groups of questions:

- *What type of service did the patient receive? Was the encounter an initial or a subsequent episode of care? Was the purpose of the encounter an initial, follow-up, or confirmatory consultative service? Did the patient receive a critical care service?*

- *Where was the service provided? A physician's office or clinic? A hospital inpatient or outpatient department? An emergency department? A nursing facility or rehabilitation unit?*

- *Was the recipient of the service a new patient or one of the physician's established patients?*

The following subsections describe the factors that should be considered in determining E/M services code assignments.

New or Established Patient

Some of the E/M categories provide separate code ranges to identify new and established patients:

Office or Other Outpatient Services	99201–99215
Domiciliary, Rest Home, or Custodial Services	99324-99337
Home Services	99341–99350
Preventive Medicine Services	99381–99429

In this context, a patient who has not received any professional services from the physician (or another physician of the same specialty who belongs to the same group practice) within the past three years is considered a *new patient.* Professional services are those face-to-face services rendered by a physician and reported by a specific CPT code or codes. An *established patient* is a patient who has received services from the physician (or another physician of the same specialty who belongs to the same group practice) within the past three years.

Concurrent Care

The CPT codebook defines concurrent care as the circumstance in which two or more physicians provide similar services (for example, hospital visits or consultations) to the same patient on the same day. Health plans often limit reimbursement to one physician per day unless the physicians have different specialties and the services of more than one physician are medically necessary. CMS assigns a specialty number that is used for this purpose.

Correct assignment of ICD-9-CM codes also plays an important role in billing and receiving payment for concurrent care services. The physicians involved in the concurrent care episode must identify the appropriate ICD-9-CM code for each service provided. Assigning the same ICD-9-CM code could result in one of the physicians being denied payment, usually the one who submitted the claim last.

Example: Patient is admitted to the hospital complaining of unstable angina and uncontrolled type II diabetes mellitus. Dr. Smith treats the patient's angina, and Dr. Reynolds follows the patient's diabetes. The following codes should be reported:

Dr. Smith: 411.1, Intermediate coronary syndrome, and the appropriate E/M level of service code from the hospital inpatient services category

Dr. Reynolds: 250.02, Diabetes mellitus, uncontrolled, and the appropriate E/M level of service code from the hospital inpatient services category

Seven Factors in Evaluation and Management Services

Three key factors and four contributing factors determine appropriate E/M code assignment. The key factors are history, examination, and medical decision making. The contributing factors include counseling, coordination of care, presenting problem, and time. Information about the three key factors should be documented in the patient's health record as should information pertaining to any or all of the other four factors when they apply to a case. All applicable factors must be considered in code assignment.

History, examination, and medical decision making are essential factors because they represent the amount of resources expended by a provider in rendering a service to a patient. For example, when counseling and coordination comprise more than 50 percent of a physician–patient or physician–family encounter, time is considered the controlling fact for determining the correct code.

Example: Established patient seen in the physician's office for disease management. The physician documents that 40 minutes of the 60-minute visit was devoted to counseling and coordination. With time as the controlling factor, the appropriate code assignment would be 99215.

Documentation in the health record must support code-level selection by describing the key components and the pertinent contributing factors. Physician selection of E/M codes is recommended to ensure clinical validity for service levels. Coders may validate code selection with documentation and assist physicians in meeting the current guidelines for code selection. Facility use of E/M coding is usually assigned via a chargemaster, which is a computerized program that contains codes, abbreviated definition descriptions, and charges. (Chargemaster programs are discussed further in chapters 5 and 6.)

Appendix C of the CPT codebook includes a supplement of clinical examples illustrating the appropriate selection of E/M services codes for specific medical specialties. However, these examples are only guidelines and the documentation in the health record remains the most authoritative and final source when assigning a code for a particular level of service.

The CPT codebook defines each level of E/M services by basing it on a unique combination of the three essential factors. The key elements that define E/M services, and the variation within these elements, are reflected in table 7.1.

History

The following types of histories are recognized. The level of complexity is based on the amount of information (number of elements) obtained by the physician:

- *Problem focused:* Limited to a chief complaint and a brief history of the present illness or condition

Table 7.1. Key elements that define E/M services

History	Examination	Medical Decision Making
Problem focused	Problem focused	Straightforward
Expanded problem focused	Expanded problem focused	Low complexity
Detailed	Detailed	Moderate complexity
Comprehensive	Comprehensive	High complexity

- *Expanded problem focused:* A chief complaint, brief history, and a problem-pertinent system review

- *Detailed:* A chief complaint, expanded history of the present illness, a system review, and one item from any of the following: past, family, or social history

- *Comprehensive:* A chief complaint, extended history of present illness, extended system review, and one item from at least two (or in some cases three, depending on the E/M category) of the following: past, family, and/or social history

Each type of history includes some or all of the following elements:

- Chief complaint

- History of present illness

- Review of systems

- Past, family, and/or social history

Chief Complaint

The chief complaint (CC) is a concise statement describing the symptom, problem, condition, diagnosis, a return visit recommended by the physician, or other factor as the reason for the visit.

History of Present Illness

The history of present illness (HPI) describes the patient's developing condition/problem from the first sign and/or symptom in chronological order, starting from the initial visit to the present. Table 7.2 reflects the elements included in the HPI.

There are two types of HPI: a brief HPI and an extended HPI. A *brief HPI* refers to the documentation of no more than one to three HPI elements. It may involve a single problem without any complicating factors or symptoms. An *extended HPI* refers to the documentation of four or more HPI elements. It may be appropriate when multiple, confusing, or complex symptoms are present; when the symptoms are prolonged in development; when the history is obtained from an individual other than the patient; and when other complicating factors are present.

> **Example:** A patient is seen in the physician's office with flu-like symptoms (chief complaint). For the past two days (duration), she has had chills, fever, and muscle aches (associated signs). She feels worse in the evening (timing).

In the above example, three HPI elements are documented (duration, associated signs, and timing). Therefore, this would be considered a brief HPI.

Table 7.2.   Elements included in the HPI

HPI Element	Examples
Location	Abdomen, chest, leg, head
Severity	Bad, intolerable, minimal, slight
Timing	Two hours after eating, one hour after waking
Quality	Burning, dull, puffy, pus-filled, red
Duration	For two months, since prescription began
Associated signs/manifestations	Rash with blistering, nausea and vomiting, abdominal pain
Context	When walking in company of smokers
Modifying factors	Improves when lying down, worse after eating

Review of Systems

A review of systems (ROS) is an inventory of body systems obtained by the physician through a series of questions seeking to identify signs and/or symptoms the patient may be experiencing or has experienced. An ROS includes the following fourteen systems:

- Constitutional symptoms (fever, weight loss, and so on)
- Eyes
- Ears, nose, mouth, throat
- Cardiovascular
- Respiratory
- Gastrointestinal
- Genitourinary
- Musculoskeletal
- Integumentary (skin and/or breast)
- Neurological
- Psychiatric
- Endocrine
- Hematologic/lymphatic
- Allergic/immunologic

Three types of ROS are recognized:

- A *problem-pertinent ROS* is directly related to the problem(s) identified in the HPI. The patient's positive responses and pertinent negatives for the system related to the problem should be documented.

- An *extended ROS* is directly related to the problem(s) identified in the HPI and a limited number of additional systems. The patient's positive responses and pertinent negatives for two to nine systems should be documented.

- A *complete ROS* is directly related to the problem(s) identified in the HPI and all additional body systems. At least ten organ systems must be reviewed. Those systems with positive or pertinent negative responses should be documented individually. For the remaining systems, a notation indicating that all other systems are negative is permissible. In the absence of such a notation, at least ten systems must be documented individually.

> **Example:** A patient presents with nausea (chief complaint). She has lost 7 pounds in the past month (constitutional). She denies abdominal pain, diarrhea, and vomiting (gastrointestinal).

According to documentation guidelines, the preceding example would demonstrate an extended ROS because two systems are documented.

Past, Family, and/or Social History

The past, family, and/or social history (PFSH) element is broken down as follows:

- A *past history* consists of the patient's past experiences with illnesses, operations, injuries, and treatments (including medications). For pediatric populations, the past history also should include prenatal and birth history, feedings, food intolerance, and immunization history.

- A *family history* consists of a review of medical events in the patient's family, including diseases that may be hereditary or may place the patient at risk, as well as the age and status (alive or dead) of blood relatives.

- A *social history* consists of an age-appropriate review of past and current social activities. It also may include the patient's marital status and number of children, present and past employment, exposure to environmental agents, religion, hobbies, living conditions, water supply, and daily habits such as alcohol, tobacco, drug, and caffeine use. For veterans, it includes military service history. For pediatric populations, it may include school grades, sleep, and play habits.

There are two types of PFSH:

- A *pertinent PFSH* includes the documentation of at least one specific item from any of the three history areas.

- A *complete PFSH* refers to the documentation of at least one specific item from two of the three history areas for the following E/M categories: office or other outpatient services, established patient; emergency department; subsequent nursing facility care; domiciliary care, established patient; and home care, established patient.

At least one specific item from each of the three history areas must be documented for a complete PFSH for the following E/M categories: office or other outpatient services, new patient; hospital observation services; hospital inpatient services, initial care; consultations; comprehensive nursing facility assessments; domiciliary care, new patient; and home care, new patient.

Table 7.3 incorporates all the elements of a history. All three levels must be met to qualify for a specific level. A CC is required for all levels.

Table 7.3. Elements of a history

History Component (equal to lowest category documented)	Problem Focused	Expanded Problem Focused	Detailed	Comprehensive
Chief Complaint _____ HPI—History of Present Illness __ Location __ Duration __ Severity __ Quality __ Context __ Timing __ Modifying factors __ Associated signs and symptoms	Brief: one to three HPI elements documented	Brief: one to three HPI elements documented	Extended: four or more HPI or status of three or more chronic conditions documented	Extended: four or more HPI or status of three or more chronic conditions documented
ROS—Review of System(s) __ Constitutional (wt loss, etc.) __ Integumentary __ Endocrine __ Eyes __ GI __ Hem/lymph __ ENT, mouth __ GU __ Allergy/ __ Respiratory __ MS Immun __ Cardiovascular __ Neuro __ Psychiatric	None	Problem specific: one system	Extended: two to nine systems	Complete: more than ten systems or some with all others negative
PFSH (past medical, family, and social histories) __Previous medical (past experience with illness, injury, surgery, medical treatments, and so on) __Family medical history (diseases, which may be hereditary or with increased risk of occurrence) __Social (relationships, diet, exercise, occupation, and so on)	None	None	Pertinent: at least one item from at least one history	Complete: specifics of at least two history areas documented

Note: A chief complaint (CC) is required for all history types.

Following are some history documentation guidelines:

- The CC, ROS, and PFSH may be listed as separate elements of the history or included in the description of the HPI.

- An ROS and/or PFSH obtained during an earlier encounter do not need to be redocumented if there is evidence that the physician has reviewed and updated the previous information. The review and update may be documented by:

  —Describing any new ROS and/or PFSH information or noting that no change in the previous information has occurred

  —Noting the date and location of the earlier ROS and/or PFSH

- The ROS and/or PFSH may be recorded by ancillary staff or the patient on a completed form. To indicate that the physician has reviewed the information, a notation must supplement or confirm the documentation recorded by the other parties.

- If the physician is unable to obtain a history from the patient or other source, the documentation in the record should describe the patient's condition or other circumstance that precludes obtaining a history.

Exercise 7.1   Evaluation and Management (History)

Using table 7.3 (p. 173) and applying the documentation guidelines, assign the history level (problem focused, expanded problem focused, detailed, comprehensive) to the following scenarios.

1.   Patient seen in the physician's office complaining of a right eye that is itchy, watery, and red. Symptoms began on Saturday. Patient denies any loss of vision.

   _____

2.   Patient seen in the clinic complaining of irritated throat, runny nose, and pressure in the cheek area for the past three days. Pressure seems to be worse today. Patient reports some coughing but denies headaches, just pressure in cheeks. Temperature has been normal. No daily meds. Takes Claritin 10 mg as needed.

   _____

3.   Patient seen in the urgent care center for back pain extending down in both legs and feeling numb at times. This has been going on for about five months but has become intolerable. She notices it more when she is driving the car. The patient denies any trauma. She recently started a new job. She denies any sense of weakness. No bowel or bladder habit changes. She is not allergic to any medications. Has a history of diabetes and takes glucose tablets. She smokes two packs of cigarettes a day and drinks alcohol occasionally.

   _____

Examination

The physical examination is the objective description of the patient's chief complaint, illness, or injury. Four types of examination are recognized:

- *Problem focused:* Exam limited to the affected body area or organ system

- *Expanded problem focused:* Exam of affected body area or organ system, as well as symptomatic or related organ systems

- *Detailed:* Extended exam of affected body area(s) and other symptomatic or related organ system(s)

- *Comprehensive:* A general multisystem examination or complete examination of a single-organ system and other symptomatic or related body area(s) or organ system(s)

The types of examination have been defined by the revised guidelines for general multi-systems as well as the following single-organ systems:

- Cardiovascular

- Ears, nose, mouth, and throat

- Eyes

- Genitourinary (female)

- Genitourinary (male)

- Hematologic/lymphatic/immunologic

- Musculoskeletal

- Neurological

- Psychiatric
- Respiratory
- Skin

The following areas of the body are examined:

- Head, including the face
- Genitalia, groin, buttocks
- Neck
- Back, including spine
- Chest, including breasts and axillae
- Each extremity
- Abdomen

The following systems are examined:

- Constitutional (vital signs, general appearance)
- Genitourinary
- Eyes
- Musculoskeletal
- Ears, nose, mouth, and throat
- Skin
- Cardiovascular
- Neurologic
- Respiratory
- Psychiatric
- Hematologic/lymphatic/immunologic
- Gastrointestinal

Table 7.4 lists all the components of an examination.

Table 7.4. Components of an examination

Exam Component			Problem Focused	Expanded Problem Focused*	Detailed	Comprehensive
Body Areas __ Head, face __ Neck __ Chest, breasts __ Abdomen __ Genit, groin __ Back, spine __ Each extremity	**Organ Systems** __ Const. (vitals, general appearance) __ Eyes __ ENT, mouth __ Respiratory __ Cardiovascular __ Gastrointestinal __ Lymph/hem/immun	__ GU __ Skin __ Integumentary __ MS __ Neurological __ Psychiatric	One body area or system	Two to four body systems or two to seven basic systems, including affected area	Two to seven detailed systems, including affected area	Eight or more systems

*Some texts use two to four body systems for expanded problem focused and five to seven body systems for detailed. Both methods have been published in CMS publications. This is a controversy in the industry, and CMS will not give an opinion on whether one method is more acceptable than the other. Physicians frequently find that the two–four and five–seven distinction is easier to understand and follow.

Exercise 7.2   Evaluation and Management (Physical Examination)

Using table 7.4 (p. 175) as a guide, assign the level of exam based on the documentation in the following scenarios.

1. Vital signs: temperature is 98.4, respirations 16, and blood pressure is 119/81. General: well-nourished, well-developed female in no apparent distress. HEENT: normocephalic, atraumatic. Mucous membranes appear moist. Lungs: clear. Heart: regular rate and rhythm. Abdomen: positive bowel sounds, soft, nontender, and nondistended. Back: no swelling, bruising, or erythema. Extremities: lower extremities show no muscle wasting. Patient has 2+ patellar and ankle jerks, 5/5 muscle strength bilaterally, and a negative straight leg raise bilaterally.

   _____

2. Alert 16-year-old male. Temperature: 98.6; pulse: 86; respirations: 14; blood pressure: 126/80. Has 2-cm laceration of chin.

   _____

3. Temperature: 98; pulse 86; respirations 16; blood pressure 150/65. General: Patient is a well-nourished female who is wearing corrective lenses and looks to be somewhat uncomfortable. HEENT: head exam is normocephalic, atraumatic. Eyes: clear. Pupils equally round and reactive to light and accommodate. Discs sharp bilaterally. Ears, tympanic membranes pearly white bilaterally. Negative fluid. Neck: trachea midline, supple, no adenopathy. Cervical spine shows no swelling, bruising, or erythema. She had tenderness in the sternocleidomastoid muscle. C-spine itself was nontender to palpation.

   _____

Medical Decision Making

Medical decision making involves the complexity of establishing a diagnosis and/or selecting a management opinion or treatment plan as measured by the following:

- The number of possible diagnoses and/or management options or treatment plans to be considered

- The amount and/or complexity of the data (health records, diagnostic tests, and/or other information) to be obtained, reviewed, and analyzed

- The risk of significant complications, morbidity, and/or mortality associated with the patient's presenting condition, the diagnostic procedure(s), and/or the possible management options or treatment plans

Number of Possible Diagnoses and/or Management Options

The number of possible diagnoses and/or management options is based on the number and types of problems addressed during the encounter, the complexity of establishing a diagnosis, and the management decisions made by the physician.

The following documentation guidelines apply:

- For each encounter, an assessment, clinical impression, or diagnosis should be documented. It may be stated explicitly or implied in documented decisions regarding management plans and/or further evaluation.

- For a presenting problem with an established diagnosis, the record should reflect whether the problem is improving, well controlled, resolving, or resolved; or inadequately controlled, worsening, or failing to change as expected.

- For a presenting problem without an established diagnosis, the assessment or clinical impression may be stated in the form of a differential diagnosis, or as a possible, probable, or rule-out diagnosis.

- The initiation of, or changes in, treatment should be documented clearly. Treatment involves a wide range of management options, including patient instructions, nursing instructions, therapies, and medications.

- The record should indicate whether referrals are made and where, whether consultations are requested and with whom, and whether advice is sought and from whom.

Amount and/or Complexity of Data for Review

The amount and/or complexity of data for review is based on the types of diagnostic testing ordered or reviewed. A decision to obtain and review old health records and/or to obtain history from sources other than the patient increases the amount and complexity of data to be reviewed.

The following documentation guidelines apply:

- When a diagnostic service (test or procedure) is ordered, planned, scheduled, or performed at the time of the E/M encounter, the type of diagnostic service should be documented.

- The review of laboratory, radiology, and/or other diagnostic tests should be documented. An entry in a progress note (for example, "WBC elevated" or "chest x-ray unremarkable") is acceptable. Alternatively, the review may be documented by initialing and dating the report containing the test results.

- Relevant findings from any review of old records and/or the receipt of additional history from the family, caretaker, or other sources should be documented. If nothing exists beyond the relevant information that already has been obtained, that fact should be documented. A notation of "old records reviewed" or "additional history obtained from family" without further specification is insufficient.

- Documentation of discussions with the physician(s) who performed or interpreted laboratory, radiology, or other diagnostic tests should be included.

- The direct visualization and independent interpretation of an image, tracing, or specimen previously or subsequently interpreted by another physician should be documented.

Risk of Significant Complications, Morbidity, and/or Mortality

The risk of significant complications, morbidity, and/or mortality is based on the risks associated with the presenting problem(s), the diagnostic procedure(s), and the possible management options. The determination of risk is complex and not readily quantifiable.

The risk assessment of the presenting problem(s) is based on the risk related to the disease process anticipated between the present and the next encounter. The risk assessment of selecting diagnostic procedures and management options is based on the risk during and immediately following any procedures or treatment. The highest level of risk in any one category (presenting problem, diagnostic procedure, or management option) determines the overall risk.

Figure 7.1 outlines the factors that determine medical decision making. Two of the three elements in table 7.5 must be met or exceeded before selecting a type of medical decision making.

Figure 7.1.   Decision-making process

Number of Diagnosis or Treatment Options

$A \times B = C$

Problem Status	Number	Point	Result
Self-limited or minor	(max. two)	1	
Established problem; stable, improving		1	
Established problem; worsening		2	
New problem; no additional workup planned	(max. one)	3	
New problem; additional workup planned		4	

Total _____

Amount and/or Complexity of Data Reviewed

Reviewed Data	Points
Review and/or order clinical lab tests	1
Review and/or order tests in the radiology section of CPT	1
Review and/or order tests in the medicine section of CPT	1
Discussion of test results with performing provider	1
Decision to obtain old records/obtain history from other than patient/discuss case with other provider	2
Independent visualization of image, tracing, or specimen itself (not simply review of report)	2

Total _____

Risk Factors

Level of Risk	Presenting Problem	Dx Procedures Ordered	Management Options
Minimal	One self-limited or minor problem	Lab tests, x-rays, EKG, EEG	Rest, superficial dressings, none required
Low	• Two or more self-limited or minor problems • One stable chronic illness • Acute uncomplicated illness or injury	• Physiologic tests w/o stress • Imaging studies w/contrast • Superficial needle biopsy • Skin biopsy • Arterial blood draw	• Over-the-counter remedy • Minor surgery w/o risk factor • Physical, occupational therapy • IV fluids w/o additive
Moderate	• One or more chronic illness with exacerbation, progression, or treatment side effects • Undiagnosed new problem with uncertain prognosis • Acute complicated injury • Acute illness with systemic symptoms	• Stress tests • Endoscopies w/o risk factor • Cardiovascular imaging study w/o identified risk factors • Deep needle or incisional biopsy • Centesis of body cavity fluid	• Minor surgery with identifiable risk factors • Elective major surgery without identifiable risk factors • Prescription drug management • Therapeutic radiology • IV fluids with additives • Closed treatment of skeletal injury
High	• One or more chronic illness with severe exacerbation, progression, or Tx side effects • Acute or chronic illness or injury that may pose a threat to life or bodily function • An abrupt change to mental status	• Cardiovascular imaging studies with identifiable risk factors • Cardiac electrophysiological tests • Endoscopy with identifiable risk factors	• Elective major surgery with identifiable risk factors • Emergency major surgery • Parenteral-controlled substances • Drug therapy requiring intensive monitoring • DNR status

Tabulation of Medical Decision-Making Elements: Highest Two of Three

Diagnosis/Management Options	Minimal (one or none)	Limited (two)	Multiple (three)	Extensive (four or more)
Amount/Complexity of Data	Minimal/Low (one or none)	Limited (two)	Moderate (three)	Extensive (four or more)
Highest Risk (from any category)	Minimal	Low	Moderate	High
Medical Decision Making	**Straightforward**	**Low Complexity**	**Moderate Complexity**	**High Complexity**

Table 7.5. Selection of level of E/M service

All three of the key components must meet or exceed the stated requirements to qualify for a particular level of E/M services code.	Two of the three components must meet or exceed the stated requirements to qualify for a particular level of E/M services code.	Time
Office or other outpatient services, new patient Initial observation care Initial hospital care Office or other outpatient consultations Initial inpatient consultations Confirmatory consultations ED services Comprehensive nursing facility assessments Domiciliary, rest home, or custodial care, new patient Home services, new patient	Office or other outpatient services, established patient Subsequent hospital care Follow-up inpatient consultations Subsequent nursing facility care Domiciliary, rest home, or custodial care, established patient Home services, established patient	When counseling and/or coordination of care dominates, or is more than 50 percent of, the face-to-face physician–patient encounter, time is considered the key factor to qualify for a particular level of E/M services code.

Counseling and Coordination of Care

Both counseling and coordination of care are contributing factors in the selection of an E/M level of service. Counseling involves discussion of the patient's care with the patient and/or his or her family. Coordination of care is a contributing factor in the majority of encounters for E/M services. When coordination of care with other providers or agencies occurs without a patient encounter on the same day, the case management codes (99361–99373) should be reported.

When counseling and/or coordination of care dominates, or comprises more than 50 percent of, the physician–patient and/or physician–family encounter (face-to-face time in the office or other outpatient setting or floor/unit time in the hospital or nursing facility), time is considered the key or controlling factor to qualify for a particular level of E/M services. Typical times are listed in the descriptions of each code. These times are used in code selection based on counseling and/or coordination of care, including time spent with parties who have assumed responsibility for the care of the patient or decision making, whether or not they are family members (for example, foster parents, person acting in loco parentis, legal guardian).

Documentation guideline: If the physician elects to report the level of service based on counseling and/or coordination of care, the total length of time of the encounter (face-to-face or floor time, as appropriate) should be documented and the record should describe the counseling and/or activities to coordinate care.

Nature of Presenting Problem

CPT defines presenting problems as diseases, conditions, illnesses, injuries, symptoms, signs, findings, complaints, or other reasons for an encounter, regardless of whether a diagnosis is established at the time of the encounter.

Five types of presenting problems are identified:

- *Minimal:* A problem that does not require the presence of a physician, although care is provided under a physician's supervision (for example, a blood pressure check).

- *Self-limited or minor:* A temporary problem with a definite and prescribed course and good prognosis (for example, an upper respiratory infection). The conditions are typically transient in nature.

- *Low severity:* With no treatment, this problem carries a low risk of morbidity and little or no risk of mortality (for example, a teenager with acne that does not respond to over-the-counter medications). A patient with this type of problem can expect full recovery without impairments.

- *Moderate severity:* With no treatment, this problem carries a moderate risk of morbidity and mortality (for example, Dupuytren's contracture of the hand involving several fingers). The patient's prognosis may be uncertain, or the probability of prolonged functional impairment is increased.

- *High severity:* With no treatment, the risk of morbidity is high and a high probability exists for severe, prolonged functional impairment or moderate to high risk of mortality (for example, Type I diabetes mellitus, uncontrolled, with chronic renal failure requiring dialysis).

Exercise 7.3 Evaluation and Management (Medical Decision Making)

Using table 7.5 (p. 179) as a reference, assign the level of medical decision making for the following case studies.

1. Patient seen in the emergency department after an automobile accident. She is complaining of pain in her back and right leg. X-rays, UA, and CBC were normal. Discharge Diagnosis: Thoracic/rib cage strain and contusion. Right leg contusion. Discharged on Voltaren 50 mg three times a day for pain and Robaxin 750 mg three times a day for muscle spasms. She is to return to work in a couple of days and follow up with her family doctor as necessary.

2. Physician office progress note: Follow-up appointment for bronchitis. Patient reports that she feels tired and weak and the bronchitis is lingering. Impression: Questionable resolution of her bronchitis. Plan: Refill Tessalon Perles and continue with amoxicillin. Will call if not improved.

3. Mother brings 4-year-old child to urgent care after sustaining a cut on the bottom of the foot. 2-inch laceration was cleaned and sutured. Tylenol given for pain. Referred to family physician.

Exercise 7.4   Evaluation and Management Case Study

Case Study: Established Patient

This 56-year-old female has been my patient for three years. She complains of cough, congestion, stuffy nose over the past 3 to 4 days; feels worse today. Denies any fever, chills, but has occasional yellow productive sputum. Denies any chest pain, nausea, vomiting, or diarrhea.

Past Medical History: Cholecystectomy

Medications: None

Allergies: None

Social History: Smoker

Physical Examination:

General: Alert woman in no apparent distress

Vital signs: Blood pressure 152/84, temperature 99.2, pulse 84, respirations 18

HEENT: Pupils equal, round and reactive to light and accommodation. Extraocular movements intact.

Neck: Supple, nontender

Lungs: Breath sounds are equal. No rales or wheezes.

Heart: S1, S2, no murmur

Abdomen: Soft, nontender. Bowel sounds present in all quadrants.

Extremities: Pulses equal

Skin: Warm and dry

Studies: Chest x-ray is negative.

Diagnosis: Acute bronchitis

Plan: Zithromax Z-Pak. Follow-up in one week. Call if symptoms worse.

1. Refer to previous tables and apply the documentation guidelines to assign the E/M code for the preceding case.

Time

The 1992 edition of *Current Procedural Terminology* introduced the notion of time as a separate contributing factor for selecting the appropriate E/M level of service codes. Prior editions had been based on the idea that time was an implicit factor in the definition of each level of service. In the current system, the specific times included in the level of service codes are averages and, as such, may vary according to the actual clinical circumstances.

Face-to-Face Time

Face-to-face time is the amount of time the physician spends face-to-face with the patient and/or his or her family. This includes the period during which the physician obtains a history, performs an examination, and counsels the patient. Face-to-face time applies to the following subsections and subcategories: Office and Other Outpatient Visits and Office Consultations.

Unit/Floor Time

Unit/floor time is the amount of time the physician is present on the patient's hospital unit and rendering services for the patient at the bedside. This includes the period when the physician establishes and/or reviews the patient's health record, examines the patient, writes notes, and communicates with other professionals and the patient's family regarding the patient's care. Unit/floor time applies to the following four subsections and subcategories: Hospital Observation Services, Inpatient Hospital Care, Initial and Follow-up Hospital Consultations, and Nursing Facility Care.

Instructions for Selection and/or Validation of E/M Service Levels

The following steps should be followed in selecting and/or validating a level of E/M services:

1. Identify the category and subcategory of service. Is this an office visit with an established patient? Initial inpatient consultation? Comprehensive nursing facility assessment? New patient home services? Individual counseling for preventive medicine services? Visit to the emergency department? Hospital outpatient service?

2. Review specific notes and instructions for the selected category and subcategory.

3. Review the narrative descriptors within the category and subcategory of the E/M services. The seven components should be reviewed in selecting the appropriate level of service code.

4. Using the definitions provided under each level of service, determine the extent of history obtained.

5. Determine the extent of examination performed using the definitions provided under each level of service.

6. Determine the complexity of medical decision making.

7. Select or verify the appropriate level of E/M services based on the information provided in table 7.5.

Selection of Modifiers

Under certain circumstances, a listed service may be modified slightly without changing its basic definition. In these situations, several modifiers are available for use with E/M services codes. Modifiers are reported as two-digit numbers attached to the main code.

The following modifiers available for use with E/M codes:

21 **Prolonged Evaluation and Management Services:** Modifier –21 may be reported only by physicians with the highest level of E/M service within a specified category. Use of this modifier informs the third-party payer that the physician's service surpassed the one described in the highest level of service.

> **Example:** Office consultation when the physician's care exceeded the criteria listed under code 99245. The physician may submit 99245–21 on the claim.

Most third-party payers require submission of a written report to support the use of modifier –21. In selected circumstances, the prolonged services codes 99354 through 99359 may be more accurate than using a modified code.

24 **Unrelated Evaluation and Management Service by the Same Physician during a Postoperative Period:** Modifier –24 can be reported by physicians with an E/M service provided during the postoperative period by the same physician who performed the original procedure.

The E/M service must be unrelated to the condition for which the original procedure was performed.

> **Example:** Office visit provided to a patient who is in the postoperative period for a cholecystectomy performed three weeks earlier. The patient's current complaint is a possible infection of a finger that was lacerated four days ago. The physician may report the appropriate office visit code and attach modifier –24 to identify this activity as an unrelated service provided during the postoperative period of the cholecystectomy.

25 **Significant, Separately Identifiable Evaluation and Management Service by the Same Physician on the Day of a Procedure or Other Service:** Modifier –25 may be reported by hospitals and physicians to indicate that the patient's condition required a separate E/M service on the day a procedure or other service was performed because the care provided went beyond the usual procedures associated with the activity. Modifier –25 is appropriate with procedures that Medicare designates as minor, which are generally those with a 10-day global fee period or 0-day global fee.

> **Example:** Office visit is provided to a patient for evaluation of diabetes and associated chronic renal failure, as well as a mole on the arm that has increased in size. Suspecting the mole is malignant, the physician excises it. The pathology report confirms a 1.1-cm malignant lesion. The physician can bill for the malignant lesion removal and use the office visit code accompanied by modifier –25 to identify that, during the visit, a separate condition was addressed (in this example, the diabetes and the renal failure). Generally, two diagnosis codes are required to explain the reporting of two separate services during the same encounter, although CPT guidelines do not require it.

Hospitals are instructed by CMS to use modifier –25 when E/M services (from only the following CPT/HCPCS codes: 92002–92014, 99201–99499, G0101, and G0175) are performed with diagnostic and/or therapeutic medical or surgical procedures.

> **Example:** A patient is seen in the emergency department for chest pains. An EKG is performed. The hospital would report the emergency department E/M code of 99283–25 with 93005 (EKG).

27 **Multiple Outpatient Hospital E/M Encounters on the Same Date:** Modifier –27 was developed to allow hospitals to report multiple outpatient hospital E/M encounters on the same date. The modifier is appended to the second encounter and each subsequent E/M code.

> **Example:** Patient is seen in the dermatology clinic in the morning and the orthopedic clinic in the afternoon. A level III clinic visit is performed at both visits. The hospital would report 99213 with 99213–27.

CMS has instructed hospitals to assign E/M codes for facility billing based on their own system, which reflects the facility's resources to give care to the patient.

32 **Mandated Services:** Modifier –32 can be reported by physicians when an entity such as a third-party payer or a quality improvement organization mandates a service. Most often, this modifier is reported with the consultation codes.

52 **Reduced Services:** Modifier –52 can be reported by both hospitals and physicians when a physician decides to partially reduce or eliminate a service. Although its purpose is to identify a reduction in the service provided, modifier –52 is used by some physicians to report a reduction in the charges for a particular service because the complete service was not carried out.

> **Example:** Patient is seen in the ophthalmologist's office for an eye exam (92002). The patient only has one eye; thus, the correct code assignment would be 92002–52.

Hospitals have been instructed by CMS to append modifier –52 to an incomplete procedure when the procedure does not involve anesthesia (local, regional, or general). Coders should reference current directives from CMS for use of modifiers. It is not unusual for guidelines to be changed.

> **Example:** Patient is taken to the endoscopy suite for a flexible sigmoidoscopy, but the scope could not be passed because of poor preparation. The patient is given conscious sedation (not considered anesthesia). For the surgeon's services, the correct code assignment would be 45330–52.

57 Decision for Surgery: Modifier –57 can be reported by physicians only along with the appropriate E/M services code when an E/M service was the result of an initial decision to perform surgery on a patient. Modifier –57 is appropriate with procedures that Medicare designates as major, which typically are those with a 90-day global fee period assigned. Generally, it is not required when the decision for surgery occurs at a time earlier than the day of or before surgery. Some insurance plans include consultation and/or visit codes where the decision is made in the global fee for surgery and do not provide separate payment.

> **Example:** An office visit is provided to a Medicare patient complaining of acute right, upper-quadrant pain and tenderness referred to the right scapula, nausea and vomiting, and anorexia. A low-grade fever and an elevated white blood count are noted. An ultrasound confirms the diagnosis of acute cholecystitis with cholelithiasis. The physician recommends that surgery be performed later that day. The physician can report the appropriate office visit code along with modifier –57 to identify that, during this office visit, it was decided to perform a cholecystectomy.

Exercise 7.5 Evaluation and Management

Circle the correct answer for each of the following statements.

1. The AMA and CMS developed documentation guidelines for use with the CPT codebook.

    True   False

2. All seven of the following are considered key components in selecting an E/M level of service: history, examination, medical decision making, coordination of care, counseling, nature of presenting problem, and time.

    True   False

3. CMS mandates use of the E/M documentation guidelines.

    True   False

4. The review of systems is a chronological description of the development of the patient's presenting symptoms.

    True   False

5. The element of time is never considered a factor in selecting an E/M level of service.

    True   False

Based on 1995 documentation guidelines, write the answer to each of the following questions in the spaces provided.

6. An 86-year-old patient presents with a CC of vomiting and dizziness. Yesterday, she became dizzy while getting ready to go to church. In addition, she vomited bile several times and complained of deafness in her left ear at the start of the dizziness. Based on this information, is this history of present illness (HPI) brief or extended?

    _____

    _____

7. The CC is chest pain. The examination determined: respiration quiet and unlabored; skin with good color, warm and dry, and no rashes; mucous membranes moist; ears and throat clear; lungs with good breath sounds in all fields; rare expiratory wheeze, no rales, no rhonchi; heart regular rate and rhythm with normal heart sounds, no murmur; abdomen soft with no liver or spleen enlargement; and bowel sounds active. Based on this information, what is the level of examination?

    _____

    _____

8. New patient presents to the office with a CC of nasal congestion and headache. ROS: Denies shortness of breath or fever, stiffness of neck, or visual disturbances. Past history: No drug allergies or other allergies were noted, nor any history of TB, COPD, or asthma. Last physical exam one year ago was unremarkable. Based on this information, is this past, family, and/or social history (pertinent or complete?

    _____

    _____

Categories of E/M Services

Evaluation and management services are divided into many different types of services as listed previously.

Office or Other Outpatient Services (99201–99215)

The office or other outpatient services category may be used to describe services provided in the physician's office, the outpatient clinic, or some other ambulatory facility. This category is divided into two subcategories: new patient and established patient. It is important to remember that the basic difference between a new and established patient is whether the patient received professional services within the past three years from the same physician or another physician within the same group practice. Whereas the new patient level of services requires meeting all three of the key components prior to assigning a code, the established patient level of services requires meeting only two of the three key components.

Reporting an office visit code is inappropriate if, during the course of events within a specific encounter, the physician admits the patient to the hospital as an inpatient or observation patient or to a nursing care facility. Only the resulting admission service should be reported in such a situation, which should incorporate the level of care provided in the office. There may be a rare circumstance where the patient receives office services early in the day and then returns later and must be admitted to the hospital from the office. Such a situation would merit use of modifier –25 to show that the services were separately identifiable.

Hospital Observation Services (99217–99220) and Hospital Observation or Inpatient Care Services (99234–99236)

The hospital observation services category identifies patients who are admitted to a hospital or are placed in observation status in a hospital and the services span more than one calendar date. For observation and inpatient care where admission and discharge occur on the same date, codes 99234 through 99236 would be used.

Consulting physicians providing services while patients are in observation status would use either outpatient consultation (99241–99245) or inpatient consultation codes (99251–99255), depending on the patient's status at the time of service. Only attending physicians should use the observation codes. When a patient is admitted to the hospital (and not discharged on the same date), the initial hospital or inpatient consultation codes will be used, as appropriate.

The initial encounter with a patient in observation status is reported with a code from 99218 to 99220. Coders should note that all three key components must be met to assign a particular level of service. In the rare circumstance that a patient remains in observation status after the date of admission, but is removed before the date of discharge, codes 99211–99215 may be used to report a physician visit on the intervening dates between removal from observation status and discharge.

Code 99217 (Observation care discharge services) is used to describe the services provided to a patient on discharge from observation status, but only if the discharge was not on the same date as the initial care. These services include a final examination of the patient, discussion of the hospital stay, instructions for continuing care, and completion of the health record.

Hospital Inpatient Services (99221–99239)

The hospital inpatient services category includes codes for initial hospital care (99221–99223), subsequent hospital care (99231–99233), and hospital discharge services (99238–99239).

These codes also may be used to describe services provided to patients in a so-called partial hospital setting. Partial hospitalization is used for crisis stabilization, intensive short-term daily treatment, or intermediate-term treatment of psychiatric disorders.

The initial hospital care codes (99221–99223) are used to report the physician's first inpatient hospital visit with a new or established patient. Coders should note that all three of the key components must be met to assign a particular level of service.

Codes 99231–99233 are reported for subsequent hospital services provided by the physician. Changes in the patient's medical status and the related documentation in the health record allow the physician to report various levels of service for the subsequent hospital care. It should be noted that only two of the three key components must be met to assign a specific level of service for subsequent hospital care services.

Codes 99238–99239 are used to report the services related to discharging a patient from the hospital. This reflects the added work the physician must perform, such as final examination of patient, discussion of hospital stay, instructions for home care, and completion of the health record. Code selection is based on time. For example, code 99238 describes discharge services requiring 30 minutes or less, and code 99239 identifies those services requiring more than 30 minutes.

Patients receiving inpatient or observation services when admission and discharge occur on the same date are reported using codes 99234 through 99236.

Consultations (99241–99255)

The CPT codebook defines a consultation as a type of service provided by a physician when his or her opinion or advice on a specific problem is requested by another physician or other appropriate source. Although consulting physicians may initiate diagnostic and/or therapeutic services, they cannot assume responsibility for any portion of that patient's care. If responsibility is assumed, the service is no longer considered a consultation and the appropriate code should be assigned for hospital care or office or other outpatient services.

Documentation to support a consultation is essential and should include the request and need for a consultation, the opinion of the consultant, and any services ordered and/or performed. All this information should be documented in the health record and communicated by written report to the requesting physician or other appropriate source.

When a consultation is requested by the patient and/or his or her family, but not by another physician, the consulting physician should report the service using the office visit or confirmatory consultation codes. Reporting the initial consultation codes would be inappropriate in this case because the consultation was not performed at the request of another physician.

Office or Other Outpatient Consultations (99241–99245)
Codes 99241–99245 describe office or other outpatient consultation services provided to new or established patients. These services may be provided in an office, outpatient or other ambulatory facility, hospital observation services program, home services program, domiciliary, rest home, custodial care program, or emergency department. Subsequent visits to the consulting physician's office are reported using the office visit codes for established patient (99211–99215). All three key components must be met in the selection of a level of service code from 99241 to 99245.

Initial Inpatient Consultations (99251–99255)
Initial inpatient consultation codes (99251–99255) are used to report consulting services provided to hospital inpatients, residents of nursing facilities, or patients in a partial hospital

setting. All three key components must be met in the selection of a level of service code from 99251 to 99255. In addition, a consultant can report only one initial consultation code per admission.

Emergency Department Services (99281–99288)

Emergency department services category codes are used to report E/M services that a physician provides when treating a patient in the emergency department. The CPT codebook defines the emergency department as an organized hospital-based facility for the provision of unscheduled episodic services to patients who present for immediate medical attention. Moreover, the facility must be available twenty-four hours a day. All three of the key components, as stated within each level, must be met prior to selection of an emergency services code.

Special attention should be given to the description of code 99285, "which requires these three key components within the constraints imposed by the urgency of the patient's clinical condition and mental status." This description allows the code to be assigned, even when not all the documentation meets the criteria so stated. For example, when the patient is unconscious, it may be impossible to document a comprehensive history.

Again, code selection by physicians rather than coders or billing services is important because a physician is the only one in a position to determine clinical condition and mental status. Nonphysicians may verify compliance of the code selection to the current guidelines, but the provider of service best determines the level of code selection.

When a patient receives critical care services in the emergency department, codes 99291 and 99292 may be reported for these services, provided the requirements for critical care are met.

Pediatric Critical Care Patient Transport (99289 and 99290)

The pediatric critical care patient transport services codes are used to report face-to-face critical care services delivered by a physician during the interfacility transport of a critically ill or injured pediatric patient, 24 months of age or less.

Code 99289 is used to report the first 30 to 74 minutes, and code 99290 is an add-on code for each additional 30 minutes. Transport time less than 30 minutes is not reported. Guidelines direct the coder to report only these codes once on any given date.

A physician's attendance during the transport of critically ill or injured patients over the age of 24 months should be reported with code 99291 or 99292.

Critical Care Services (99291–99292)

The critical care services category involves the care of critically ill patients in a medical emergency that requires the constant attention of the physician. However, the physician's constant attendance/monitoring does not have to be continuous on a given date. Types of medical emergencies can include cardiac arrest, shock, bleeding, respiratory failure, and postoperative complications. Although usually provided in critical care areas such as a coronary care unit, intensive care unit (ICU), or emergency department, this type of care may be offered in other settings as well.

Critical care provided to neonatal and pediatric inpatients is reported with codes 99293 through 99296.

Critical care services include the following procedures, which should not be reported separately:

- Interpretation of cardiac output measurements (93561, 93562)

- Chest x-rays (71010, 71015, 71020)

- Pulse oximetry (94760, 94761, 94762)

- Blood gases and information data stored in computers (99090)

- Gastric intubation (43752, 91105)

- Temporary transcutaneous pacing (92953)

- Ventilator management (94656, 94657, 94660, 94662)

- Vascular access procedures (36000, 36410, 36415, 36540, 36600)

Other services performed that are not included in the preceding list may be reported separately.

Time is a key factor when selecting a critical care code. Code 99291 is reported for the first 30 to 74 minutes of critical care on a given date and may be reported only once per date. Code 99292 is reported for each additional 30 minutes of care beyond the first 74 minutes. As mentioned above, coders should note that the constant attention the physician provides need not be continuous on a given date. Critical care of less than 30 minutes on a given date should be reported with an appropriate E/M services code, such as subsequent hospital inpatient services, rather than a critical care code. A comprehensive explanation of time as an element in code selection can be found in the note under the critical care services subcategory.

Neonatal and Pediatric Critical Care Services (Inpatient) (99293–99296)

These codes are used to report services performed by a physician to direct the care of a critically ill neonate or infant. Code 99295 should be assigned for the initial critical care services provided to a neonatal patient (birth through 28 days of age), and code 99296 should be assigned for subsequent critical care. Code 99293 should be assigned for the initial critical care services provided to a pediatric patient (29 days to 24 months of age), and code 99294 should be assigned for subsequent critical care.

Coding guidelines dictate that these codes may be reported only once by a single physician per patient per day. The same definitions for critical care services apply for adult, pediatric, and neonatal patients.

Continuing Intensive Care Services (99298–99300)

Codes in this category are used by physicians to report intensive (noncritical) care given to infants with low birth weights. These infants require intensive services that do not meet the definition of critical care. For very low-birth-weight (less than 1500 gm) infants, a code from initial hospital care (99221–99223) should be assigned for initial intensive care services, and code 99298 should be assigned for subsequent intensive care services. For low-birth-weight (between 1500 and 2500 gm) infants, a code from initial hospital care (99221–99223) should be assigned for initial intensive care services and code 99299 for subsequent intensive care services. CPT code 99300 is assigned for those infants who weigh between 2501 and 5000 grams. Physicians may report these codes only once per patient per day.

Nursing Facility Services (99304–99310)

The codes in the nursing facility services category are used to report services in the following facilities:

- Skilled nursing facilities, including hospital-based skilled care or swing beds in rural hospitals

- Intermediate care facilities

- Long-term care facilities

Nursing facilities (NFs) are required by law to perform a comprehensive assessment of each resident's functional capacity upon admission. Additional assessments must be conducted immediately after significant changes in a resident's condition, or at least every twelve months. The assessments are documented in a form called the resident assessment instrument (RAI), which is composed of a uniform Minimum Data Set (MDS) and resident assessment protocols (RAPs). The MDS includes a minimum set of assessment elements to evaluate SNF and NF residents. SNFs and NFs are responsible for completing the RAI, although specific portions of the form must be completed by a physician only.

CPT recognizes two types of NF services: initial nursing facility care and subsequent nursing facility care. Both subcategories apply to new or established patients. All three of the key components must be met in these cases before code selection.

Subsequent NF care (99307–99310) includes reviewing the health record, noting changes in the resident's status since the last visit, and reviewing and signing orders. Subsequent NF care requires that only two of the three key components be met before assigning a specific level of service code.

NF discharge day management codes are used to report the total duration of time spent by a physician for the final NF discharge of a patient. These include final examination of the patient and discussion of the NF stay, even when the time spent on that date is not continuous. Instructions are given for continuing care to all relevant caregivers and for preparation of discharge records, prescriptions, and referral forms. These codes are 99315 for services of 30 minutes or less and 99316 for services of more than 30 minutes.

Domiciliary, Rest Home, or Custodial Care Services (99324–99337)

Physician visits to patients being provided room, board, and other personal assistance services (usually on a long-term basis) are reported using codes 99324–99337. A medical component is not part of the facility's services. Such facilities may include group homes or correctional facilities. All three key components, as defined in the levels of service, must be met before code assignment in the new patient subcategory (99324–99328). However, only two of the three key components must be met in the established patient subcategory (99334–99337).

Home Services (99341–99350)

Home services codes 99341–99350 are used to report E/M services provided in a private residence. As stated in the levels of service, all three key components are required prior to code assignment in the new patient subcategory (99341–99345). However, only two of the three key components must be met in the established patient subcategory (99347–99350).

Prolonged Services/Standby Services (99354–99360)

The first set of codes (99354–99357) is used when a physician provides prolonged service involving direct, face-to-face contact with the patient that is beyond the usual service. The time the physician spends providing prolonged service on a given date need not be continuous. Coders should note that these codes may be reported in addition to other services, including E/M services at any level. Moreover, other procedures or supplies provided during the same encounter should be reported according to payer directions or guidelines.

The codes are further subdivided to identify prolonged services provided in the outpatient setting (99354–99355) and the inpatient setting (99356–99357). Codes 99354 and 99356 describe the first hour of prolonged service and should be reported only once per any given date. Codes 99355 and 99357 describe each additional 30 minutes of prolonged service. Coders should note that prolonged service of less than 30 minutes should not be reported separately.

Codes 99358–99359 describe prolonged physician service without direct or face-to-face contact with the patient that is beyond the usual service. This type of service can involve prolonged communication with other healthcare professionals, prolonged review of extensive health record and diagnostic tests, and prolonged communication with the patient and/or family regarding the patient's prognosis. These codes may be reported along with other services, including E/M services at any level. Code 99358 is used to report the first hour of prolonged service, and code 99359 describes each additional 30 minutes of service. Prolonged service of less than 30 minutes should not be reported separately.

Code 99360 is used to report physician standby services requested by another physician that require prolonged physician attendance without direct or face-to-face contact. This type of service may involve a physician who stands by for assistance in surgery or high-risk delivery for care of a newborn. Code 99360 may be reported for each full 30-minute period the physician stands by. Less than 30 minutes of standby service may not be reported separately.

Case Management Services (99361–99373)

The case management services category includes services when a physician is responsible for providing direct care for a patient, as well as coordinating and controlling access to other healthcare services or initiating and/or supervising them. This category includes two subcategories: team conferences and telephone calls.

Codes 99361 through 99362 describe a team conference that includes a physician, an interdisciplinary health team, or representatives of community agencies for the purpose of coordinating the activities of the patient. Codes 99371 through 99373 describe telephone calls a physician makes to consult with a patient or to coordinate medical management with other healthcare professionals. The content of the call determines the code assignment: simple/brief, intermediate, or complex/lengthy. Many health plans consider telephone communication bundled with other E/M services and do not provide additional reimbursement for this service.

Care Plan Oversight Services (99374–99380)

The care plan oversight services category describes the services a physician provides when supervising and coordinating the patient's care within a 30-day period, but not actually seeing the patient face-to-face. These codes are appropriate when a physician provides recurrent supervision of therapy for patients in NFs, home health agencies, or hospice beds. Care plan oversight services for patients in home, domiciliary, or rest home (for example, assisted living facility) are assigned codes in the 99339–99340 range.

Code 99374 (home health), code 99377 (hospice), or code 99379 (NF) is reported for services lasting between 15 and 29 minutes, whereas codes 99375, 99378, and 99380 cover services lasting longer than 30 minutes. Only one physician may report this type of service within a 30-day period. Work involved in providing very low-intensity services or infrequent supervision is included in the pre- and postencounter work for the home, office/outpatient, and NF or domiciliary visit codes and should not be reported with care plan oversight codes.

Preventive Medicine Services (99381–99429)

The preventive medicine services category codes are used to report the preventive medicine evaluation and management of infants, children, adolescents, and adults. When an abnormality is discovered or a preexisting condition is addressed during this service, the appropriate office visit code also should be reported if the condition/abnormality proves significant enough to require additional workup. Moreover, modifier –25 should be added to the office visit code to indicate that the same physician provided a significant and separate E/M service and on the same date as the preventive medicine service. Any insignificant conditions/abnormalities discovered during the preventive medicine services that do not require additional workup should not be reported separately.

Ancillary procedures (such as laboratory or radiological procedures), screening tests identified with a specific CPT code, and immunizations provided during the preventive medicine encounter should be coded and reported separately.

The subcategories of preventive medicine services distinguish between new and established patients, with the individual codes identifying specified age ranges. Codes 99401 through 99412 are used to report services provided to individuals at a separate encounter for the purpose of promoting health and preventing illness or injury. Counseling and/or risk factor reduction intervention vary with age and should address issues such as family problems, diet and exercise, substance abuse, sexual practices, injury prevention, dental health, and diagnostic and laboratory test results available at the time of visit.

A separate code is not needed for counseling (99401–99412) when provided as part of preventive medicine services (99381–99397) or during an E/M service. The preventive medicine codes (99381–99397) include counseling, anticipatory guidance, and risk factor reductions in the service provided. An additional code is not required to identify them. The E/M services codes also include counseling in the care provided.

Newborn Care (99431–99440)

The newborn care codes are used to report services provided to normal or high-risk newborns in different settings. Code 99431 is reported for history and examination of the normal newborn, initiation of diagnostic and treatment programs, and preparation of hospital records. This code is appropriate for birthing room deliveries. Code 99433 is reported to indicate subsequent hospital care for the evaluation and management of a normal newborn on a per day basis. Code 99435 should be reported for discharge services provided to the newborn admitted and discharged on the same date. Code 99436 is used to report attendance at a delivery at the request of the delivering physician for initial stabilization of the newborn. Newborn resuscitative services are reported with code 99440, which includes the provision of positive pressure ventilation and/or chest compressions in the presence of acute inadequate ventilation and/or cardiac output. Code 99440 cannot be reported with 99436. When other procedures are performed in addition to the resuscitative services, additional codes should be reported.

Special Evaluation and Management Services (99450–99456)

The special evaluation and management services category codes were developed to report services that can be performed in the office setting or other setting to establish baseline information before life or disability insurance certificates are issued. Coders should note that no active management of the patient's problem is performed during this visit. If other E/M services and/or procedures are performed on the same date, the appropriate E/M services codes also should be reported, with modifier –25 appending them.

Other Evaluation and Management Services (99499)

The other evaluation and management services category code is used to report an unlisted E/M service that does not fit into the previous categories.

Exercise 7.6   Chapter 7 Review

Assign only the appropriate E/M services code(s) for the following cases.

1. An established patient with hypertension visits a physician's office for a blood pressure check. The nurse performs the service under the physician's supervision.

   _____

2. A new patient was seen in the physician's office for abdominal pain. The physician performs a detailed history and comprehensive examination. Medical decision making is of moderate complexity.

   _____

3. A patient with rectal bleeding was seen in the office of a gastroenterologist. The patient's primary care physician requested that the gastroenterologist provide advice about this case. The specialist conducted a comprehensive history and exam, and medical decision making was high. The consultant documented his findings and communicated them via written report to the primary care physician.

   _____

4. A new patient is seen in the physician's office for a cough, sore throat, and fever. The physician performs an expanded problem-focused history and a detailed exam, and medical decision making was of low complexity.

   _____

5. Dr. Jones provides critical care services in the emergency department for a patient in respiratory failure and with congestive heart failure. Ventilator management is initiated. Dr. Jones spends an hour and 10 minutes providing critical care for this patient.

   _____

6. Dr. Michaels provides E/M services for a patient in acute hysteria who has been admitted to the emergency department. After performing a problem-focused history and examination with straightforward medical decision making, he determines that the patient is suffering from acute grief reaction secondary to the death of her granddaughter due to sudden infant death syndrome. At discharge, the patient is in complete control of her actions and is referred to a SIDS organization.

   _____

(Continued on next page)

Exercise 7.6 (Continued)

7.   Dr. Gerald provides preventive medicine services to an established 45-year-old patient who is in good health and has no complaints. Dr. Gerald obtains a comprehensive history, performs a comprehensive examination, and counsels the patient on proper diet and exercise.

_____

8.   Dr. Hawthorne sees an established patient in his office for evaluation of insulin-dependent diabetes mellitus with nephropathy. In addition to a problem-focused history, he performs an expanded problem-focused examination that includes a limited exam of the genito-urinary, immunologic, skin, and musculoskeletal systems, and documents all positive and negative findings. The patient's status does not seem to have changed, and medical decision making is of low complexity. Dr. Hawthorne discusses the patient's insulin dosage, diet, and exercise, and plans to see the patient in six months.

_____

9.   An established patient sees Dr. Ryan in his office with complaints of chest pain. Dr. Ryan decides to admit the patient to Central Hospital on March 2 under observation status. He obtains a comprehensive history that includes a complete review of body systems and complete past, family, and social histories. The patient reveals that he has been under emotional stress the past month due to his recent divorce and that this is the first time he has experienced chest pain. Dr. Ryan performs a comprehensive examination that includes a complete evaluation of the respiratory and cardiovascular systems. Pertinent diagnostic tests reveal no coronary artery disease. Dr. Ryan performs medical decision making of moderate complexity and determines the origin of the pain to be musculoskeletal secondary to stress. He discharges the patient on March 2 and recommends that he join a stress management group.

_____

10.   In her office, Dr. Childers sees an established patient who complains of abdominal pain. She provides a problem-focused history and examination, which reveals the onset of abdominal pain beginning early that morning and characterized by a sharp, crampy feeling with some radiation to the back. Nausea and dry heaves are present, but no vomiting. The patient had a normal bowel movement in the morning. No fever or chills are noted, and bowel sounds are active. A rectal examination reveals hard stool in the rectal vault, guaiac negative. An x-ray of the abdomen is negative except for extensive gas. Dr. Childers tells the patient to take an enema and return if the pain is not relieved. A change in diet would involve increasing the intake of fiber. The impression is that the patient's pain is the result of impacted feces.

_____

11.   A new patient sees Dr. Reynolds in his office complaining of diarrhea and watery stool the previous night, as well as nausea, vomiting, and crampy, lower abdominal pain. Dr. Reynolds provides a detailed history and examination, and medical decision making of moderate complexity.

_____

Chapter 7 Test

Choose or write the appropriate answer.

1. Select the appropriate evaluation and management code for a new patient office visit in which a comprehensive history and comprehensive physical examination were performed and medical decision making was of high complexity. 99205

2. Select the appropriate evaluation and management code for a new patient office visit in which a comprehensive history and comprehensive physical examination were performed and medical decision making was of straightforward complexity. 99202

3. Select the appropriate evaluation and management code for an established patient visit in which a comprehensive history and expanded problem-focused examination was performed and medical decision making was of low complexity. 99213

4. Observation evaluation and management codes (99218–99220) are used when:
    a. A patient is admitted and discharged on the same date.
    b. A patient is admitted for routine nursing care following surgery.
    c. A patient does not meet admission criteria.
    d. A patient is placed in designated observation status.

5. History, physical examination, and medical decision making are the __Key__ components considered in assigning an evaluation and management code.

6. Per CPT guidelines, a concise statement describing the symptom, problem, condition, diagnosis, or other factor that is the reason for the encounter, usually stated in the patient's words, is the definition of the:
    a. History of present illness
    b. Chief complaint
    c. Admission diagnosis
    d. Past history

7. Which of the following are parts of medical decision making?
    a. Number of possible diagnoses or management options that must be considered
    b. Amount or complexity of medical record, diagnostic tests, or other information that must be obtained, reviewed, and analyzed
    c. Risk of significant complications, morbidity, and/or mortality associated with the patient's presenting problem, the diagnostic procedures, and/or the management options
    d. All of the above

8. Which evaluation and management codes are used to report services to patients in a facility that provides room, board, and other personal assistance services, generally on a long-term basis?
    a. Outpatient services
    b. Nursing facility care
    c. Domiciliary, rest home, or custodial care services
    d. Care plan oversight services

9. Preventive medicine services are based upon which of the following criteria?
    a. Documentation of history, physical examination, and medical decision making
    b. Age of the patient
    c. Amount of time spent with the patient
    d. The final diagnosis for the visit

10. In order to report a critical care code, a physician must spend at least __30__ minutes with a critically ill patient.

Chapter 8

Medicine

The medicine section of the CPT codebook comprises a wide variety of specialty services and procedures such as psychiatric therapy, chemotherapy, rehabilitation, and immunization. The modifiers that apply to medicine codes were discussed extensively in earlier chapters of this workbook.

The medicine section includes the following subsections:

Subsection	Code Range
Immune Globulins	90281–90399
Immunization Administration for Vaccines/Toxoids	90465–90474
Vaccines and Toxoids	90476–90749
Hydration, Therapeutic, Prophylactic, and Diagnostic Injections and Infusions (Excludes Chemotherapy)	90760-90779
Psychiatry	90801–90899
Biofeedback	90901–90911
Dialysis	90918–90999
Gastroenterology	91000–91299
Ophthalmology	92002–92499
Special Otorhinolaryngologic Services	92502–92700
Cardiovascular	92950–93799
Non-Invasive Vascular Diagnostic Studies	93875–93990
Pulmonary	94010–94799
Allergy and Clinical Immunology	95004–95199
Endocrinology	95250–95251
Neurology and Neuromuscular Procedures	95805–96004
Central Nervous System Assessments/Tests	96101–96120
Health and Behavior Assessment/Intervention	96150–96155
Chemotherapy Administration	96401–96549
Photodynamic Therapy	96567–96571
Special Dermatological Procedures	96900–96999
Physical Medicine and Rehabilitation	97001–97799
Medical Nutrition Therapy	97802–97804
Acupuncture	97810–97814

Osteopathic Manipulative Therapy	98925–98929
Chiropractic Manipulative Treatment	98940–98943
Education and Training for Patient Self-Management	98960–98962
Special Services, Procedures, and Reports	99000–99091
Qualifying Circumstances for Anesthesia	99100–99140
Moderate (Conscious) Sedation	99143–99150
Other Services and Procedures	99170–99199
Home Health Procedures/Services	99500–99602

Specific subsections are discussed later in this chapter. In some cases, the services listed in the medicine section may be performed in conjunction with services or procedures listed elsewhere in the CPT codebook. It may be appropriate to use multiple codes from different sections of the codebook to identify the particular circumstances.

Example: An established patient was seen in the physician's office for DTP immunization injection. In addition to the immunization, the physician provides documentation for a minimal-level office visit. The following codes are reported: 90701, 90471, and 99211–25 (E/M code).

Immunization Injections

Separate codes exist for the administration (immunization procedure) of vaccines and toxoids and for the toxoid products themselves. Codes 90471–90474 are used to report the administration of a toxoid substance, and a code or codes from the 90476–90749 range identify the type of immunization or vaccine (measles, polio, DTP, and so on). Codes 90465 through 90468 are available for immunization administration for patients under eight years of age when the physician counsels the patient's family.

When a significant, separately identifiable E/M service (for example, office or other outpatient services or preventive medicine services) is performed, the appropriate E/M services code appended with modifier 25 should be reported in addition to the immunization administration and toxoid substance codes. For some health plans, other types of injections, including immunization administration, are bundled with E/M services and not reported separately.

Exercise 8.1   Immunizations

Assign the appropriate code(s) for each of the following procedures/services.

1.   Immunization injection for measles, mumps, rubella, and varicella vaccine (MMRV)

_____

2.   IM injection for tetanus

_____

3.   50-year-old male traveling abroad requires IM injection for hepatitis A; IM flu shot also administered during this encounter

_____

Hydration, Therapeutic, Prophylactic, and Diagnostic Injections and Infusions (Excludes Chemotherapy)

The physician services included in codes 90760–90779 are related to affirmation of treatment plan and direct supervision of staff. Note that the following services are included if performed to facilitate the infusion or injection:

- Use of local anesthesia

- IV start

- Access to indwelling IV, subcutaneous catheter or port

- Flush at conclusion of infusion

- Standard tubing, syringes, and supplies

If it is elected during the patient encounter to administer multiple infusions, injections, or combinations, only one "initial" service code should be reported, unless medical protocol requires that two separate IV sites be used. It is important to note that the initial code describes the primary reason for the encounter as well as the amount of time required for the injection/ infusion. CPT guidelines state that if an injection or infusion is of a "subsequent" or "concurrent nature," even if it is the first such service within that group of services, a subsequent or concurrent code from the appropriate section should be reported. For example, if the first IV push is given subsequent to an initial one-hour infusion, this service is reported using a subsequent IV push code.

Hydration (90760–90761)

Two codes are provided for hydration IV infusion, code 90760 for the initial (up to 1 hour) infusion and 90761 for each additional hour, up to eight hours. Hydration IV infusion consists of pre-packaged fluid and electrolytes (for example, normal saline).

Therapeutic, Prophylactic, and Diagnostic Injections and Infusions (90765–90779)

CPT codes from this section are used to describe administration of substances and/or drugs. The fluid used to administer the drug(s) is incidental hydration and is not reported with a separate CPT code.

As with immunization injections, the specific substance injected must be reported with another code. For Medicare cases, a Level II HCPCS code (J series) is reported with the identification of the specific substance or drug; for non-Medicare cases, code 99070 may be reported. (HCPCS Level II codes [J codes] are discussed in chapter 10 of this workbook.) This series of codes is not to be used for allergy injections or immunizations; specific CPT codes are available for these services.

The payment policies of individual payers (including Medicare) differ and should be reviewed carefully to ensure appropriate payment. For example, some payers reimburse for an office visit code only when an injection was performed during that visit; others reimburse only for the drug administered (J code), as well as the method of administration (for example, intravenous injection). When there is a need for data collection, most health plans do not object to a nonpayable code being reported with a zero or no-charge amount.

Exercise 8.2   Injections and Infusions

Assign the appropriate code(s) for each of the following procedures/services.

1.   Immunization injection of cholera vaccine

   _____

2.   IV infusion hydration for one hour

   _____

3.   IM injection of hepatitis B and Hemophilus influenza B vaccine

   _____

4.   Intramuscular B_{12} injection

   _____

Psychiatry

The psychiatric services included in codes 90801 through 90899 may be provided in an outpatient or inpatient setting or in a partial hospital setting. The Centers for Medicare and Medicaid Services (CMS) defines psychiatric facility partial hospitalization as a facility for the diagnosis and treatment of mental illness that provides a planned therapeutic program for patients who do not require full-time hospitalization, but who need broader programs than are possible from outpatient visits in a hospital-based or hospital-affiliated facility. Partial hospitalization may be used for crisis stabilization, intensive short-term daily treatment, or intermediate-term treatment of psychiatric disorders.

When E/M services such as hospital or office visits are provided along with services from the psychiatry subsection, a code from the E/M section and a code from the psychiatry subsection are usually reported. However, some codes in the psychiatry subsection combine the psychiatric services and the E/M services into one code. In this situation, only the code from the psychiatry subsection is reported.

Example #1:   A psychiatrist provided psychoanalysis along with E/M services to an established patient in the office setting. The office visit included an expanded, problem-focused history and an examination and medical decision making of low complexity. The following codes should be reported: 90845 and 99213–25.

Example #2:   A patient in a clinic receives individual insight-oriented psychotherapy for more than 25 minutes. The physician also provides E/M services that include a problem-focused history, a problem-focused examination, and a straightforward level of medical decision making. Code 90805 should be reported.

Note that some third-party payers, including Medicare, do not reimburse for an E/M service and psychotherapy when both are performed on the same day.

The psychiatry subsection is further divided to identify consultative and therapeutic services such as psychotherapy, electroconvulsive therapy, and hypnotherapy.

General Diagnostic and Evaluative Interview Procedures

Code 90801, Psychiatric diagnostic interview examination, typically is reported during the initial phases of psychiatric treatment. This service includes a complete medical and psychiatric history, which may be obtained from the patient and/or the patient's family, and a complete mental status examination that focuses on the patient's condition at the time of the examination. When this service is provided in an inpatient hospital setting, it may be reported only once during the hospital stay.

Psychiatric Therapeutic Procedures

Codes 90804 through 90899 describe specific psychotherapeutic procedures in the treatment of mental disorders and behavioral disturbances, including interactive psychotherapy, supportive psychotherapy, psychoanalysis, narcosynthesis, electroconvulsive therapy, and so on. Interactive psychotherapy (90810–90815 and 90823–90829) uses physical aids and nonverbal communication as a way for physicians to communicate with patients who are unable to interact verbally. Narcosynthesis (90865) involves the administration of a medication that frees patients of their inhibitions and allows them to reveal information they might otherwise have found difficult to discuss.

It should be noted that some psychotherapy codes factor in the amount of time spent with the patient. When the amount of time spent with a patient is less or greater than the time specified in the code description, modifier –22, Unusual Procedural Services, or –52, Reduced Services, may be reported to reflect the actual situation.

Exercise 8.3   Psychiatry

Assign the appropriate code(s) for each of the following procedures/services.

1. Psychiatric evaluation of patient's health records, psychiatric reports, and tests in order to make a diagnosis

   _____

2. Psychotherapy involving patient and family members

   _____

3. Individual behavior modification and insight-oriented psychotherapy in office for 45 minutes

   _____

Dialysis

Codes 90918 through 90999 describe services related to end-stage renal disease, hemodialysis, and peritoneal dialysis. The CPT codebook indicates that all E/M services related to the patient's renal disease that are provided on the same day as the dialysis should be included in the dialysis procedure code (90935–90947) and should not be reported separately. However, E/M services unrelated to the patient's renal disease that cannot be performed during the dialysis session may be reported separately.

The first series of codes (90918–90925) describes the physician services provided to patients with end-stage renal disease, including outpatient visits, telephone calls, and general management. Codes 90918 through 90921 describe services provided for a full month and are divided further by age. The second series of codes (90922–90925), also subdivided by age, is reported for services provided for less than one full month. A code from this series is assigned each day the physician provides the service.

Two methods are used to treat patients with end-stage renal disease: hemodialysis and peritoneal dialysis. Hemodialysis can be defined as the process of removing metabolic waste products, toxins, and excess fluid from the blood. Codes 90935 and 90937 are reported to identify the physician service(s) provided on the day of hemodialysis. Code 90935 is reported when the physician provides a single evaluation of the patient during the hemodialysis, and code 90937 is reported when the physician is required to evaluate the patient more than once during the procedure. When the physician is required to provide prolonged services, a code from the range 99354 through 99360 may be reported along with the hemodialysis code. Codes describing development of a shunt, cannula, or fistula for hemodialysis are categorized in the surgery section of the CPT codebook.

Peritoneal dialysis involves the insertion of a catheter into the abdominal cavity and infusion of a fluid (dialysate) into the peritoneum that allows for diffusion between the dialyzing fluid and the body fluids containing the waste products. The fluid containing the waste products then is removed from the peritoneum through the catheter. Codes 90945 and 90947 are reported to identify the physician service(s) provided on the day of peritoneal dialysis. Code 90945 is reported when the physician provides a single evaluation of the patient during the peritoneal dialysis, and code 90947 is reported when the physician is required to evaluate the patient more than once during the dialysis procedure. When the physician is required to provide prolonged services, a code from the range 99354 through 99360 may be reported along with the dialysis code. The codes describing the insertion of the peritoneal dialysis catheter are categorized in the surgery section of the CPT codebook.

Exercise 8.4   Dialysis

Assign the appropriate code(s) for each of the following physician procedures/services.

1.   A 50-year-old patient with end-stage renal disease treated in the outpatient dialysis unit for the past month

_____

2.   Peritoneal dialysis with a single physician evaluation

_____

Ophthalmology

The ophthalmology subsection includes codes (92002–92499) describing ophthalmologic medical services provided to both new and established patients. The definitions for new and established patient are the same as those mentioned for E/M services:

- A new patient is one who has not received any professional services (face-to-face) within the past three years from the physician or another physician of the same specialty who belongs to the same group practice.

- An established patient is one who has received professional services (face-to-face) within the past three years from the physician or another physician of the same specialty who belongs to the same group practice.

Complete definitions and examples for intermediate and comprehensive ophthalmologic services are provided in the CPT codebook. Briefly, the two types of service can be described as follows:

- *Intermediate services* involve the evaluation of a new or existing condition complicated with a new diagnostic or management problem and include a history, general medical observation, external ocular and adnexal examination, and other diagnostic procedures as indicated.

- *Comprehensive services* involve a general evaluation of the complete visual system and include a history, general medical observation, an external and ophthalmoscopic examination, gross visual fields, and a basic sensorimotor examination. Initiation of diagnostic and treatment programs is always part of a comprehensive service.

An ophthalmologic examination and evaluation performed under general anesthesia is reported with code 92018 or 92019.

The prescription of contact lenses is not part of the general ophthalmologic service and should be reported separately with a code from the series 92310 through 92326. When supplying contact lenses is part of the service of fitting them (92310–92317), a separate code should not be reported.

The prescription of glasses is considered part of a general ophthalmologic service and thus should not be reported separately. Because the actual fitting of the glasses is considered a separate procedure, the fitting should be reported with a code from the series 92340 through 92371.

Exercise 8.5   Ophthalmology

Assign the appropriate code(s) for each of the following procedures/services.

1.   Gonioscopy is performed under general anesthesia.

_____

2.   New patient has a comprehensive ophthalmologic exam and evaluation.

_____

Otorhinolaryngologic Services

Special otorhinolaryngologic services include the diagnostic and therapeutic services usually provided by ear, nose, and throat specialists. Vestibular function tests and audiological function tests are found in this section. No specific coding guidelines apply to these codes other than to use modifier –52, Reduced Services, for audiological function tests when a test is applied to only one ear.

Cardiovascular Services

The cardiovascular subsection includes codes describing diagnostic and therapeutic services such as electrocardiography, cardiac catheterization, atrial septostomy, and percutaneous transluminal coronary atherectomy. The first series of codes in this subsection (92950–92998) describes therapeutic services such as cardiopulmonary resuscitation, percutaneous transluminal coronary angioplasty (PTCA), percutaneous valvuloplasty, and coronary thrombolysis.

Stent Placement

Code 92980 is reported for transcatheter stenting of a single coronary vessel. This code is only reported once per vessel even when multiple stents are placed. Code 92981 is an add-on code that can be used for stenting of additional vessels. These codes include PTCA and/or atherectomy in the same vessel.

> **Example:** Physician performs stenting of the right coronary artery, and angioplasty and stenting of the left circumflex artery. Report the following codes: 92980-RC (stenting of right coronary artery), 92981-LC (stenting of left circumflex artery). Note that the angioplasty is not separately coded.

Drug-eluting stents coated with medication are used to prevent build-up of new tissue that would reclog the artery. Physicians report code 92980 or 92981 for placement of the drug-eluting stents. Hospitals report HCPCS Level II codes for placement of drug-eluting stents, as follows:

- G0290 Transcatheter placement of a drug-eluting intracoronary stent(s), percutaneous, with or without other therapeutic intervention, any method; single vessel

- G0291 Each additional vessel

Atherectomy

Percutaneous transluminal coronary atherectomy is reported with 92995 (for first vessel treated) and 92996 (for each additional vessel). These CPT codes include any angioplasty performed in the same vessel.

Percutaneous Transluminal Coronary Angioplasty

Percutaneous transluminal coronary angioplasties (PTCAs) are reported with 92982 (for the first vessel) and 92984 (for each additional vessel). These codes should be assigned for per vessel even when multiple strictures are treated within the same vessel. Angioplasty procedures performed with a cutting balloon are reported by assigning a PTCA procedure code (not an atherectomy code).

Thrombectomy

Code 92973 should be reported when a percutaneous transluminal coronary thrombectomy (for example, with Angiojet catheter) is performed in conjunction with stenting or angioplasty. Code 92973 is considered an add-on code.

Brachytherapy

Code 92974 should be reported for a transcatheter placement of a radiation delivery device for intravascular brachytherapy. This code can be used in conjunction with codes for stenting, angioplasty, or angiography without left-heart catheterization (CPT code 93508). This procedure is used to prevent repeat stenosing of the cardiac arteries. Code 92974 is an add-on code and does not include the radiation oncology service for brachytherapy.

It should be noted that the codes describing PTCA procedures (92982–92984), arthrectomies (92995–92996), and transcatheter placements of stent(s) (92980–92981) require the assignment of additional codes when more than one vessel is involved, as follows:

Procedure	Single Vessel	Each Additional Vessel
Stent placement	92980	92981
Coronary angioplasty	92982	92984
Coronary atherectomy	92995	92996

Example: Percutaneous transluminal coronary balloon angioplasty involving three vessels. The following codes should be reported: 92982 (first vessel), 92984 (second vessel), and 92984 (third vessel).

Codes 92995 and 92996 describe percutaneous transluminal coronary atherectomy that may or may not be accompanied by balloon angioplasty of the same vessel.

When percutaneous coronary atherectomy and balloon angioplasty are performed during the same episode on different vessels, the two treatment modes should be reported with multiple codes to describe them.

Example: Percutaneous transluminal coronary balloon angioplasty of the left anterior descending artery and percutaneous transluminal coronary atherectomy of the right anterior descending artery. The following codes should be reported: 92995 and 92982.

Cardiography

The next two series of codes involve diagnostic cardiography (93000–93278), which includes electrocardiograms (EKGs) and stress tests, and echocardiography (93303–93350), which includes echocardiograms (ultrasounds of the heart).

Coronary Angiography

CPT code 93508 identifies coronary angiography performed without heart catheterization. This technique is similar to a retrograde left-heart catheterization, but the catheter is not advanced across the aortic valve into the heart. Instead, the surgeon advances the catheter immediately into one of the coronary arteries or a vein graft. Coding guidelines state that the applicable injection code(s) (93539, 93540, 93544, 93545) and imaging code (93556) should also be assigned.

Cardiac Catheterization

Cardiac catheterization is a diagnostic procedure that can identify diseases in the coronary arteries. (See figure 8.1.) According to the CPT definition, a cardiac catheterization includes the following procedures and services:

- Introduction, positioning, and repositioning of catheter(s)
- Recording of intracardiac and intravascular pressure
- Obtaining blood samples for measurement of blood gases or dilution curves

- Cardiac output measurements (Fick or other method) with or without electrode catheter placement

- Final evaluation and report of procedure

Codes 93501 through 93562 describe cardiac catheterizations and associated procedures. Most cardiac codes require at least three CPT codes for a complete description of the cardiac catheterization procedure. The following codes are provided to describe these procedures:

- Codes 93501 through 93529 for catheter placement

- Codes 93539 through 93545 for the injection procedure

- Codes 93555 through 93556 for imaging supervision and interpretation

When only the professional component of the services was provided, modifier –26 should be applied to the catheter placement and imaging supervision and interpretation codes. The injection codes do not require modifier –26.

Figure 8.1. Cardiac catheterization

Several procedures performed during catheter placement are considered inherent to the procedure. These procedures include the following:

- Introduction, positioning, and repositioning of the catheter(s)

- Recording of pressures

- Drawing blood samples for gases and/or dilution

- Measuring cardiac output

The following cardiac catheterization procedures are the most common procedures:

- *Right-heart catheterization (93501):* The catheter is introduced into the *venous* system (femoral vein, internal jugular vein, subclavian vein) and advanced through the inferior vena cava into right atrium, right ventricle, pulmonary artery, and pulmonary capillary wedge positions.

- *Left-heart catheterization (93510):* The catheter is introduced into the *arterial* system (the brachial artery, axillary artery, femoral artery-percutaneous) and advanced through aorta into the left atrium and left ventricle. Catheter inserted by cutdown is assigned code 93511.

- *Combined right and left (93526):* This single code describes a procedure that is both a right-heart catheterization and a retrograde left-heart catheterization.

Note that there are other codes for unusual techniques, including direct ventricular puncture and puncture of the septum between the left and right atrium.

Swan-Ganz Catheterization
Code 93503 is assigned to report placement of a Swan-Ganz catheter for monitoring purposes. This procedure is typically performed on patients who are critically ill or undergoing major surgery.

Injections
Codes 93539 through 93545 are assigned for contrast injection during cardiac catheterization. It is important to note that each code can only be reported once, even when multiple vessels are injected. The following list summarizes the injection codes:

- Code 93539 for injections of one or more arterial bypass grafts (for example, internal mammary artery and radial artery)

- Code 93540 for injections of one or more venous bypass grafts (for example, saphenous)

- Code 93541 for injections of the pulmonary artery (or one of its branches)

- Code 93542 for injections of the right atrium or ventricle

- Code 93543 for injections of the left atrium or ventricle

- Code 93544 for injections of the aorta

- Code 93545 for injections of one or more of the patient's native coronary arteries (not bypass grafts)

Imaging

Only two codes are provided for reporting the imaging procedures performed during a cardiac catheterization: 93555 for atrial and/or ventricular angiography and 93556 for all other angiography (for example, coronary artery and bypass graft). Both codes should be reported when both types of imaging were performed.

Infusion during Cardiac Catheterization Procedure

Physicians often infuse medications such as nitroglycerine during cardiac catheterization procedures. The January 1998 issue of *CPT Assistant* states that infusion of medications should be considered an intrinsic part of the catheterization procedure.

Intracardiac Electrophysiological Procedures and Studies

Electrophysiological testing is performed on patients with cardiac arrhythmias that result in palpitations, near syncope, or syncope with cardiac arrest. Intracardiac electrophysiological procedures, which may be diagnostic or therapeutic, are reported with codes from the range 93600 through 93662. The services described in codes 93600 through 93652 include the insertion and repositioning of catheters.

Codes 93600 through 93612 include diagnostic electrophysiological procedures that provide only recording and pacing from a single site. Codes 93619 through 93622 describe a comprehensive electrophysiological evaluation that may be reported when recording and pacing are performed from multiple sites.

Exercise 8.6   Cardiovascular Services

Assign the appropriate code(s) for each of the following procedures/services.

1. Patient with ventricular arrhythmia undergoes a microvolt T-wave alternans test

   _____

2. Left-heart catheterization with injection of the native left and right coronary arteries and coronary angiography

   _____

3. Coronary thrombolysis by IV infusion

   _____

4. Cardiac stress test performed under physician supervision with interpretation and report

   _____

5. Laser (percutaneous) atherectomy of left circumflex and left anterior descending coronary arteries and angioplasty of left anterior descending (assign Level II modifiers)

   _____

6. PTCA of two branches of the left anterior descending artery; PTCA of the right coronary artery (assign Level II modifiers)

   _____

Pulmonary Services

Pulmonologists and hospitals use codes from the pulmonary subsection for pulmonary testing. When E/M services are provided separately, a code from the E/M section also should be assigned. Codes 94010 through 94799 include the performance of lab procedures and the interpretation of the test results.

Exercise 8.7   Pulmonary Services

Assign the appropriate codes for the following procedures/services.

1. Spirometry for bronchodilator response evaluation

    _____

2. Continuous positive airway pressure (CPAP)

    _____

3. Hypoxia response curve

    _____

Allergy and Clinical Immunology

The allergy and clinical immunology subsection includes the categories of allergy testing and allergen immunotherapy. The codes for allergy sensitivity tests include the performance and evaluation of selective skin and mucus tests in association with the patient's history and physical examination. Immunotherapy (desensitization, hyposensitization) involves the parenteral administration of allergenic extracts as antigens at periodic intervals, usually on a higher dosage than a maintenance dosage. The CPT codebook provides more complete definitions.

Codes from the E/M services section should be used to report visits with the patient involving the use of mechanical and electronic devices such as air conditioners, air filters, and humidifiers; climatotherapy; and physical, occupational, and recreational therapy.

Allergy testing (95004–95078) is further divided by type of test: percutaneous, intracutaneous, patch or application, and so on. For most of the codes in this series, the number of tests performed should be reported on the CMS-1500 form under item 24G.

> **Example:** Ten percutaneous tests with allergenic extracts were performed. The following should be reported: 95004 with 10 (to identify the number of tests) in item 24G of the CMS-1500 form.

Allergen immunotherapy (95115–95199), more commonly referred to as allergy shots, includes the professional services related to the immunotherapy. A separate office visit code(s) should not be reported unless some other identifiable service was provided during the visit.

Exercise 8.8 Allergy and Clinical Immunology

Assign the appropriate code(s) for each of the following procedures/services.

1. Scratch test performed to determine allergy to bees, wasps, and yellow jackets

   _____

2. Allergy shot for grass pollen (includes extract)

   _____

Neurology and Neuromuscular Procedures and Central Nervous System Assessments and Tests

Consulting neurologists and hospitals generally use the range of codes in the subsections classifying neurology and neuromuscular procedures and central nervous system tests to report such procedures, assessments, and tests. Sleep testing, nerve conduction studies, and developmental testing are classified to this area of the medicine section of the CPT codebook.

Health and Behavior Assessment and Intervention

The focus of health and behavior assessments and interventions (codes 96150–96155) is not on mental health, but on the biopsychosocial factors affecting physical health problems and treatments (that is, patients with chronic illnesses). The codes can be reported by clinical social workers, advanced practice nurses, psychologists, and other healthcare professionals who have training in health and behavior assessment and intervention procedures. Physicians performing these services are directed to report E/M or preventive medicine codes.

Chemotherapy Administration

The administration of chemotherapy is reported with codes 96401 through 96549. The codes further identify the mode of administration: subcutaneous or intramuscular, intralesional, intravenous, or intra-arterial. The codes describing intravenous and intra-arterial administration are further subdivided to identify the technique—infusion or push—and length of time. Codes 96440 through 96450 describe the administration of chemotherapy to specific body sites: pleural or peritoneal cavity, or central nervous system. Codes 96521 and 96522 describe the maintenance and refilling of portable or implantable pumps or reservoirs.

Although preparation of the chemotherapy agent is included in the administration, provision of the chemotherapy drug is not. For Medicare claims, a code from the J series of the Level II HCPCS should be reported to identify the specific drug administered. (The CMS Web site provides chemotherapy coding guidelines.) The individual payer should be contacted for further directions. Codes describing the placement of pumps, catheters, or reservoirs can be found in the surgery section of the CPT codebook.

> **Example:** Patient with lung cancer is seen in the hospital outpatient department for chemotherapy treatment. The patient receives Cisplatin 80 mg IV for one hour. The following should be reported:
>
> 96413 Chemotherapy administration, infusion, 1st hour
> J9060 Cisplatin, per 10 mg (bill would reflect 8 units since 80 mg was administered).

When additional services are provided on the same day as the chemotherapy and are independent of the chemotherapy, the physician may bill the additional services separately (for example, an E/M office visit).

Exercise 8.9   Chemotherapy Services

Assign the appropriate codes for the following procedures/services.

1.   IV infusion of Cisplatin administered for 2 hours   _____

2.   Intra-arterial chemotherapy administration, IV push   _____

Special Dermatological Procedures

Services such as actinotherapy and photochemotherapy are found in the special dermatological procedures subsection of CPT. Generally, these codes are used by consulting dermatologists.

Physical Medicine and Rehabilitation

The number of physical medicine and rehabilitation services available to patients continues to expand as new modalities and therapeutic procedures are developed. The CPT codes for these services (97001–97755) are used by the physiatrists and physical therapists who provide physical therapy services to patients recovering from injuries, strokes, and other debilitating conditions. Test and measurement codes can be reported to document the use of prosthetic devices and physical performance testing apparatus. No special coding guidelines apply to this section. Physiatrists use the E/M section for professional service billing.

Active wound care management (97597–97606) codes are also provided in this subsection. These codes are meant to be assigned to report active wound care performed by nonphysician healthcare professionals (for example, nurses, physician assistants, physical therapists, and occupational therapists).

According to CPT coding guidelines, the wound care management codes should not be reported in addition to the debridement codes (11040–11044) included in the integumentary system subsection of the Surgery section. The debridement codes (11040–11044) are considered surgical debridement, whereas wound care management codes are considered nonsurgical.

The nonsurgical debridement can be described as either selective or nonselective. Codes 97597 and 97598 are assigned for the selective technique, which includes the use of scalpels, scissors, and forceps to cut and remove the necrotic tissue. Other selective debridement includes the use of high-pressure water jets, enzyme applications, and autolysis. Code 97602 is assigned for nonselective techniques, which include the gradual removal of loosely adherent areas of necrotic tissue achieved by irrigating the wound and hydrotherapy.

Codes 97605 and 97606 are used to report negative pressure wound therapy, which is often described as a vacuum-assisted closure. This system encourages wound closure by applying localized negative pressure to the surface and margins of the wound. Negative pressure therapy is applied to a special dressing positioned in the wound cavity or over a flap or graft. The pressure-distributing wound dressing helps drain fluids from the wound.

Exercise 8.10   Physical Medicine and Rehabilitation

Assign the appropriate code(s) for each of the following procedures/services.

1. TENS unit applied by therapist for patient with low back pain

    _____

2. Thirty minutes of water aerobics with therapist for treatment of arthritis

    _____

3. Physician orders a reevaluation of a knee injury following a course of athletic training

    _____

4. Physical therapist provides whirlpool therapy to promote healing of a necrotic wound

    _____

Manipulative Treatment

Osteopathic physicians and chiropractic physicians as well as other physicians trained in manipulation techniques use the codes found in the osteopathic manipulative treatment and chiropractic manipulative treatment subsections. E/M service codes are to be reported separately only when the services are significant and separate from the manipulative treatments. In these cases, modifier –25, Significant, Separately Identifiable Evaluation and Management Service by the Same Physician on the Same Day of the Procedure or Other Service, may be appended to the E/M code to communicate the circumstances on a claim form.

Special Services, Procedures, and Reports

The special services and reports subsection (99000–99091) of the CPT Medicine section describes certain procedures and services or reports that the physician may add to other basic services. Codes 99050 through 99060 describe special services provided to a patient beyond the basic service, such as those requested between 10 p.m. and 8 a.m. (code 99052). Because a third-party payer may or may not reimburse these services, a review of each payer's policies might be informative. However, coded information is also used in many activities unrelated to reimbursement, and so assigning the codes for nonreimbursable services may be desirable from a data management perspective.

CPT code 99070 may be reported when the physician submits claims for supplies and other materials to an insurance plan that does not recognize Level II HCPCS codes. For Medicare claims, coders should remember that, in most cases, a more specific code describing a particular supply may exist in Level II of HCPCS, and routine supplies associated with professional services are not reimbursed separately.

Qualifying Circumstances for Anesthesia

Four CPT codes (99100–99140) may be used to report qualifying circumstances or additional information on patients undergoing anesthesia who show greater risk of complications. For example, codes describing patients of extreme age (elderly or newborn), with total body hypothermia or controlled hypotension, or with possible emergency conditions, may need to be reported in addition to the code describing the anesthesia service.

Moderate (Conscious) Sedation

The moderate sedation codes are available to report moderate (conscious) sedation, a technique used during a number of endoscopic and other procedures. The use of these codes requires the presence of an independent, trained observer to assist the operating physician in monitoring the patient's level of consciousness and physiological status. The codes represent performance and documentation of presedation and postsedation evaluations of the patient, administration of the sedation, and monitoring of cardiorespiratory functions.

Other Services and Procedures

The Medicine section of CPT also provides codes for several miscellaneous procedures that are performed by physicians but do not fit into the other sections of CPT. One example is hyperbaric oxygen therapy supervision. Another is the administration of Ipecac and observation of the patient until the stomach is emptied of poison. Such codes are located in the other services and procedures subsection.

Home Health Procedures and Services

Codes from the section on home health procedures and services (99500–99512) are used by nonphysician healthcare professionals who provide medical services in the homes of patients. Physicians use codes from the E/M section for coding the home health services they provide. Healthcare professionals who are authorized to use E/M home visit codes (99341–99350) may report codes from the range 99500 through 99512 with the E/M code when a patient's condition requires a significant evaluation and management services beyond the home health service or procedure. In such cases, modifier –25 may be appended to the E/M code.

Home Infusion Procedures

Codes from the home infusion procedures section (99601 and 99602) include a code for home visits by nonphysician healthcare professionals and a code for all the necessary solutions, equipment, and supplies required to deliver a therapeutic service in one visit. Drugs are excluded from this code and should be reported separately.

Exercise 8.11   Chapter 8 Review

Assign the appropriate code(s) from the CPT Medicine section as well as modifiers, when appropriate, for each of the following non-Medicare cases.

1. Hemodialysis with the physician evaluating the patient twice during the service

2. Active immunization with live measles, mumps, and rubella virus vaccine

3. Routine EKG with 15 leads, with the physician providing only the interpretation and report of the test

4. IV chemotherapy lasting three hours

(Continued on next page)

Exercise 8.11   (Continued)

5. His Bundle recording performed to evaluate patient with syncope

   _____

6. Speech audiometry with threshold and recognition, both ears

   _____

7. Intramuscular steroid injection

   _____

8. Individual interactive psychotherapy for 45 minutes provided in the outpatient setting

   _____

9. Percutaneous transluminal coronary atherectomy of left posterior descending and left obtuse marginal arteries

   _____

10. Comprehensive ophthalmologic services provided to an established patient with extended color vision examination

    _____

11. Angioplasty and thrombectomy of right coronary artery; angioplasty and placement of drug-eluting stent, left circumflex

    _____

12. Leg prosthetic training for 45 minutes by a physical therapist

    _____

13. In addition to E/M services, a physician provided a medical service on July 4 to fulfill a patient's request for the service

    _____

14. Complete duplex scan of the lower extremity arteries

    _____

15. EMG of three extremities and related paraspinal areas

    _____

16. Physician treats plaque psoriasis of arms and legs with use of laser (200 cm^2)

    _____

17. Osteopathic manipulation; head, cervical, thoracic, and lumbar spine

    _____

18. Nurse makes a home visit for newborn care and assessment

    _____

19. MDI (metered dose inhaler) treatment for patient with asthma

    _____

20. Sleep study performed by a technician that included an EKG, recordings of breathing, and O_2 saturation

    _____

Chapter 8 Test

Write the appropriate answer.

1. Individual psychotherapy, inpatient hospital, 50 minutes

   _____

2. Esophageal motility study with acid perfusion testing

   _____

3. Fluorescein angiography

   _____

4. Reprogramming of cochlear implant device, patient 3 years of age

   _____

5. Transcatheter placement of coronary artery stent, right coronary artery

   _____

6. EKG, physician interpretation and report, using hospital equipment

   _____

7. Combined right-heart catheterization and retrograde left-heart catheterization via femoral artery approach

   _____

8. Duplex scan of bilateral lower extremity arteries

   _____

9. Pulmonary stress testing

   _____

10. Bronchospasm evaluation

    _____

Chapter 9

Anesthesia

CPT codes in this section can be reported under the condition that the procedure/services were performed by, or under the responsible supervision of, a physician or a certified registered nurse anesthetist (CRNA). The anesthesia section of the CPT codebook includes codes that describe general, regional, and local anesthesia services. These services should be reported by the physician who provides or supervises the anesthesia. The anesthesia services (00100–01999) in this section include:

- Usual preoperative and postoperative visits
- Anesthesia provided during the procedure
- Administration of fluids and/or blood
- Usual monitoring services, such as EKG, temperature, blood pressure, oximetry, capnography, and mass spectrometry (unusual monitoring, such as intra-arterial, central venous, or Swan-Ganz, is not included and should be reported separately)

Coding anesthesia services can be challenging because reporting of services and reimbursement will vary depending upon the payer's specific guidelines. Some payers request that the provider submit time; others want the reporting of either anesthesia CPT codes (00100–01999) or surgical CPT codes (10021–99602).

The codes in the Anesthesia section are arranged first by body site and then by specific surgical procedure performed. They may be found in the alphabetic index of the CPT codebook by referencing the main entries of Anesthesia or Analgesia.

Reporting of Time

Time may be reported for reimbursement of services, if preferred, by local carrier. Counting anesthesia time should begin with preparation of the patient by the anesthesiologist for induction of anesthesia (usually in the OR) and end when the anesthesiologist no longer is in attendance. Only face-to-face time is billable (with the exception of deliveries).

The American Society of Anesthesiologists (ASA) publishes the *Relative Value Guide* each year to provide a resource for establishing basic values for anesthesia used in most surgical procedures. The basic value unit includes usual preoperative and postoperative visits by the anesthesiologist. Total time is converted to time units. The usual time unit is 15 minutes. It should be noted that the ASA guide is a relative value study and not a fee schedule, although it is widely accepted as a method of establishing fees for anesthesia services.

Anesthesia Modifiers

When reporting anesthesia services, a physical status modifier code should be used to distinguish between various levels of complexity of the anesthesia service provided. The anesthesiologist usually provides physical status modifiers on the anesthesia record. The ranking of patient physical status by the ASA is consistent with the following modifiers:

P1   A normal, healthy patient
P2   A patient with mild systemic disease
P3   A patient with severe systemic disease
P4   A patient with severe systemic disease that is a constant threat to life
P5   A moribund patient who is not expected to survive without the operation
P6   A declared brain-dead patient whose organs are being removed for donor purposes

Under certain circumstances, other modifiers may be assigned. The following modifiers are commonly used with codes from the anesthesia section.

22   **Unusual Procedural Services:** Modifier –22 may be reported to identify that the service provided was greater than that usually required for a particular service. Supportive documentation may need to be submitted to the third-party payer to justify use of modifier –22.

23   **Unusual Anesthesia:** Modifier –23 may be reported when anesthesia is administered for a procedure that usually requires local anesthesia or none at all. This modifier would be reported along with the appropriate code describing the anesthesia service.

32   **Mandated Services:** Modifier –32 may be reported when a group such as a third-party payer or a quality improvement organization (QIO) mandates a service.

51   **Multiple Procedures:** Modifier –51 may be reported to identify that multiple anesthesia services were provided on the same day or during the same operative episode. The first procedure listed should identify the major or most resource-intensive service provided. Subsequent or secondary services should be appended with modifier –51.

53   **Discontinued Procedure:** Modifier –53 is appropriate for circumstances when the physician elects to terminate or discontinue a procedure, usually because of risk to the patient's well-being. However, this modifier is not meant to report the elective cancellation of a procedure before the patient's surgical preparation or induction of anesthesia. Also, the appropriate ICD-9-CM code should be assigned to identify the reason for the procedure's termination or discontinuation.

59   **Distinct Procedural Service:** Modifier –59 may be used to identify that a procedure/service was distinct or independent from other services provided on the same day.

Modifier –47, Anesthesia by Surgeon, is never used as a modifier for the anesthesia procedures in the CPT codebook (00100–01999).

HCPCS Level II Modifiers

The following National Code modifiers are applicable to anesthesia services:

AA   **Anesthesia services performed personally by anesthesiologist**

AD   **Medical supervision by a physician: more than four concurrent anesthesia procedures**

G8   **Monitored anesthesia care (MAC) for deep complex, complicated or markedly invasive surgical procedures**

G9   Monitored anesthesia care for patient who has a history of a severe cardiopulmonary condition

QK   Medical direction of two, three, or four concurrent anesthesia procedures involving qualified individuals

QS   Monitored anesthesia care service

QX   CRNA service; with medical direction by a physician

QY   Medical direction of one certified registered nurse anesthetist (CRNA) by an anesthesiologist

QZ   CRNA service; without medical direction by a physician

The assignment of modifier –QK indicates that the anesthesiologist provided medical direction to at least two, but not more than four, certified nurse anesthetists.

Anesthesia Codes versus Surgery Codes

The codes in the anesthesia section are reported exclusively for Medicare claims, along with the appropriate physical status modifier. Selected third-party payers require anesthesiologists to report their services with the appropriate code from the surgery section that describes the procedure performed. The surgery code should be appended with the appropriate physical status modifier.

> **Example:** Anesthesia services provided to a normal, healthy patient for transurethral resection of the prostate
>
> Medicare Claim: 00914–P1
> Non-Medicare Claim: 52601–P1

Qualifying Circumstances

When anesthesia services are provided under difficult circumstances because of the patient's condition, operative conditions, or unusual risk factors, an additional code may be reported along with the code describing the basic anesthesia service. Codes 99100 through 99140 can never be reported alone. Located in the medicine section of the CPT codebook, these codes (99100–99140) are described as follows:

- 99100, Anesthesia for patient of extreme age, under one year and over seventy

- 99116, Anesthesia complicated by utilization of total body hypothermia

- 99135, Anesthesia complicated by utilization of controlled hypotension

- 99140, Anesthesia complicated by emergency conditions

When code 99140 is reported, a separate report must be submitted describing the type of emergency. According to the CPT codebook, an emergency exists when delay in treatment of the patient would significantly increase the threat to life or body part.

Application of Anesthesia Codes in the Hospital Setting

Because the anesthesia coders were developed to represent the professional services provided by anesthesiologists, the anesthesia codes cannot be reported by hospitals unless the hospitals perform billing services for the anesthesiologists.

Exercise 9.1 Chapter 9 Review

Assign the appropriate codes and physical status modifiers to describe the anesthesia services for the following Medicare claims. The anesthesia codes should be assigned from the anesthesia section when applicable.

1. Anesthesia services for radical mastectomy with internal mammary node dissection; patient has diabetes mellitus well controlled with American Dietetic Association (ADA) diet

   _____

2. Anesthesia services for closed treatment of fracture of humerus; patient is 85 years old, but healthy

   _____

3. Anesthesia services for CABG surgery of five vessels with pump oxygenator; patient has severe coronary artery disease as well as hypertensive end-stage renal disease requiring hemodialysis

   _____

4. Anesthesia services for left lobectomy due to lung carcinoma; patient also has severe chronic obstructive pulmonary disease and emphysema treated with bronchodilators

   _____

5. Anesthesia services for left carotid endarterectomy; patient is otherwise healthy

   _____

Assign the appropriate codes and physical status modifiers to describe anesthesia services for the following non-Medicare claims. The anesthesia codes should be assigned from the CPT Surgery section.

6. Anesthesia services for partial nephrectomy in a patient with renal cell carcinoma; 45-year-old patient also has mild coronary artery disease and hypertension treated with medication

   _____

7. Anesthesia services for heart transplant secondary to congenital heart defect; patient is three weeks old and requires a transplant to survive

   _____

8. Anesthesia services for carotid thromboendarterectomy with patch graft for severe carotid artery stenosis; patient is 75 years old and has had recurrent carotid artery stenosis; patient also has a pacemaker for control of atrial fibrillation

   _____

9. Anesthesia services for laparoscopic cholecystectomy with cholangiography for acute cholecystitis; patient is 35 years old and in good health

   _____

10. Anesthesia services for extracapsular cataract extraction with insertion of intraocular lens prosthesis; patient is 79 years old, with mild diabetes mellitus and hypertension

   _____

Chapter 9 Test

Choose or write the appropriate answer.

1. Per CPT guidelines, anesthesia time begins when the anesthesiologist begins to prepare the patient for induction, and ends:
   a. When the patient leaves the operating room
   b. When the anesthesiologist is no longer in personal attendance on the patient
   c. When the patient has fulfilled postanesthesia care unit criteria for recovery
   d. When the patient leaves the postanesthesia care unit

2. A physical status anesthesia modifier of P4 means that a patient:
   a. Has a mild systemic disease
   b. Has a severe systemic disease
   c. Has a severe systemic disease that is a constant threat to life
   d. Is moribund

3. Anesthesia for total repair of cleft palate, patient 4 years of age

   _____

4. Anesthesia for permanent transvenous pacemaker insertion

   _____

5. Anesthesia for ventral hernia repair, patient a 76-year-old female

   _____

6. Anesthesia for left knee arthroscopy with medial meniscectomy

   _____

7. Anesthesia for vasectomy

   _____

8. Anesthesia for cesarean section following failed attempt at vaginal delivery under spinal anesthesia

   _____

9. Anesthesia for Whipple procedure

   _____

10. Anesthesia for laparoscopically assisted vaginal hysterectomy

    _____

Chapter 10

HCPCS Level II

Developed by the Centers for Medicare and Medicaid Services (CMS), Level II HCPCS also is referred to as the National Codes. The National Codes were designed to report physician and nonphysician services such as drugs, chiropractic services, dental procedures, durable medical equipment, and other selected procedures.

Although the National Codes were developed for Medicare, they also are used by commercial payers. Coders should note that some Medicare carriers mandate the use of Level II codes rather than specific CPT codes. For example, there is a CPT code for removal of impacted cerumen (69210), but CMS will deny payment for this code. HCPCS Level II code G0268 should be reported for the earwax removal procedure. Bulletins from Medicare carriers announce such mandates. Some Medicaid programs and private insurance carriers also may accept or mandate the use of National Codes.

As mentioned in chapter 1 of this workbook, a listing of these codes may be purchased from the U.S. Government Printing Office or any local Medicare carrier (which provides them as a computer-generated list). In addition, several publishing firms offer the National Codes in book format, which can offer better indexing and cross-references. Finally, a file containing the most current versions of the HCPCS Level II codes can be found under the Utilities/Miscellaneous heading at the following CMS Web site page: cms.gov/providers/pufdownload/. The HCPCS Level II codes included in this publication are current as of October 1, 2005.

Structure of the HCPCS Level II Codes

Level II HCPCS consists of five-digit alphanumeric codes beginning with an alphabetic character (A through V, excluding S) followed by four numbers.

Example:

	A4625	Tracheostomy care kit for new tracheostomy
	D5730	Reline complete maxillary denture (chairside)
	J2360	Injection, orphenadrine, citrate, up to 60 mg
	V2500	Contact lens, PMMA, spherical, per lens

The National Codes are divided into the following sections:

Codes	Section
A codes	Transportation Services, Including Ambulance
	Medical and Surgical Supplies
	Administrative, Miscellaneous, and Investigational
B codes	Enteral and Parenteral Therapy

C codes	Temporary Codes for Use with Outpatient PPS
D codes	Dental Procedures
E codes	Durable Medical Equipment (DME)
G codes	Procedures/Professional Services (Temporary)
H codes	Alcohol and Drug Abuse Treatment Services
J codes	Drugs Administered, Other Than Oral Method, Chemotherapy Drugs
K codes	Temporary (Assigned to Durable Medical Equipment Regional Carriers [DMERC])
L codes	Orthotic Procedures, Prosthetic Procedures
M codes	Medical Services
P codes	Pathology and Laboratory Services
Q codes	Miscellaneous Services (Temporary Codes)
R codes	Diagnostic Radiology Services
S codes	Temporary National Codes (Non-Medicare)
T codes	Established for State Medicaid Agencies
V codes	Vision Services, Hearing Services

General Guidelines for HCPCS Level II Coding

The HCPCS coding guidelines, like the CPT coding guidelines, establish a four-step coding process:

1. Never code directly from the index.

2. Search for main terms and any applicable subterms.

3. Note the reference codes as given in the index.

4. Verify the codes by reading the entire description.

Table of Drugs

The HCPCS National Codes describe drugs that have been administered with codes that begin with the capital letter J. J codes describe drugs using their generic names, amounts, and routes of administration. The following abbreviations are used to designate the route of administration:

IA	Intra-arterial
IT	Intrathecal
IV	Intravenous
IM	Intramuscular
SC	Subcutaneous
INH	Inhalant solution
INJ	Injection, not otherwise specified
VAR	Various routes
ORAL	Oral
OTH	Other routes

The abbreviation VAR is used for drugs that are commonly administered into cavities, joints, or tissues or as topical applications. OTH refers to other administration methods such as suppositories or catheter injections.

HCPCS Level II Modifiers

The modifiers used in HCPCS Level II were developed to serve the same purpose that modifiers serve in the CPT codebook. The assignment of a modifier may indicate that a service or procedure was modified in some way, but with no change to its basic definition. HCPCS modifiers can be used to indicate the following types of information:

- The service was supervised by an anesthesiologist.

- The service was performed by a healthcare professional other than a physician, such as a clinical psychologist, a nurse practitioner, or a physician assistant.

- The service was provided as part of a specific government program.

- The service was provided to a specific site of the body.

- Equipment was purchased or rented.

- Single or multiple patients were seen during nursing home visits.

In the coding of Medicare claims, HCPCS Level II modifiers may be used with the National Codes or with CPT Category I codes.

The HCPCS modifiers consist of one or two characters and are appended to the appropriate HCPCS Level II or CPT Category I codes. Some of the modifiers commonly used include:

AA	Anesthesia services personally furnished by the anesthesiologist
AD	Medical supervision by a physician: more than four concurrent anesthesia procedures
AH	Clinical psychologist
AJ	Clinical social worker
AM	Physician, team member service
AP	Determination of refractive state not performed in the course of diagnostic ophthalmologic examination
AS	Physician assistant, nurse practitioner, or clinical nurse specialist services for assistant at surgery
AT	Acute treatment (should be used when reporting services 98940, 98941, and 98942)
CC	Procedure code change (use –CC when the procedure code submitted was changed either for administrative reasons or because an incorrect code was initially filed)
GA	Waiver of liability statement on file
KP	First drug of a multiple-drug unit dose formulation
LR	Laboratory round trip
NU	New equipment
QS	Monitored anesthesia care service
TD	RN

The following modifiers are reported in field items 12 and 13 on CMS form 1491 (figure 10.1). They are used to identify ambulance place of origin and destination. The first modifier listed identifies the origin and the second, the destination.

D	Diagnostic or therapeutic site other than –P or –H when these are used as origin codes
E	Residential, domiciliary, custodial facility (other than an 1819 [SNF] facility)
G	Hospital-based dialysis facility (hospital or hospital related)
H	Hospital
I	Site of transfer (for example, airport or helicopter pad) between types of ambulance vehicles
J	Non-hospital-based dialysis facility
N	Skilled nursing facility (SNF) (1819 facility)
P	Physician's office (includes HMO nonhospital facility, clinic, and so on)
R	Residence
S	Scene of accident or acute event
X	(Destination code only) Intermediate stop at physician's office on the way to the hospital (includes HMO nonhospital facility, clinic, and so on)

Figure 10.1. CMS form 1491

REQUEST FOR MEDICARE PAYMENT – AMBULANCE
MEDICAL INSURANCE BENEFITS - SOCIAL SECURITY ACT
(SEE INSTRUCTIONS ON BACK - TYPE OR PRINT INFORMATION)

FORM APPROVED
OMB NO 0938-0042

PART 1 – PATIENT TO FILL IN ITEMS 1 THROUGH 6 ONLY

No Part B Medicare Benefits may be paid unless a completed application form has been received as required by existing law and regulations (20 C.F.R. 405-251).
NOTICE – Anyone who misrepresents or falsifies essential information requested by this form may upon conviction be subject to fine and imprisonment under Federal law.

COPY FROM YOUR OWN HEALTH INSURANCE CARD *(See Example on Back)*

1 Name of Patient (First Name, Middle Initial, Last Name)

2 Health Insurance Claim No.　　　☐ Male　　☐ Female

3 Patient's complete mailing address *(including Apt. No.)* City, State, ZIP code　　|　Telephone Number ( )

4 Was your illness or injury:

	Yes	No
a. Connected with your employment?		
b. Result of an auto accident?		
c. Result of other type accident?		

5 If any of your medical expenses will be or could be paid by another insurance organization or government agency, show below

Name and address of organization or agency　　|　Policy or Identification Number

Note: If you **Do Not** want information about this Medicare claim released to the above upon request, check (X) the following block ☐

6 I authorize any holder of medical or other information about me to release to the Social Security Administration and Centers for Medicare & Medicaid Services or its intermediaries or carriers any information needed for this or a related Medicare claim. I permit a copy of this authorization to be used in place of the original, and request payment of medical insurance benefits either to myself or to the party who accepts assignment below.

Signature of patient *(See instructions on reverse where patient is unable to sign)*　　|　Date signed
SIGN HERE ▶

PART II – AMBULANCE SUPPLIER TO FILL IN 7 THROUGH 25

7. Date of Service　☐ Emergency　☐ Admission　☐ Discharge　☐ Outpatient visit　|　8. Ordered By

9. Description of Illness or Injury *(Describe factors which made ambulance transportation necessary)*

10. Name of Treating Doctor　|　11. Address and Telephone Number of Doctor

12. Origin of Service　|　13. Destination of Service

14. Number of Miles　|　15. Cost per Mile　|　16. Mileage Charge

22. Describe special service *(no none leave blank)*　|　17. Base Rate

18. Spec. Serv. Chg. *(Desc. Item 22)*

23. Name and Address of Supplier *(Number and Street, City, State, ZIP Code)*　|　Supplier Code　|　19. Total Charges

20. Amount Paid

Telephone Number ( )　|　21. Any Unpaid Balance Due

24. Assignment of Patient's Bill　☐ I accept assignment *(See reverse)*　☐ I do not accept assignment

25. Signature of Supplier　|　Date Signed

CMS-1491 (SC) (1/89)

Department of Health and Human Services
Centers for Medicare & Medicaid Services

Exercise 10.1   Chapter 10 Review

Use the HCPCS Level II codebook to answer the following questions.

1. What is the code for a gel mattress?

   _____

2. What code would be assigned if the surgeon provided a surgical tray for a procedure?

   _____

3. If a patient was given a B_{12} injection in the office, what HCPCS code would be assigned for the actual substance?

   _____

4. What Level II code would indicate that the patient received an above-the-knee surgical stocking?

   _____

5. If a patient was given an IM injection of 400,000 units of penicillin G benzathine, what HCPCS code would be assigned for this drug?

   _____

Assign HCPCS Level I (CPT) code(s) and HCPCS Level II code(s) to the following procedures.

6. The physician implanted contraceptive capsules in a 23-year-old female patient.

   CPT code for procedure: _____

   HCPCS code for contraceptive supplies: _____

7. Patient was treated for a sprained ankle; strapping was applied, and the patient was given crutches (a pair of adjustable, underarm, wood with pads, tips, and handgrips).

   CPT code for procedure: _____

   HCPCS code for crutches:_____

In addition to HCPCS Level I (CPT) codes, assign HCPCS Level II modifiers for the following procedures, if applicable.

8. Patient is seen in the emergency department for a 1.5-cm laceration of the lower right eyelid. Physician performs a simple wound repair.

   _____

9. Avulsion of nail bed of left great toe and left second toe

   _____

10. Release of trigger finger, right ring finger

   _____

Chapter 10 Test

Write the appropriate answer.

1. Temporary crown for a fractured tooth

   _____

2. Injection of 40 mg of theophylline

   _____

3. 6-month-old patient requires a Benesch boot

   _____

4. Motorized wheelchair with detachable arms and elevating leg rests

   _____

5. Box of alcohol wipes

   _____

Chapter 11

Reimbursement in the Ambulatory Setting

The purpose of this chapter is to provide an overview of reimbursement systems in ambulatory care settings. Coding professionals must be aware of, and apply skills to, the reimbursement systems used by government payers and other health plans. Because these systems utilize codes as the basis for calculating payment amounts, complete and accurate coding is a key element in the financial performance of healthcare organizations. Thus, coding professionals must understand the coding guidelines currently in use and how to apply them to ensure that their facilities receive appropriate reimbursement for their services.

Although all the reimbursement systems use codes, the ways in which payments to healthcare facilities are determined can vary greatly. For example, guidelines for reimbursement for ambulatory services provided to Medicare patients changed with implementation of ambulatory payment classifications, which divide outpatient services into fixed-payment groups. On the other hand, ambulatory surgery centers receive reimbursement for their services at fixed prices determined by nine different payment groups. Fees for services provided to Medicare patients by physicians are determined by a fee schedule based on the resource-based relative value scale designed to provide a systematic and more equitable approach to compensation.

Managed care organizations often contract with physicians and facilities for a fee schedule that lists CPT codes with the corresponding amount of payment. When they participate in these plans, physicians and/or healthcare facilities agree that they will not expect or require more than this amount in compensation for the services provided to patients covered by the plan. Paying attention to reporting requirements for codes, as well as to rules on bundling of services, is essential for optimizing reimbursement in a managed care environment or within a government-mandated prospective payment system (PPS).

Reimbursement for Ambulatory Services Provided to Medicare Patients

Reimbursement for ambulatory services provided to Medicare patients changed significantly in 2000 with implementation of ambulatory payment classifications (APCs) in hospital settings.

Hospital Outpatient Prospective Payment System

In 2000, the Centers for Medicare and Medicaid Services (CMS) issued its final rule on an outpatient prospective payment system (OPPS). This payment system is based on groups of services called ambulatory payment classifications (APCs), which divide outpatient services into fixed-payment groups. Each APC may include multiple CPT/HCPCS codes but is clinically similar and requires comparable resources. National payment rates were established with an adjustment for geographical factors. Table 11.1 contains an excerpt from the list of ambulatory payment classes. Table 11.2 is an excerpt from the *Federal Register* that shows APCs 0001 through 0004 with the associated HCPCS codes, descriptions, status indicators, relative weights, and payments.

Case Study

Using APC 0004 from table 11.1 as a reference, follow this simulated case study. Assume a patient with Medicare insurance was seen in the outpatient surgery suite for a puncture aspiration of a cyst of the breast. CPT code 19000 was assigned for the procedure. Note that from the reference above, CPT code 19000 is assigned to APC 0004. According to table 11.1, the hospital will be reimbursed $104.72 for providing the services applicable to this procedure. The APC payment will include packaged items such as room charges, medical–surgical equipment, surgical dressings and supplies, and pharmaceuticals. The APC payment methodology is only applicable to the hospital services; the physician will be reimbursed under another method.

Now look at the status indicators in table 11.1. Every APC has a status indicator code. Code T for APC 0004 designates that the APC payment is subject to payment reduction when multiple procedures are performed during the same visit. In the above case study, there were no additional procedures so the status indicator does not affect payment. A complete list of status indicators is found in table 11.2.

Table 11.1. APCs 0001–0004

APC #	HCPCS	APC Title	HCPCS Short Description	Status Indicator	Relative Weight	Payment Rate
0001		Level I photochemotherapy		S	0.4213	$25.00
0001	96900		Ultraviolet light therapy			
0001	96910		Photochemotherapy with UV-B			
0001	96912		Photochemotherapy with UV-A			
0002		Level I fine needle biopsy/aspiration		T	0.9559	$56.73
0002	10021		Fna without image			
0002	47399		Liver surgery procedure			
0003		Bone marrow biopsy/aspiration		T	2.6530	$157.44
0003	38220		Bone marrow aspiration			
0003	38221		Bone marrow biopsy			
0004		Level I needle biopsy/ aspiration except bone marrow		T	1.7646	$104.72
0004	19000		Drainage of breast lesion			
0004	19001		Drain breast lesion add-on			

Key to Status Indicators
S: Payment discount does not apply
T: Multiple-procedure payment discount applies

Table 11.2. APC status indicators

Indicator	Item/Code/Service	Status
A	Services furnished to a hospital outpatient that are paid under a fee schedule/payment system other than OPPS; examples: • Ambulance services • Clinical diagnostic laboratory services • Nonimplantable prosthetic and orthotic devices • EPO for ESRD patients • Physical, occupational, and speech therapy • Routine dialysis services for ESRD patients provided in a certified dialysis unit of a hospital • Diagnostic mammography • Screening mammography	Not paid under OPPS; paid by intermediaries under a fee schedule/payment system other than OPPS
B	Codes that are not recognized by OPPS when submitted on an Outpatient Hospital Part B bill type (12x, 13x, and 14x)	Not paid under OPPS; may be paid by intermediaries when submitted on a different bill type (e.g., 75x [CORF]), but not paid under OPPS. An alternate code that is recognized by OPPS when submitted on an Outpatient Hospital Part B bill type (12x, 13x, 14x) may be available.
C	Inpatient procedures	Not paid under OPPS; patient admitted; bill as inpatient
D	Discontinued codes	Not paid under OPPS
E	Items, codes, and services: • That are not covered by Medicare based on statutory exclusion • That are not covered by Medicare for reasons other than statutory exclusion • That are not recognized by Medicare, but for which an alternate code for the same item or service may be available • For which separate payment is not provided by Medicare	Not covered under OPPS
F	Corneal tissue acquisition; certain CRNA services and hepatitis B vaccines	Not paid under OPPS; paid at reasonable cost
G	Pass-through drugs, biologicals, and radiopharmaceutical agents	Paid under OPPS; separate APC payment that includes pass-through amount
H	Pass-through device category; brachytherapy sources paid at cost	Paid under OPPS; (a) separate cost-based pass-through payment; (b) separate cost-based non-pass-through payment
K	Non-pass-through drugs, biologicals, and radiopharmaceutical agents	Paid under OPPS; separate APC payment
L	Influenza vaccine; Pneumococcal pneumonia vaccine	Not paid under OPPS; paid at a reasonable cost; not subject to deductible or coinsurance
M	Items and services not billable to the fiscal intermediary	Not paid under OPPS.
N	Items and services package into APC rates	Paid under OPPS. However, payment is packaged into payment for other services, including outliers; therefore, there is no separate APC payment.
P	Partial hospitalization	Paid under OPPS; per diem APC payment
Q	Packaged services subject to separate payment under OPPS payment criteria	Paid under OPPS; separate APC payment, based on criteria. IF criteria not met, payment is packaged
S	Significant procedure, separately payable	Paid under OPPS; separate APC payment
T	Significant procedures, multiple reduction applies	Paid under OPPS; separate APC payment
V	Clinic or emergency department visit	Paid under OPPS; separate APC payment
Y	Nonimplantable durable medical equipment	Not paid under OPPS. All institutional providers other than home health agencies bill to DMERC.
X	Ancillary service	Paid under OPPS; separate APC payment

Some outpatient facility services are not paid under OPPS. Medicare has a variety of payment methods for a range of outpatient services. Every HCPCS code is assigned a status indicator, as shown in table 11.2. The indicator shows how each service is to be reimbursed. For example, ambulance services are reimbursed by the ambulance fee schedule.

Drug and Device Pass-through Payments

Under the APC system, additional reimbursement may be made for certain drugs and devices. Certain high-cost drugs are not packaged into the APC groups. Additional information can be found on the CMS Web site at cms.hhs.gov.

Reimbursement for Ambulatory Surgery Centers

An ambulatory surgery center (ASC) is a state-licensed supplier of surgical healthcare services. It is a separate entity from any other facility, such as a hospital. ASCs are reimbursed at fixed prices according to one of nine payment groups. Medicare maintains a list showing the appropriate CPT code for each procedure and the payment group to which each procedure is assigned. The ASC list and its payment methodology apply only to Medicare claims.

The procedures mentioned in the ASC list are classified on the basis of complexity and resource intensity. The fixed rate covers the cost of nursing services, supplies, equipment, and use of the facility. The physician's fee for performing the procedure is reported separately. More information about ASCs can be found at the CMS Web site.

Reimbursement for Ambulatory Services Provided to Non-Medicare Patients

Ambulatory services provided to non-Medicare patients may be reimbursed based on ambulatory payment groups (APGs). APGs are used by many third-party payers, including Blue Cross/Blue Shield plans and state Medicaid agencies. They use CPT codes to place procedures in specified groups with an assigned relative weight. Because APG system rules may vary by health plan, no general rules currently apply. Packaging and discounting depend on the plan or version of the APG grouper used.

Reimbursement for Physician Services Provided to Medicare Patients

In 1985, the Health Care Financing Administration (now the CMS) awarded a contract to W. C. Hsiao and his colleagues at the Harvard School of Public Health to develop a resource-based relative value scale (RBRVS) for application in a reimbursement system for physician services. The goals of the project were (1) to provide a systematic, rational approach to establishing physician payments for services provided to Medicare beneficiaries, (2) to establish a fair and equitable approach to compensating physicians, (3) to eliminate distortions in current fees, and (4) to enhance cost-effective medical care.

In September 1990, the *Federal Register* published the initial RBRVS values. With payment reforms implemented through the Omnibus Reconciliation Acts of 1989 and 1990, the RBRVS fee schedule was phased in over a five-year period. RBRVS was implemented on January 1, 1992, along with the newly developed E/M services codes in the CPT codebook. Before this time, physicians were paid for Medicare claims on the basis of customary, prevailing, and reasonable charges.

The standard relative values per procedure include the following elements:

- *Physician work:* Technical skill, physical and mental effort; level of risk; and related stress

- *Practice expense:* The cost of supplies and equipment, wages for employees, and other overhead expenses, such as rent and utilities (there are currently values for facility and nonfacility physician practice expense in the RBRVS system; services rendered at a facility have a lower RVU associated with them than nonfacility or office-based services)

- *Malpractice expense:* The average cost of malpractice insurance

For determining payment, the geographic practice cost index value considers similar factors:

- *Physician work:* Percentage of difference between the physician's work effort in a geographic area and the national average for the work effort

- *Practice expense:* Relative cost of the mix of goods and services in a geographic area

- *Malpractice expense:* Relative cost of malpractice insurance in a geographic area

The following formula is used to determine the RBRVS for a specific CPT code:

$$(RVUw \times GPCIw) + (RVUpe \times GPCIpe) + (RVUm \times GPCIm) = RBRVS$$
$$\text{Total RBRVs} \times CF = fee$$

In the preceding equation, RVU stands for the relative value of the procedure; w stands for physician work; GPCI stands for geographic practice cost index value; pe stands for practice expense; m stands for malpractice expense; and CF stands for conversion factor (a variable).

The RVUs for CPT codes are updated every year, as reported in the *Federal Register*. Payment files can be located on the CMS Web site: cms.hhs.gov/physicians. For example, the RVU for CPT code 19000 in 2005 was calculated using 0.84 for the physician's work, 1.98 for the physician's practice expense, and 0.08 for the physician's malpractice expense.

Then, assuming a simulated geographic practice expense of 0.938 (Ohio), a malpractice expense of 0.976), and work of 1.00 and a conversion factor of \$37.90, one can calculate the payment for this procedure as follows:

$$(0.84 \times 1.00) + (1.98 \times 0.938) + (0.08 \times 0.976) \times \$37.90 = \$105.28$$
$$(RVUw \times GPCIw) + (RVUpe \times GPCIpe) + (RVUm \times GPCIm) = RBRVS = \text{Total RBRVs} \times CF = fee$$

You may recall in an earlier case study that the APC payment rate for the hospital (for the same procedure) was calculated as \$104.72.

Medicare Outpatient Code Editor

CMS carefully evaluates the procedural and diagnostic data submitted with ambulatory claims. The agency requires Medicare carriers and fiscal intermediaries (FIs) (organizations that process Medicare claims under contracts with CMS) to use a tool known as the Medicare Outpatient Code Editor (OCE). The goal is to weed out incomplete or incorrect claims. With

CMS's emphasis on detecting potential cases of fraud and abuse, coding professionals are expected to exhibit a high degree of competency in CPT coding. CMS also is particularly interested in the correct application of coding guidelines.

Since implementation of the Medicare OPPS, the functionality of the OCE has been greatly expanded. The OCE performs four basic functions:

- Editing the data on the claim for accuracy

- Specifying the action the FI should take when specific edits occur

- Assigning APCs to the claim (for hospital outpatient services)

- Determining payment-related conditions that require direct reference to HCPCS codes or modifiers

Routine edits for age and sex inconsistencies are performed on all claim forms. In addition to editing HCPCS codes, the hospital billing form (UB-92) is checked for revenue codes, modifier use, and service units. All claims are subject to National Correct Coding Initiative (NCCI) edits. The NCCI edits identify combinations of procedures that are mutually exclusive. If an NCCI edit occurs, payment for the component code is denied. When an OCE edit occurs, the fiscal intermediary may take one of six different actions:

- *Claim rejection:* When a claim is rejected, the provider may correct and resubmit the claim, but it cannot appeal the FI's decision.

- *Claim denial:* The provider cannot resubmit the claim, but it may appeal the FI's decision.

- *Claim returned to provider (RTP):* The provider may correct and resubmit the claim.

- *Claim suspension:* Payment is delayed for FI determination; the FI may need additional information before it can make a decision.

- *Line item rejection:* The claim is paid, but one of the line items is rejected; the provider may correct and resubmit the claim, but the FI's decision cannot be appealed.

- *Line item denial:* The claim is paid, but some line items are denied; the provider cannot resubmit the claim, but the FI's decision can be appealed.

Reimbursement and record-processing efficiency are seriously compromised when incomplete or error-ridden claims are returned to the provider for correction and resubmission. Most insurance carriers accept only "clean claims," that is, claims that have passed OCE scrutiny.

Quality Controls

Every healthcare facility, clinic, hospital, physician practice, and ambulatory service should implement quality controls to limit coding and claim errors so as to ensure that no fraudulent or abusive coding practices occur. ICD-9-CM and CPT codebooks must be updated annually to ensure that the most current and complete codes are available for reporting purposes. Coding professionals should receive routine training to promote skill development and increase knowledge of new payment guidelines and rules. A regular coding review is a key element in any Medicare compliance program.

Updated CPT codebooks are available late in the year (usually November or December), and the updated codes go into effect sometime after January 1. The actual implementation dates vary among third-party payers. The updated ICD-9-CM codebooks are available in late summer or early fall, and changes take effect on October 1 every year.

Exercise 11.1   Chapter 11 Review

Review the following scenarios and the codes suggested for reporting the services on the CMS-1500 billing form. Determine whether the CPT codes are correct or incorrect, and circle your answer. For those codes that are incorrect, identify the coding error. The ICD-9-CM codes are provided for reference only.

1. The patient was seen in the emergency department for facial lacerations. Simple repairs were performed on a 3.0-cm laceration on the forehead, a 2.8-cm laceration of the left upper eyelid, and a 1.0-cm laceration of the right upper eyelid.

    Correct   Incorrect

    Comments: _____

    21. DIAGNOSIS OR NATURE OF ILLNESS OR INJURY, (RELATE ITEMS 1,2,3 OR 4 TO ITEM 24E BY LINE)

    1. 873.42   3.

    2. 870.0   4.

24.	DATE(S) OF SERVICE From MM DD YY	To MM DD YY	B Place of Service	C Type of Service	D PROCEDURES, SERVICES, OR SUPPLIES (Explain Unusual Circumstances) CPT/HCPCS	MODIFIER	E DIAGNOSIS CODE
1	01-19				12013		1
2	01-19				12013	LT	2
3	01-19				12011	RT	2
4							
5							
6							

2. The patient was seen in the dermatologist's office, where seven skin tags were removed.

    Correct   Incorrect

    Comments: _____

    21. DIAGNOSIS OR NATURE OF ILLNESS OR INJURY, (RELATE ITEMS 1,2,3 OR 4 TO ITEM 24E BY LINE)

    1. 701.9   3.

    2.   4.

24.	DATE(S) OF SERVICE From MM DD YY	To MM DD YY	B Place of Service	C Type of Service	D PROCEDURES, SERVICES, OR SUPPLIES (Explain Unusual Circumstances) CPT/HCPCS	MODIFIER	E DIAGNOSIS CODE
1	01-19				17000		1
2	01-19				17003		1
3							
4							
5							
6							

(Continued on next page)

Exercise 11.1 (Continued)

3. The patient underwent a diagnostic colonoscopy to determine the etiology of bleeding. Using the snare technique, the physician removed a benign polyp of the cecum.

   Correct   Incorrect

   Comments: _____

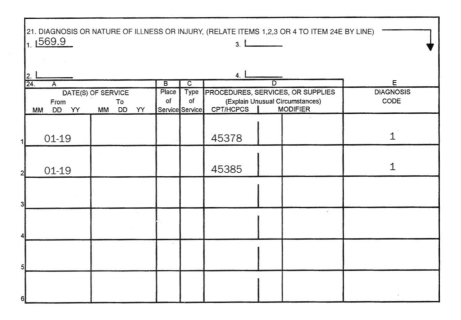

21. DIAGNOSIS OR NATURE OF ILLNESS OR INJURY, (RELATE ITEMS 1,2,3 OR 4 TO ITEM 24E BY LINE)					
1. 569.9			3.		
2.			4.		

24. A DATE(S) OF SERVICE		B Place of Service	C Type of Service	D PROCEDURES, SERVICES, OR SUPPLIES (Explain Unusual Circumstances)	E DIAGNOSIS CODE
From MM DD YY	To MM DD YY			CPT/HCPCS | MODIFIER	
1 01-19				45378	1
2 01-19				45385	1
3					
4					
5					
6					

4. The patient's chief complaint was dysuria. The physician performed a cystourethroscopy, ureteroscopy, and fulguration of ureteral polyp.

   Correct   Incorrect

   Comments: _____

21. DIAGNOSIS OR NATURE OF ILLNESS OR INJURY, (RELATE ITEMS 1,2,3 OR 4 TO ITEM 24E BY LINE)					
1. 893.89			3.		
2.			4.		

24. A DATE(S) OF SERVICE		B Place of Service	C Type of Service	D PROCEDURES, SERVICES, OR SUPPLIES (Explain Unusual Circumstances)	E DIAGNOSIS CODE
From MM DD YY	To MM DD YY			CPT/HCPCS | MODIFIER	
1 01-19				52214	1
2					
3					
4					
5					
6					

Exercise 11.1   (Continued)

5. A gynecologist performed a total abdominal hysterectomy with bilateral salpingo-oophorectomy. The pathological diagnosis was submucous leiomyoma of the uterus.

Correct   Incorrect

Comments: _____

21. DIAGNOSIS OR NATURE OF ILLNESS OR INJURY, (RELATE ITEMS 1,2,3 OR 4 TO ITEM 24E BY LINE)					
1. 218.0			3.		
2.			4.		

24. A DATE(S) OF SERVICE From / To		B Place of Service	C Type of Service	D PROCEDURES, SERVICES, OR SUPPLIES CPT/HCPCS | MODIFIER	E DIAGNOSIS CODE
1	01-19			58150	1
2	01-19			58720	1
3					
4					
5					
6					

6. A lab performed a hepatic function test, including albumin, total bilirubin, direct bilirubin, Alkaline phosphatase, and SGOT for a patient with jaundice.

Correct   Incorrect

Comments: _____

21. DIAGNOSIS OR NATURE OF ILLNESS OR INJURY, (RELATE ITEMS 1,2,3 OR 4 TO ITEM 24E BY LINE)					
1. 782.4			3.		
2.			4.		

24. A DATE(S) OF SERVICE From / To		B Place of Service	C Type of Service	D PROCEDURES, SERVICES, OR SUPPLIES CPT/HCPCS | MODIFIER	E DIAGNOSIS CODE
1	01-19			80076	1
2					
3					
4					
5					
6					

(Continued on next page)

Exercise 11.1 (Continued)

7. A gynecologist performed a hysteroscopy with biopsy of endometrium and dilatation and curettage.

Correct   Incorrect

Comments: _____

21. DIAGNOSIS OR NATURE OF ILLNESS OR INJURY, (RELATE ITEMS 1,2,3 OR 4 TO ITEM 24E BY LINE)					
1. 626.8			3.		
2.			4.		

24. A DATE(S) OF SERVICE From MM DD YY	To MM DD YY	B Place of Service	C Type of Service	D PROCEDURES, SERVICES, OR SUPPLIES (Explain Unusual Circumstances) CPT/HCPCS | MODIFIER	E DIAGNOSIS CODE
1 01-09				58558	1
2 01-09				58120	1
3					
4					
5					
6					

8. A physician performed an excision of breast mass.

Correct   Incorrect

Comments: _____

21. DIAGNOSIS OR NATURE OF ILLNESS OR INJURY, (RELATE ITEMS 1,2,3 OR 4 TO ITEM 24E BY LINE)					
1. 611.72			3.		
2.			4.		

24. A DATE(S) OF SERVICE From MM DD YY	To MM DD YY	B Place of Service	C Type of Service	D PROCEDURES, SERVICES, OR SUPPLIES (Explain Unusual Circumstances) CPT/HCPCS | MODIFIER	E DIAGNOSIS CODE
1 01-09				19120	1
2					
3					
4					
5					
6					

Exercise 11.1   (Continued)

9. A surgeon reported that he removed a 1.0-cm lesion of the chin with 0.5-cm margins around the diameter. Pathology report revealed basal cell carcinoma.

    Correct   Incorrect

    Comments: _____

21. DIAGNOSIS OR NATURE OF ILLNESS OR INJURY, (RELATE ITEMS 1,2,3 OR 4 TO ITEM 24E BY LINE)
1. 173.3   3.
2.   4.

24. A DATE(S) OF SERVICE						B Place of Service	C Type of Service	D PROCEDURES, SERVICES, OR SUPPLIES (Explain Unusual Circumstances)		E DIAGNOSIS CODE
From MM DD YY			To MM DD YY					CPT/HCPCS	MODIFIER	
1	01-09							11442		1
2										
3										
4										
5										
6										

10. A surgeon performed a flexible bronchoscopy with cell washings and brushings for a patient with acute bronchitis.

    Correct   Incorrect

    Comments: _____

1. 466.0   3.
2.   4.

24. A DATE(S) OF SERVICE						B Place of Service	C Type of Service	D PROCEDURES, SERVICES, OR SUPPLIES (Explain Unusual Circumstances)		E DIAGNOSIS CODE
From MM DD YY			To MM DD YY					CPT/HCPCS	MODIFIER	
1	01-09							31622		1
2	01-09							31623		1
3										
4										
5										
6										

(Continued on next page)

Chapter 11 Test

Choose or write the appropriate answer.

1. A patient with Medicare insurance presents in a local hospital's outpatient surgery center for an inguinal hernia repair. What method of reimbursement would apply to this case?

   _____

2. What three key elements comprise RBRVS?

   _____

3. Which of the following services will not be reimbursed under OPPS?
   a. Excision of breast mass
   b. Radiopharmaceutical agents
   c. Ambulance services
   d. Brachytherapy

4. Referencing Table 11.1 from the workbook, what is the payment rate for CPT code 38221?

   _____

5. Referencing Table 11.2 from the workbook, what APC status indicator would be assigned for a screening mammogram?

   _____

Appendix A

References, Bibliography, and Web Resources

References and Bibliography

American Health Information Management Association. 1990–2005. Coding Notes and Clinical Notes. *Journal of American Health Information Management Association.* Chicago: AHIMA.

American Medical Association. 2006. *Current Procedural Terminology 2006.* Chicago: AMA.

American Medical Association. 1989–2005. *CPT Assistant.* Chicago: AMA.

Fordney, M.T. 2005. *Insurance Handbook for the Medical Office*, 6th ed. Philadelphia: W.B. Saunders.

Ingenix. 2005. *HCPCS Level II Expert.* Salt Lake City: Ingenix.

Ingenix. 2006. *Coder's Desk Reference for Procedures.* Salt Lake City: Ingenix.

Ingenix. 2005. *Understanding Modifiers.* Salt Lake City: Ingenix.

Rakel, R. 2005. *Saunders Manual of Medical Practice*, 2nd ed. Philadelphia: W.B. Saunders.

Rogers, V.L. 2004. *Applying Inpatient Coding Skills under Prospective Payment.* Chicago: American Health Information Management Association.

Schraffenberger, L.A. 2006. *Basic ICD-9-CM Coding.* Chicago: AHIMA.

Society of Cardiovascular and Interventional Radiology, et al. 2005. *Interventional Radiology Coding User's Guide*, 5th ed. Fairfax, VA: Society of Cardiovascular and Interventional Radiology, American College of Radiology, Radiology Business Management Association, American Health Radiology Administrators.

Web Resources

Aetna IntelliHealth: intelihealth.com
Aetna IntelliHealth is a partnership between Harvard Medical School and Aetna. It includes search tests/procedures, a medical dictionary, lists of drugs, and so on. It also is simple to navigate.

American Academy of Dermatology: aad.org
Click on "Public Resources" for links to sites about diseases of skin.

American Academy of Facial Plastic and Reconstructive Surgery: aafprs.org
Click on "Procedures" for links. A glossary and a page featuring common surgeries are included.

American Academy of Family Physicians: aafp.org
This Web resource includes articles on documentation guidelines.

American Academy of Orthopaedic Surgeons: aaos.org

Click on "Patient Information" to find fact sheets on many diseases and procedures.

American College of Cardiology: acc.org

Click on "Payer Advocacy" for information about CPT.

American College of Gastroenterology: acg.gi.org

Click on "Patient Information" for links of interest.

American College of Obstetricians and Gynecologists: acog.org

This site has information on patient education and provides links to coding/nomenclature.

American Gastroenterological Association: gastro.org

Click on "Patient Center" and "Procedures" for explanation of common gastroenterological procedures.

American Health Information Management Association: ahima.org

This site provides coding products and an educational forum for coders called Communities of Practice (members only).

American Medical Association: ama-assn.org

This site contains information about coding products, *CPT Assistant*, and CPT updates and errata.

American Society of Plastic Surgery: plasticsurgery.org

Click on "Procedures."

Anatomy: innerbody.com

This site contains diagrams and definitions.

Anatomy: medtropolis.com

This site uses audio and visual effects to explain basic human anatomy. Visit the "Virtual Body."

Cancer: cancer.gov

Click on "Cancer Information" and then choose from the various types.

Cardiology: hgcardio.com

This site offers diagrams and descriptions of cardiac procedures.

Centers for Medicare and Medicaid Services (CMS):   cms.hhs.gov

This site provides information about coding and reimbursement for Medicare and Medicaid services. Go to cms.hhs.gov/paymentsystem/ for information about Medicare payment systems and coding files. Go to cms.hhs.gov/providers/hopps/ for information about hospital outpatient prospective payment system. Go to cms.gov/providers/pufdownload/ to download information pertaining to the Medicare payment systems. Go to cms.hhs.gov/medlearn/ for reference guides and training modules. Go to cms.hhs.gov/manuals/ to find Medicare transmittals and program memos. Go to cms.hhs.gov/medlearn/emdoc.asp for information on the 1995 and 1997 E/M documentation guidelines. Go to cms.hhs.gov/medlearn/icd9code.asp for coding education resources and information on new and revised ICD-9-CM codes.

Discovery Health: discoveryhealth.com

This site has numerous links and is very searchable.

Encyclopedia of Medicine: findarticles.com

Clink on "Health" for a variety of links to health information articles.

Health Central: healthcentral.com

Health Central is a consumer-friendly site.

Healthfinder: healthfinder.gov

This consumer-friendly site offers a free guide for health and human services.

Heart Center: heartcenteronline.com

Click on "Patients" on this consumer-friendly site for quizzes and descriptions of cardiac procedures.

How Stuff Works: howstuffworks.com

Click on "Health Stuff."

Kidney: thekidney.com

This is an education site with links.

Knee: knee1.com

This site provides descriptions of various knee surgeries.

MayoClinic: mayoclinic.com

This site provides consumer-oriented information about illnesses.

MedLearn: medlearn.com

MedLearn sells coding products, including a guide for interventional radiology coding.

MEDLINEplus: medlineplus.gov

Operated by the U.S. National Library of Medicine, MEDLINEplus includes encyclopedic background on all diseases, definitions of medical terms, and referrals to other organizations that deal with specific illnesses.

National Library of Medicine: anatquest.nlm.nih.gov/Anatline/index.html

This site provides an anatomy reference and a query database.

Society of Interventional Radiology: sirweb.org

The society sells coding products (for example, *Interventional Radiology Coding Users' Guide*).

Stanford Health Library: healthlibrary.stanford.edu/resources/internet/bodysys.html

This site offers links providing information on diseases, disorders, and treatment.

Surgical Procedures: mic.ki.se/Diseases/e4.html

This site offers numerous links to surgical procedures.

WebMD: webmd.com

WebMD provides basic facts on any condition. The site guides the user from general topics to more specific facts.

Appendix B

Evaluation and Management Documentation Guidelines

The following information was excerpted from the 1997 document developed by CMS and the AMA. A complete copy of this document and up-to-date information on the status of revised guidelines can be found on the CMS Web site at www.cms.gov/medlearn/emdoc.asp.

To qualify for a given level of multisystem examination, the following content and documentation requirements should be met:

- A problem-focused examination should include performance and documentation of one to five elements identified by a bullet (•) in one or more organ system(s) or body area(s).

- An expanded problem-focused examination should include performance and documentation of at least six elements identified by a bullet (•) in one or more organ system(s) or body area(s).

- A detailed examination should include at least six organ systems or body areas. For each system/area selected, performance and documentation of at least two elements identified by a bullet (•) are expected. Alternatively, a detailed examination may include performance and documentation of at least twelve elements identified by a bullet (•) in two or more organ systems or body areas.

- A comprehensive examination should include at least nine organ systems or body areas. For each system/area selected, all elements of the examination identified by a bullet (•) should be performed, unless specific directions limit the content of the examination. For each area/ system, documentation of at least two elements identified by a bullet is expected.

Examination Documentation Guidelines

- Specific abnormal and relevant negative findings of the examination of the affected or symptomatic body area(s) or organ system(s) should be documented. A notation of "abnormal" without elaboration is insufficient.

- Abnormal or unexpected findings of the examination of any asymptomatic body area(s) or organ system(s) should be described.

- A brief statement or notation indicating "negative" or "normal" is sufficient to document normal findings related to unaffected area(s) or asymptomatic organ system(s).

Content and Documentation Requirements

General Multisystem Examination

System/Body Area	Elements of Examination
Constitutional	• Measurement of *any three of the following seven vital signs:* (1) sitting or standing blood pressure; (2) supine blood pressure; (3) pulse rate and regularity; (4) respiration; (5) temperature; (6) height; and (7) weight (may be measured and recorded by ancillary staff) • General appearance of patient (e.g., development, nutrition, body habitus, deformities, attention to grooming)
Eyes	• Inspection of conjunctivae and lids • Examination of pupils and irises (e.g., reaction to light and accommodation, size, and symmetry) • Ophthalmoscopic examination of optic discs (e.g., size, C/D ratio, appearance) and posterior segments (e.g., vessel changes, exudates, hemorrhages)
Ears, Nose, Mouth, and Throat	• External inspection of ears and nose (e.g., overall appearance, scars, lesions, masses) • Otoscopic examination of external auditory canals and tympanic membranes • Assessment of hearing (e.g., whispered voice, finger rub, tuning fork) • Inspection of nasal mucosa, septum, and turbinates • Inspection of lips, teeth, and gums • Examination of oropharynx: oral mucosa, salivary glands, hard and soft palates, tongue, tonsils, and posterior pharynx
Neck	• Examination of neck (e.g., masses, overall appearance, symmetry, tracheal position, crepitus) • Examination of thyroid (e.g., enlargement, tenderness, mass)
Respiratory	• Assessment of respiratory effort (e.g., intercostal retractions, use of accessory muscles, diaphragmatic movement) • Percussion of chest (e.g., dullness, flatness, hyperresonance) • Palpation of chest (e.g., tactile fremitus) • Auscultation of lungs (e.g., breath sounds, adventitious sounds, rubs)
Cardiovascular	• Palpation of heart (e.g., location, size, thrills) • Auscultation of heart with notation of abnormal sounds and murmurs Examination of: • Carotid arteries (e.g., pulse amplitude, bruits) • Abdominal aorta (e.g., size, bruits) • Femoral arteries (e.g., pulse amplitude, bruits) • Pedal pulses (e.g., pulse amplitude) • Extremities for edema and/or varicosities
Chest (Breasts)	• Inspection of breasts (e.g., symmetry, nipple discharge) • Palpation of breasts and axillae (e.g., masses or lumps, tenderness)
Gastrointestinal (Abdomen)	• Examination of abdomen with notation of presence of masses or tenderness • Examination of liver and spleen • Examination for presence or absence of hernia • Examination of anus, perineum, and rectum, including sphincter tone, presence of hemorrhoids, rectal masses • Obtain stool sample for occult blood test when indicated

System/Body Area	Elements of Examination
Genitourinary	*Male:* • Examination of the scrotal contents (e.g., hydrocele, spermatocele, tenderness of cord, testicular mass) • Examination of the penis • Digital rectal examination of prostate gland (e.g., size, symmetry, nodularity, tenderness) *Female:* Pelvic examination (with or without specimen collection for smears and cultures), including: • Examination of the external genitalia (e.g., general appearance, hair distribution, lesions) and vagina (e.g., general appearance, estrogen effect, discharge, lesions, pelvic support, cystocele, rectocele) • Examination of urethra (e.g., masses, tenderness, scarring) • Examination of bladder (e.g., fullness, masses, tenderness) • Cervix (e.g., general appearance, lesions, discharge) • Uterus (e.g., size, contour, position, mobility, tenderness, consistency, descent, or support) • Adnexa/parametria (e.g., masses, tenderness, organomegaly, nodularity)
Lymphatic	Palpitation of lymph nodes in two or more areas: • Neck • Axillae • Groin • Other
Musculoskeletal	• Examination of gait and station • Inspection and/or palpation of digits and nails (e.g., clubbing, cyanosis, inflammatory conditions, petechiae, ischemia, infections, nodes) Examination of joints, bones, and muscles of **one or more of the following six areas:** (1) head and neck; (2) spine, ribs, and pelvis; (3) right upper extremity; (4) left upper extremity; (5) right lower extremity; and (6) left lower extremity. The examination of a given area includes: • Inspection and/or palpation with notation of presence of any misalignment, asymmetry, crepitation, defects, tenderness, masses, or effusions • Assessment of range of motion with notation of any pain, crepitation, or contracture • Assessment of stability with notation of any dislocation (luxation), subluxation, or laxity • Assessment of muscle strength and tone (e.g., flaccid, cog wheel, spastic) with notation of any atrophy or abnormal movements
Skin	• Inspection of skin and subcutaneous tissue (e.g., rashes, lesions, ulcers) • Palpation of skin and subcutaneous tissue (e.g., induration, subcutaneous nodules, tightening)
Neurologic	• Test cranial nerves with notation of any deficits • Examination of deep tendon reflexes with notation of pathological reflexes (e.g., Babinski) • Examination of sensation (e.g., touch, pin, vibration, proprioception)
Psychiatric	• Description of patient's judgment and insight Brief assessment of mental status, including: • Orientation to time, place, and person • Recent and remote memory • Mood and affect (e.g., depression, anxiety, agitation)

(Continued on next page)

Content and Documentation Requirements

Level of Exam	Perform and Document:
Problem focused	**One to five** elements identified by a bullet
Expanded problem focused	**At least six** elements identified by a bullet
Detailed	**At least two** elements identified by a bullet **from each of six areas/systems** *or* **at least twelve** elements identified by a bullet **in two or more areas/systems**
Comprehensive	Perform **all elements** identified by a bullet in **at least nine** organ systems or body areas and document **at least two** elements identified by a bullet **from each of nine areas/systems**

Appendix C

Additional Practice Exercises

The following surgical cases were performed in an ambulatory setting of Central Hospital. Determine the appropriate CPT code(s) for each case so that the hospital can receive the correct reimbursement. It is important to practice using the CPT index and to note how, in many instances, the codes may be found using more than one index entry. The appropriate modifiers should be assigned, when applicable, and the index entry(s) used to locate the code(s) should be noted.

If you wish to practice assigning codes by body system, the following reference will help.

Practice Exercises Indexed by Surgical Section

Integumentary System
Case #17
Case #25
Case #26
Case #27
Case #33
Case #39
Case #43
Case #50
Case #54
Case #57

Musculoskeletal System
Case #4
Case #10
Case #12
Case #20
Case #42
Case #44
Case #45
Case #47
Case #60

Respiratory System
Case #6
Case #13 (also Digestive System)
Case #18
Case #41
Case #55

Cardiovascular System
Case #15
Case #31
Case #48
Case #52

Hemic and Lymphatic Systems
Case #38

Digestive System
Case #1
Case #3
Case #11
Case #13 (also Respiratory System)
Case #14
Case #19
Case #21
Case #22
Case #23
Case #24
Case #30
Case #32
Case #53
Case #56

Urinary System
Case #2
Case #9
Case #51
Case #59

Male/Female Genital System
Case #7
Case #8
Case #16
Case #28
Case #29
Case #36

Nervous System
Case #35
Case #37
Case #58

Eye and Ocular Adnexa
Case #5
Case #34
Case #40
Case #46
Case #49

Surgical Case #1

Operative Report

Procedure: Tonsillectomy *42820-42826*

Diagnosis: Recurrent tonsillitis

Indications: This 10-year-old patient was found to have recurrent tonsillitis, and a tonsillectomy was planned.

Technique: The patient was placed in the supine position, and general endotracheal anesthesia was begun. The nasopharynx was inspected, revealing only a very small amount of adenoid, which was not removed. The tonsils were noted to be very large and obstructive, and were removed by dissection and snare technique. The bleeders were electrocoagulated. The inferior cuff was suture ligated with 2-0 plain catgut. The patient tolerated the procedure well and was brought to the recovery room in satisfactory condition.

Assign appropriate CPT code(s) for the preceding procedures and indicate the index entries that were used to identify the codes. Assign only CPT codes (no E/M codes) and append any applicable modifiers.

Code(s): *42825*

Index entries:

Tonsillectomy

Surgical Case #2

Operative Report

Procedure: Extracorporeal shock wave lithotripsy of right kidney stone *50590, 52353*

Diagnosis: Right kidney stone

Anesthesia: IV sedation

Technique: Under IV sedation, the patient was placed in the supine position. The stone in the upper right kidney was positioned at F2. The extracorporeal lithotripsy was started at 19 KV, which subsequently was increased to a maximum of 26 KV at 1,600 shocks. The stone was revisualized, and repositioning was done considering the transverse colon passing right anterior to the stone. Because the stone appeared to be in the same place after the repositioning, shocks were delivered. Apparent adequate fragmentation was obtained after a total of 2,400 shocks had been administered. The patient tolerated the procedure quite well.

Assign appropriate CPT code(s) for the preceding procedures and indicate the index entries that were used to identify the codes. Assign only CPT codes (no E/M codes) and append any applicable modifiers.

Code(s): *50590 - RT*

Index entries: *Lithotripsy, Kidney*

Surgical Case #3

Operative Report

Procedure: Esophagogastroduodenoscopy with biopsy   43239

Diagnosis: Gastritis and duodenitis

Technique: The patient was premedicated and brought to the endoscopy suite where his throat was anesthetized with Cetacaine spray. He then was placed in the left lateral position and given 2 mg Versed, IV.

An Olympus gastroscope was advanced into the esophagus, which was well visualized with no significant segmental spasms. Subsequently, the scope was advanced into the distal esophagus, which was essentially normal. Then the scope was advanced into the stomach, which showed evidence of erythema and gastritis. The pylorus was intubated and the duodenal bulb visualized. The duodenal bulb showed severe erythema, suggestive of duodenitis. Multiple biopsies were taken. The scope was withdrawn, and the patient tolerated the procedure well.

Assign appropriate CPT code(s) for the preceding procedures and indicate the index entries that were used to identify the codes. Assign only CPT codes (no E/M codes) and append any applicable modifiers.

Code(s):_____43239_____

Index entries:

_____Endoscopy, gastrointestinal, upper_____

_____

Surgical Case #4

Emergency Department Record

Chief Complaint:	Right shoulder dislocation
History of Present Illness:	The patient is a 53-year-old male who has dislocated his right shoulder three previous episodes. Today, he was kayaking and dislocated his shoulder while paddling.
Past Medical History:	Previous right shoulder dislocation
Medications:	Vitamins
Allergies:	Sulfa
Physical Examination:	Alert male in no acute distress
Right Upper Extremity:	He has obvious deformity with loss of the right shoulder prominence with a palpable anterior dislocation of the humeral head. He has good distal pulses with the remainder of his arm being nontender.
Emergency Department Course:	X-ray of his right shoulder shows an anterior dislocation.
Procedure:	Reduction of the shoulder dislocation. The patient was placed on a monitor with continuous pulse oximetry. He was given Demerol and Phenergan IV for pain control. In-line traction and reduction was accomplished after three attempts. Reduction films showed good position of the shoulder. He had good distal neurovascular status after reduction. He tolerated the procedure well.
Diagnosis:	Anterior dislocation, right shoulder
Disposition and Plan:	Sling and swathe for two to three days. Vicodin #30. Follow up with Dr. Smith in one to two days or call for an orthopedic referral. The patient states he has been avoiding any potential surgery at this point and would prefer to avoid it. I explained to him that he should follow up with Dr. Smith or an orthopedist. He should not use the shoulder in the next several days until reevaluation.

Assign appropriate CPT code(s) for the preceding procedures and indicate the index entries that were used to identify the codes. Assign only CPT codes (no E/M codes) and append any applicable modifiers.

Code(s):_____ 23655 ~ RT _____

Index entries:

_____ Dislocation Shoulder _____

_____

23650-23655

Surgical Case #5

Operative Report

Procedure: Extracapsular cataract extraction with intraocular lens implantation, right eye

Diagnosis: Cataract of the right eye

Technique: The patient was given a retrobulbar injection of 2.5 to 3.0 cc of a mixture of equal parts of 2% lidocaine with epinephrine and 0.75% Marcaine with Wydase. The area around the right eye was infiltrated with an additional 6 to 7 cc of this mixture in a modified Van Lint technique. A self-maintaining pressure device was applied to the eye, and a short time later, the patient was taken to the OR.

The patient was properly positioned on the operating table, and the area around the right eye was prepped and draped in the usual fashion. A self-retaining eyelid speculum was positioned and 4-0 silk suture passed through the tendon of the superior rectus muscle, thereby deviating the eye inferiorly. A 160° fornix-based conjunctival flap was created followed by a 150° corneoscleral groove with a #64 Beaver blade. Hemostasis was maintained throughout with gentle cautery. A 6-0 silk suture was introduced to cross this groove at the 12 o'clock position and looped out of the operative field. The anterior chamber was then entered superiorly temporally, and after injecting Occucoat, an anterior capsulotomy was performed without difficulty. The nucleus was easily brought forward into the anterior chamber. The corneoscleral section was opened with scissors to the left and the nucleus delivered with irrigation and gentle lens loop manipulation. Interrupted 10-0 nylon sutures were placed at both the nasal and lateral extent of the incision. A manual irrigating aspirating setup then was used to remove remaining cortical material from both the anterior and posterior chambers.

At this point, a modified C-loop posterior chamber lens was removed from its package and irrigated and inspected. It then was positioned into the inferior capsular bag without difficulty, and the superior haptic was placed behind the iris at the 12 o'clock location. The lens was rotated to a horizontal orientation in an attempt to better enhance capsular fixation. Miochol was used to constrict the pupil, and a peripheral iridectomy was performed in the superior nasal quadrant. In addition, three or four interrupted 10-0 nylon sutures were used to close the corneal scleral section. The silk sutures were removed, and the conjunctiva advanced back into its normal location and was secured with cautery burns at the 3 and 9 o'clock positions. Approximately 20 to 30 mg of both Gentamicin and Kenalog were injected into the inferior cul-de-sac in a subconjunctival and sub-Tenon fashion. After instillation of 2% Pilocarpine and Maxitrol ophthalmic solution, the eyelid speculum was removed and the eye dressed in a sterile fashion. The patient was discharged to the recovery room in good condition.

Assign appropriate CPT code(s) for the preceding procedures and indicate the index entries that were used to identify the codes. Assign only CPT codes (no E/M codes) and append any applicable modifiers.

Code(s):_____

Index entries:

_____

_____

Surgical Case #6

Operative Report

Procedure: Fiberoptic bronchoscopy

Diagnosis: Hemoptysis with easily bruisable mucosa and bronchiectasis

Technique: The patient was brought to the endoscopy suite and placed on a stretcher. Oxygen was given via nasal cannula at three liters per minute. Local anesthetic lidocaine was given to anesthetize the upper airway. Because the nostrils had considerable blockage secondary to trauma, the oral route was used for the bronchoscopy. Following placement of a bite block and application of Cetacaine to the posterior pharynx, the fiberoptic bronchoscope was placed without difficulty into the upper airway.

The epiglottis appeared somewhat prominent, but normal. In addition, the vocal cords appeared normal. The bronchoscope was passed easily through the cords into the trachea, which also appeared normal, although somewhat easily bruisable. The carina appeared normal. The right side was entered first. The right upper lobe and its subsegments were seen very clearly, and there appeared to be bronchiectasis. The 6-mm bronchoscope would go very easily into the subsegments. No mass lesions were seen. The bronchus intermedius, right middle lobe, lower lobe, and its subsegments also were entered; and, again, bronchiectasis was noted. There appeared to be no abnormal mucosal lesions and no abnormal secretions; however, the bronchial tree was easily bruisable. The bronchoscope then was withdrawn to the carina and the left side entered.

The left main bronchus, upper lobe, lower lobe, and its subsegments were seen. There appeared to be an extrinsic compression of a subsegment of the left lower lobe; however, no mucosal lesions were seen and this area appeared pulsatile, which suggested extrinsic compression from the descending aorta. Once again, easy bruisability of the mucosa was noted. The bronchoscope was withdrawn. There were no apparent complications.

Assign appropriate CPT code(s) for the preceding procedures and indicate the index entries that were used to identify the codes. Assign only CPT codes (no E/M codes) and append any applicable modifiers.

Code(s):_____

Index entries:

_____

_____

Surgical Case #7

Operative Report

Procedure:	Colposcopy
Diagnosis:	Class II Pap; cervicitis
History of Present Illness:	The patient is a 27-year-old female who had previously undergone a Pap smear showing class II Pap. She is admitted today for a colposcopy.
Technique:	The patient was placed in the lithotomy position. Her vagina and cervix were examined and a speculum inserted; dying was done with acetic acid followed by gram iodine and methylene blue. Cervical biopsies were performed at indicated areas, with Monsel solution applied for cautery. There were no complications, and the patient tolerated the procedure well.
Plan:	The patient is to call the office within one week for her biopsy report.

Assign appropriate CPT code(s) for the preceding procedures and indicate the index entries that were used to identify the codes. Assign only CPT codes (no E/M codes) and append any applicable modifiers.

Code(s):_____

Index entries:

_____

_____

Surgical Case #8

Operative Report

Procedure: Laparoscopic tubal ligation with application of Falope rings; dilatation and curettage (D&C) and removal of intrauterine device

Diagnosis: Multiparity, voluntary sterilization; removal of retained intrauterine device

Anesthesia: General

Technique: Placed in the supine lithotomy position, the patient was prepped and draped in the usual manner for a laparoscopic and D&C procedure. A D&C was performed to gain access to a deeply embedded IUD. This was curetted up and eventually removed with some difficulty. Both the IUD and the curetted endometrial tissue were submitted to pathology.

A two-puncture laparoscopy was performed in the usual manner of insufflation through a Veress needle inserted infraumbilically. Through a first puncture, a trocar insertion infra-umbilically was followed by the laparoscope and a second trocar insertion suprapubically in the midline was followed by, first, a probe and, then, a Falope ring applicator. Both tubes were ligated in their midsegment. On the right side, two rings were applied because of the round position of the Falope ring director. The left tube was ligated singly. The procedure was performed with no complications. After the operation, the trocar sites were closed with subcuticular sutures of 2-0 Vicryl and the patient was transferred to the recovery room in satisfactory condition.

Assign appropriate CPT code(s) for the preceding procedures and indicate the index entries that were used to identify the codes. Assign only CPT codes (no E/M codes) and append any applicable modifiers.

Code(s):_____

Index entries:

_____

_____

Surgical Case #9

Operative Report

Procedure: Transurethral resection of the prostate

Diagnosis: Bladder outlet obstruction; benign prostatic hypertrophy

Anesthesia: General

Technique: The patient was placed under general anesthesia and in the dorsolithotomy position. Two grams of Claforan parenterally were used. The Iglesias resectoscope was introduced through the obturator, and this was followed by the working element connected to the Olympus video camera. The obstructive prostatic tissue was appreciated mainly anteriorly and to the left lateral lobe. Resection was started at the bladder neck down to the level of the verumontanum and toward the capsule, as necessary, in all directions. Bleeders were fulgurated, with satisfactory patency with coagulation having been secured. Dissected tissues were removed using the Ellik evacuator. A size 24 three-way Foley catheter was retained with a 30-cc balloon inflation. Minimal blood loss was appreciated. The patient tolerated the procedure well and was transferred to the recovery room in stable condition.

Assign appropriate CPT code(s) for the preceding procedures and indicate the index entries that were used to identify the codes. Assign only CPT codes (no E/M codes) and append any applicable modifiers.

Code(s):_____

Index entries:

_____

_____

Surgical Case #10

Operative Report

Procedure: Open reduction of left zygomatic arch fracture

Diagnosis: Left zygomatic arch fracture

Anesthesia: General

Technique: The patient was placed on the operating table in the supine position and administered general endotracheal anesthesia. He was prepped and draped in the usual fashion. A small incision was made in the temporal scalp area and carried down through the superficial temporal fascia until the deep temporal fascia was identified. This was incised, and an elevator was passed beneath the deep fascia until it was below the zygomatic arch. The arch was reduced manually and elevated back into its anatomical position noted by palpation. The wound was irrigated, and hemostasis was obtained with cautery.

The superficial temporal fascia was reapproximated using interrupted 4-0 Monocryl sutures. The skin was closed with interrupted 4-0 nylon sutures, and a sterile dressing was applied along with a metal cup to protect the zygomatic arch. The patient was extubated and transferred to the recovery room in stable condition.

Assign appropriate CPT code(s) for the preceding procedures and indicate the index entries that were used to identify the codes. Assign only CPT codes (no E/M codes) and append any applicable modifiers.

Code(s):_____

Index entries:

_____

_____

Surgical Case #11

Operative Report

Procedure: Lateral lobe parotidectomy with facial nerve preservation

Diagnosis: Warthin's tumor of the parotid gland

Anesthesia: General

Findings: The patient has a long history of a right parotid mass that apparently has grown and fluctuated in size. An office examination revealed the nose, nasopharynx, larynx, and neck to be normal. She is status post thyroidectomy with a well-healed thyroidectomy incision. The parotid mass is overlying the mandible approximately 2 to 2.5 × 3 cm in diameter, and there is a possibility of another mass or lymphadenopathy in the lower aspect of the parotid gland. Facial nerve functions are normal.

Technique: Placed in the supine position, the patient was given general endotracheal anesthesia. Her neck was positioned, and the whole right side of her face and neck was prepped and draped in the usual manner.

The modified Blair type of incision was made in the preauricular area vertically, and then curved behind and below the earlobe and extended as a curved submandibular incision. The bleeders were electrocoagulated and the dissection deepened in the lower part to the platysma. The dissection and front of the tragus were done by both sharp and blunt dissection until the external ear canal cartilage was identified and palpated. The dissection was pushed through this and inferiorly, identifying the anterior border of the sternocleidomastoid muscle, mastoid process, and, subsequently, the main trunk of the facial nerve, which was preserved from trauma. The major lower and inferior subdivisions were followed, identifying the cervical, mandibular, and buccal branches, as well as the upper division.

The cystic mass was bluish in color. The lateral lobe of the parotid gland was removed and given for frozen section, and this was reported as a benign cystic mass. No lobe was encountered with suspicion of malignancy, and no other masses were in the deep lobe. Hemostasis was obtained by electrocautery on the superficial oozing points and ligature of the small vessels. The wound was washed, and afterward the main trunk and subdivisions of the facial nerve again were identified and verified to be intact.

The lower Hemovac drain was placed. The wound was closed with 3-0 chromic catgut interrupted involving both the subcutaneous tissue and the platysma muscle with continuous and interrupted mattress sutures using 5-0 silk. The wound was cleaned, Bacitracin ointment was applied, and a dry sterile occlusive dressing was placed over it. After the procedure was terminated, the patient was extubated and brought to the recovery room in good condition.

Assign appropriate CPT code(s) for the preceding procedures and indicate the index entries that were used to identify the codes. Assign only CPT codes (no E/M codes) and append any applicable modifiers.

Code(s):_____

Index entries:

_____

_____

Surgical Case #12

Operative Report

Procedure: Arthroscopic partial medial meniscectomy

Diagnosis: Torn left medial meniscus

Anesthesia: General

Technique: After induction with general anesthesia, a standard three-portal approach of the knee was evaluated. Mild synovitic changes were noted in the suprapatellar pouch. No chondromalacia changes were noted in all three compartments. The anterior cruciate ligament was intact, as was the lateral meniscus; and there were only slight synovitic changes in the anterior compartment. The anterior portion of the medial meniscus had a flap tear, which was debrided with an aggressive resector.

After all instruments were withdrawn, 4-0 nylon horizontal mattress stitches were used to close the wound and pressure dressings were applied. The patient was awakened and removed to the recovery room in good condition.

Assign appropriate CPT code(s) for the preceding procedures and indicate the index entries that were used to identify the codes. Assign only CPT codes (no E/M codes) and append any applicable modifiers.

Code(s):_____

Index entries:

_____

_____

Surgical Case #13

Operative Report

Preoperative Diagnosis: Bilateral vocal cord neoplasm

Postoperative Diagnosis: The same with right postprocedural pharyngeal bleed

Procedures:
1. Laryngoscopy with bilateral vocal cord stripping with use of operating microscope
2. Control of oral pharyngeal hemorrhage, less than 20 cc

Indications for Surgery: This 65-year-old female presented to the ENT Service with a two-year history of hoarseness. Upon evaluation, she was noted to have bilateral vocal cord neoplasms. The patient also has a history of smoking. A decision for the above-stated procedure was made for definitive diagnosis.

Procedure: The patient was brought to the Operating Suite, given a general anesthetic, and properly prepped and draped. It was noted that her teeth were not in good repair and that the lateral incisor was already loose on the right side. However, teeth guards were put into place. The Jako laryngoscope was carefully introduced into the oral cavity with attention not to injure the lips, gums, or teeth. The base of the tongue, vallecula, epiglottis, paraform sinuses, and false and true vocal cords were all visualized. The laryngoscope was fixed into place with microsuspension. The vocal cords were well visualized. There were polypoid-type neoplasms bilaterally. These were grasped anteriorly, stripped to the posterior bilaterally, and sent to Pathology. Hemostasis was obtained with an adrenaline cotton ball and silver nitrate. After good hemostasis was obtained, the scope was removed. However, upon removal, she was noted to have a pooling of blood in the posterior pharynx and that the blood was coming from the right tonsillar fossa. Apparently, this had been abraded with the laryngoscope upon insertion. Therefore, a self-retaining mouth gag was carefully introduced into the oral cavity. The patient did not have good extension of the mandible, but after this was visualized, the right pharyngeal wall was noted to have oozing and some irritation. This was controlled with the help of silver nitrate and suction cautery. After good hemostasis was obtained, the oral cavity was irrigated with a saline solution. When the patient exhibited good hemostasis, she was taken out of anesthetic and transferred to the Recovery Room in stable condition.

Assign appropriate CPT code(s) for the preceding procedures and indicate the index entries that were used to identify the codes. Assign only CPT codes (no E/M codes) and append any applicable modifiers.

Code(s):_____

Index entries:

_____

_____

Surgical Case #14

Operative Report

Procedure: Percutaneous endoscopic gastrostomy (PEG) tube placement

Diagnosis: Old cerebrovascular accident with inanition and need for supplemental nutritional support with no contraindication to enteral access

Technique: After anesthetization of the gag reflex, the gastroscope was introduced. There was no abnormality of the esophagus, stomach, pylorus, or duodenum. The abdomen had been prepped and draped as a sterile field. The light was found to transilluminate in the left upper quadrant. The skin was anesthetized with 1% Xylocaine. A blunt needle was used to access the stomach percutaneously and a guide wire inserted. The guide wire was grasped with a snare and brought through the mouth, along with the gastroscope. The feeding tube was threaded over the guide wire and brought through the abdominal wall with a small stab incision made along the guide wire. The gastroscope was reinserted and the PEG tube photo documented. There was no evidence of bleeding or undue tension as a result of tube placement. Air was suctioned from the stomach, and the gastroscope was removed with no other findings. The Silastic fastener was placed on the PEG tube near the skin entrance. The PEG tube then was connected to dependent drainage. The patient tolerated the procedure well and was taken to the recovery area with stable vital signs.

Assign appropriate CPT code(s) for the preceding procedures and indicate the index entries that were used to identify the codes. Assign only CPT codes (no E/M codes) and append any applicable modifiers.

Code(s):_____

Index entries:

_____

_____

Surgical Case #15

Operative Report

Procedure: Right carotid thromboendarterectomy and vein patch angioplasty

Diagnosis: Right carotid artery stenosis with hemorrhagic plaque

Anesthesia: General

Technique: Under general anesthesia, the right side of the patient's neck was prepped and draped in a sterile fashion. An incision was made along the sternocleidomastoid muscle, and a sharp dissection was carried down to expose the common internal and external carotid arteries. Care was taken to avoid injury to the hypoglossal, vagus, and ansa cervicalis nerves. The vessels were inserted with elastic tapes. The patient was heparinized, and an arteriotomy was made. A very high-grade stenosis estimated at 1.5-mm opening was present at the origin of the internal carotid artery, and there was evidence of significant hemorrhage and degeneration in the plaque. A shunt was placed for cerebral perfusion, and then the endarterectomy was done in the usual fashion. The vessel was picked free of any debris or other plaque and then closed with a patch angioplasty using saphenous vein from the left groin. This was sutured in place with 6-0 Prolene. Flow was first directed into the external carotid to allow any possible air or debris to escape and then restored to the internal carotid. The wound was packed open until the end of the procedure and after the heparin was reversed. Then the wound was closed with 3-0 Vicryl in the subcutaneous and platysma muscle and 4-0 Vicryl for a subcuticular skin closure. The patient left the operating room in satisfactory condition.

Assign appropriate CPT code(s) for the preceding procedures and indicate the index entries that were used to identify the codes. Assign only CPT codes (no E/M codes) and append any applicable modifiers.

Code(s):_____

Index entries:

_____

_____

Surgical Case #16

Operative Report

Procedure:	McDonald's cerclage placement
Diagnosis:	Intrauterine pregnancy at 12 weeks, history of cervical incompetence
Anesthesia:	Epidural
History:	The patient is a 36-year-old gravida 3 para 2 with a last menstrual period (LMP) on January 28. Positive HCG was noted on March 1. Intrauterine pregnancy was determined to be at 12 weeks by last LMP and at first trimester by ultrasound. She has a history of cervical incompetence in a previous pregnancy that was brought to term with a cerclage. She also has a history of diethylstilbestrol (DES) exposure and of cerclage placement times 2, D&C times 2, and umbilical herniorrhaphy.
Findings and Technique:	Preoperatively, her internal os was approximately 1 cm dilated. The posterior cervix was approximately 2 cm long, and the interior cervix was approximately 1 cm long. At the end of the procedure, the knot could be felt at the 12 o'clock position and the internal os was closed to digital examination.
	The patient was in the dorsal lithotomy position. She had internal and external perineal preps and was draped for the procedure. A Mersilene band on two needles was used with one needle placed in at the 6 o'clock position and brought out at 3 o'clock, and replaced at the same position and brought out at 12 o'clock. The other needle was taken in at 3 o'clock and brought out at 9 o'clock, and then replaced and brought out at 12 o'clock. The Mersilene band then was tied at the 12 o'clock position until the internal os was closed. It was palpable at the end of the procedure, and the two ends were cut long. The patient received perioperative antibiotics, and her heart tones were Dopplerable before the procedure. The procedure was without complications, and the patient was taken to the recovery room in stable condition.

Assign appropriate CPT code(s) for the preceding procedures and indicate the index entries that were used to identify the codes. Assign only CPT codes (no E/M codes) and append any applicable modifiers.

Code(s):_____

Index entries:

_____

_____

Surgical Case #17

Operative Report

Procedure: Modified radical mastectomy

Diagnosis: Infiltrating ductal carcinoma, left breast

Indications: The patient is a 79-year-old female who recently noticed a left breast mass. A subsequent mammogram revealed a spiculated suspicious lesion. On examination, she had a 2.5 to 3 cm palpable mass with no obvious axillary adenopathy. After an outpatient breast biopsy performed a week ago showed the mass was positive for carcinoma, she was admitted for a mastectomy.

Technique: Under general anesthesia, the patient's left breast was prepped. A transverse elliptical incision, including the nipple, areolar complex, and the previous biopsy site were utilized. Flaps were elevated medially to the sternum, superiorly to the clavicle, laterally to the latissimus, and inferiorly to the rectus. The depressed and anteropectoral fascia were dissected from medial to lateral with cautery dissection. The axilla was entered and the axillary vein identified. The venous tributaries were clipped inferiorly and divided. The long thoracic and thoracodorsal nerves were identified and traced to their insertions; and the axillary contents were swept inferiorly and laterally out with the breast specimen.

Hemostasis was obtained with a Bovie in addition to clips and sutures. Two Jackson Pratt drains were placed. The subcutaneous tissue was reapproximated with interrupted 3-0 Vicryl, and the skin was closed with clips. Some of the skin flaps were trimmed to make the closure more acceptable cosmetically. The patient tolerated the procedure well and was returned to the recovery area in satisfactory condition.

Assign appropriate CPT code(s) for the preceding procedures and indicate the index entries that were used to identify the codes. Assign only CPT codes (no E/M codes) and append any applicable modifiers.

Code(s):_____

Index entries:

_____

_____

Surgical Case #18

Operative Report

Procedure: Direct microlaryngoscopy under general anesthesia

Diagnosis: Dysphonia

Technique: A 40-year-old patient was taken to the OR where, under general anesthesia, the Jako laryngoscope was inserted with the operating microscope to perform a laryngoscopy. The vocal cords were found to be totally normal on both sides with no evidence of nodules or granuloma formation. The entire endolarynx was well visualized. Moreover, there was no evidence of subglottic stenosis; and as the patient was awakening, vocal cord mobility appeared to be normal. The procedure was terminated, and the patient awakened and taken to the recovery room in good condition with stable vital signs.

Recommendation: Speech therapy

Assign appropriate CPT code(s) for the preceding procedures and indicate the index entries that were used to identify the codes. Assign only CPT codes (no E/M codes) and append any applicable modifiers.

Code(s):_____

Index entries:

_____

_____

Surgical Case #19

Operative Report

Procedure: Colonoscopy

History and Indications: The patient is a 30-year-old female who has had complaints of abdominal pain, altered bowel habits, and a 2- to 3-gram documented decline in her hemoglobin. Her stools have been heme negative, but there is significant suspicion that she may have pathology in the colon.

Technique: The patient was sedated with 1.5 mg Versed and received antibiotics prior to the procedure per the recommendations of the cardiology service. She is status post heart transplant with significant cardiac complications.

In the endoscopy suite with appropriate monitoring of pulse, oxygenation, temperature, blood pressure, and other vital signs, a digital rectal examination was performed. Following the exam, the Pentax video colonoscope was inserted through the anus and advanced to the cecum. There was no evidence of malignancy. The scope was withdrawn.

Assign appropriate CPT code(s) for the preceding procedures and indicate the index entries that were used to identify the codes. Assign only CPT codes (no E/M codes) and append any applicable modifiers.

Code(s):_____

Index entries:

_____

_____

Surgical Case #20

Operative Report

Preoperative Diagnosis: Sebaceous cyst, right posterior neck

Postoperative Diagnosis: Lipomatous lesion, approximately 1.5 cm, right posterior neck, intramuscular

Procedure: Excision of lipoma, right posterior neck

Technique: The patient was brought to the operating suite and was placed in the prone position on the operating table. The patient's right neck was then prepped and draped in a sterile fashion. At this point, we suspected the patient to have a cyst. We subsequently decided to do a circumferential incision around what was thought to be the puncta. The incision was marked, and the area was prepped and draped with a local anesthetic. A skin incision was made. The incision was carried down to the subcutaneous tissue. At this point, we realized that it was not a cyst but, rather, a lipoma, which was actually deep into the muscle area. We excised the skin, dissected down through the capsule of the lipoma, and then were able to harvest this from its capsule within the muscle fibers. This was done with sharp dissection. Bleeding was controlled with cautery. The wound was closed with 3-0 Vicryl subcutaneous sutures, and a 4-0 Vicryl subcuticular stitch was placed. The wound edges were painted with Benzoin and Steri-Strips applied. The patient tolerated the procedure well and was taken to the recovery area in stable condition.

Assign appropriate CPT code(s) for the preceding procedures and indicate the index entries that were used to identify the codes. Assign only CPT codes (no E/M codes) and append any applicable modifiers.

Code(s):_____

Index entries:

_____

_____

Surgical Case #21

Operative Report

Procedure:	Colonoscopy
Indications for Procedure:	This is a 65-year-old female with a family history of colonic malignancy who is being evaluated for altered bowel function. When evaluated in my office prior to the procedure, her vital signs, cardiac status, pulmonary status, and mental status were stable and adequate for conscious sedation.
Description of Procedure:	The patient was given Demerol 50 mg IV and Versed 3 mg IV, and the CF100L video colonoscope was inserted and passed without difficulty to the cecum. Its position was confirmed by the ileocecal valve. Diverticulosis was observed in the left colon. A 5 to 7 mm circular, semipedunculated polyp was observed in the cecal area. It was secured with the snare and recovered. The patient tolerated the procedure well.
Impression:	She has a small cecal polyp, which has been removed. She has diverticulosis and will need reevaluation in three years.
Clinical Diagnosis:	Polyp, cecum
Pathological Diagnosis:	Polyp, cecum: Villotubular adenoma

Assign appropriate CPT code(s) for the preceding procedures and indicate the index entries that were used to identify the codes. Assign only CPT codes (no E/M codes) and append any applicable modifiers.

Code(s):_____

Index entries:

_____

_____

Surgical Case #22

Operative Report

Preoperative Diagnosis:	Cholecystitis with cholelithiasis
Postoperative Diagnosis:	Cholecystitis with cholelithiasis
Procedure Performed:	Laparoscopic cholecystectomy with operative cholangiogram
Anesthesia:	General
Bleeding:	None
Complications:	None

Description of Procedure: The patient was brought to the OR, placed in the supine position, and given general anesthesia. The skin over the abdomen was prepped with Duraprep and draped in the sterile fashion. A 1-cm incision was made above the umbilicus, and the Veress needle was introduced into the abdomen cavity obtaining pneumo-peritoneum. A 10-mm trocar was inserted and a laparoscope introduced. The patient had significant cholecystitis. Direct exploration of the abdomen was normal. Other trocars were inserted into subcostal space under direct vision. Lysis of adhesions was performed. Exposure to the gallbladder bed was obtained, and the cystic artery and the cystic duct were isolated. The common duct was of normal size. The cystic duct was ligated distally and proximally and was opened. We inserted the biliary catheter and obtained a cholangiogram that showed a normal biliary tree. The catheter was removed and the cystic duct double-ligated with hemoclips and divided. The gallbladder was removed through the upper trocar and dissected with electrocautery. The area was irrigated with saline solution. The trocars were removed under vision and pneumoperitoneum decompressed. The skin was closed with subcuticular 4-0 Vicryl, and a sterile dressing was applied. The patient tolerated the procedure well.

Assign appropriate CPT code(s) for the preceding procedures and indicate the index entries that were used to identify the codes. Assign only CPT codes (no E/M codes) and append any applicable modifiers.

Code(s):_____

Index entries:

_____

_____

Surgical Case #23

Operative Report

Procedure: Endoscopy

Preoperative Diagnosis: Abdominal pain, possible peptic ulcer disease.
Patient has upper abdominal pain, unresponsive to H2 blockers.

Postoperative Diagnosis:
1. Hiatal hernia
2. Moderate reflux esophagitis
3. Healing prepyloric gastric ulcer
4. Normal sigmoidoscopy

Findings: Endoscopy was performed with the Olympus video panendoscope, which was easily introduced into the esophagus. This was normal to the proximal midportion of the esophagus, but at the GE junction, there was evidence of a moderate degree of reflux esophagitis with several small superficial erosions at the location and also isolated erosions several centimeters above. The endoscope was advanced into the stomach and turned in a retrograde direction. The cardiac and fundic areas were examined and found to be otherwise normal. The antrum showed normal peristalsis and mucosa. In the immediate prepyloric area, a small defect was thought to represent scarring from a previous ulcer, which was still healing. Biopsies were obtained. The duodenum, including the second portion, was normal. Subsequently, the endoscope was withdrawn and the patient turned onto his left side. Flexible sigmoidoscopy then was carried out to the lower descending colon. A biopsy of the sigmoid was obtained. Patient tolerated the procedure well.

Assign appropriate CPT code(s) for the preceding procedures and indicate the index entries that were used to identify the codes. Assign only CPT codes (no E/M codes) and append any applicable modifiers.

Code(s):_____

Index entries:

_____

_____

Surgical Case #24

Operative Report

Procedure: Esophagogastroduodenoscopy

Instrument Used: Olympus GIF-100

Premedication: The patient was premedicated with a total of Fentanyl, 50 mcg, and Versed, 4 mg, intravenously.

Indications: The patient has presented with recurrent dysphagia. She has a history of a Schatzki's ring, which has been dilated in the past.

Procedure: The endoscope was inserted into the esophagus without difficulty. The esophageal mucosa was normal. A reformed Schatzki's ring was located at the Z line, which was at approximately 29 cm. The endoscope could be inserted through this area with no resistance. The ring was located above a 3-cm hiatal hernia. The stomach, duodenal bulb, and descending duodenum were all normal. After the endoscope was withdrawn, a #60 French Maloney dilator was passed with very mild resistance. The patient tolerated the procedure well, and there were no immediate complications.

Impression: 1.   A reformed Schatzki's ring, which was dilated
                   2.   A 3-cm hiatal hernia

Assign appropriate CPT code(s) for the preceding procedures and indicate the index entries that were used to identify the codes. Assign only CPT codes (no E/M codes) and append any applicable modifiers.

Code(s):_____

Index entries:

_____

_____

Surgical Case #25

Emergency Department Report

Chief Complaint:	Lacerations, left face
History of Present Illness:	Patient is a 26-year-old male who was driving a car with the window down when another car moving in the opposite direction hit his mirror. Glass from the broken mirror flew into his face, and he sustained two small lacerations. There were no other injuries.
Past Medical History:	Unremarkable
Medications:	None
Allergies:	None
Physical Examination:	
General:	Alert male in no acute distress
HEENT:	Pupils are equal and reactive to light. Extraocular muscles intact. Nose is clear. Oropharynx negative. Two lacerations are on left cheek region. The uppermost laceration is about 2 cm below the eye laterally and is about 0.75 cm in length. Full-skin thickness. The second laceration is about 1.5 cm below the first and is 1.25 cm in length. Full-skin thickness. No palpable foreign bodies.
Procedure:	Local injection with a total of 3 cc 1% lidocaine with epinephrine. Prepped and routine exploration performed. The upper laceration is only about 5 mm deep. No foreign bodies noted. No neurovascular injuries. It was closed with three 6-0 Nylon sutures. The lower laceration was approximately 12 to 15 mm deep. I could not palpate any foreign bodies. There are no obvious neurovascular injuries. Closed in single layer with five 6-0 nylon sutures. Polysporin ointment was applied.
Laboratory Data:	X-ray to rule out foreign body negative
Diagnosis:	1. Simple facial laceration, 1.25 cm 2. Simple facial laceration, 0.75 cm
Disposition and Plan:	Wound care instructions given; sutures out in 5 to 7 days

Assign appropriate CPT code(s) for the preceding procedures and indicate the index entries that were used to identify the codes. Assign only CPT codes (no E/M codes) and append any applicable modifiers.

Code(s):_____

Index entries:

_____

_____

Surgical Case #26

Operative Report

Preoperative Diagnosis: Dermal cyst of right breast

Postoperative Diagnosis: Dermal cyst of right breast

Procedure Performed: Excision of dermal cyst of right breast

Description of Procedure: Erythematous dermal cystic area of the right breast was marked out with an elliptical incision, anesthetized with local anesthesia, and prepped and draped sterilely.

Incision was made elliptically, including the whole cyst down through the fatty tissue. On palpation afterward no abnormalities were noted. Then the area had hemostasis obtained with electrocautery. The incision was closed with interrupted 3-0 Vicryl sutures.

The skin was closed with interrupted 5-0 nylon sutures. Steri-Strips and a sterile dressing were applied over it. The patient tolerated the procedure well and was sent to the recovery room with instructions to be discharged home with follow-up appointment given.

Assign appropriate CPT code(s) for the preceding procedures and indicate the index entries that were used to identify the codes. Assign only CPT codes (no E/M codes) and append any applicable modifiers.

Code(s):_____

Index entries:

_____

_____

Surgical Case #27

Operative Report

Preoperative Diagnosis: Right arm lipoma

Postoperative Diagnosis: Same

Procedure Performed: Excision of right arm lipoma

Anesthesia: Local

Indications for Procedure: The patient is a 48-year-old female who presents with a 4.0-cm mass on her right arm. She has had the mass for several months, and it is getting larger. She now presents for an excisional biopsy.

Description of Procedure: The patient was brought to the OR and placed on the operating table in the supine position. Her right arm was prepped and draped in the usual sterile fashion, and anesthetized with 1% lidocaine with bicarbonate. A longitudinal incision was made measuring 3 cm and carried down through the skin and subcutaneous tissues, and the underlying lipoma was dissected away from the surrounding tissues and removed. Parts of the lipoma were intermingled with surrounding tissues, requiring these areas to be pulled out. Hemostasis then was assured and the wound closed with layered Vicryl, followed by Benzoin, Steri-Strips, and a Tegaderm dressing. The patient tolerated the procedure well and was taken to the recovery room in stable condition.

Pathological Diagnosis: Forearm, right: lipoma

Gross: The specimen consists of nine pieces of soft, predominantly fatty yellow tissue ranging from 0.9 cm to 3 cm in greatest diameter; representative sections submitted in one cassette.

Assign appropriate CPT code(s) for the preceding procedures and indicate the index entries that were used to identify the codes. Assign only CPT codes (no E/M codes) and append any applicable modifiers.

Code(s):_____

Index entries:

_____

_____

Surgical Case #28

Operative Report

Preoperative Diagnosis: Elevated PSA of 16.6 and bladder outlet obstruction

Postoperative Diagnosis: Same

Procedure: Cystoscopy and transrectal needle biopsy of the prostate

Anesthesia: General

Procedure: This man was taken to the Operative Suite, placed in the dorsolithotomy position after being administered anesthesia, and sterilely prepped and draped in the normal fashion. A needle was used to take multiple transrectal biopsies of his prostate. After this, a cystoscopy was performed and bladder outlet obstruction and BPH were noted. The urethra was normal, and the bladder was moderately trabeculated. There was no evidence of neoplasm, infection, or calculus; and the ureters were normal in position, effluxing clear urine. The bladder was emptied, and the patient was sent to the Recovery Room in satisfactory condition.

Assign appropriate CPT code(s) for the preceding procedures and indicate the index entries that were used to identify the codes. Assign only CPT codes (no E/M codes) and append any applicable modifiers.

Code(s):_____

Index entries:

_____

_____

Surgical Case #29

Operative Report

Preoperative Diagnosis:	Incomplete abortion
Postoperative Diagnosis:	Same
Operation:	Dilatation & curettage
History:	This 22-year-old female, gravida IV, para II, AB I, comes in today because of abdominal pain and passing fetus on the sidewalk just outside the hospital. Apparently, her last menstrual period was two months ago. She had been doing well, and this problem just started today.
Procedure:	The patient was placed on the operating table in the lithotomy position, and prepped and draped in the usual manner. Under satisfactory intravenous sedation, the cervix was visualized by means of a weighted speculum and grasped in the anterior lip with a sponge forceps. Cord was prolapsed through the cervix and vagina, and a considerable amount of placental tissue was in the vagina and cervix. This was removed. A sharp curet was used to explore the endometrial cavity, and a minimal amount of curettings was obtained. The patient tolerated the procedure well.

Assign appropriate CPT code(s) for the preceding procedures and indicate the index entries that were used to identify the codes. Assign only CPT codes (no E/M codes) and append any applicable modifiers.

Code(s):_____

Index entries:

_____

_____

Surgical Case #30

Operative Report

Procedure: Sigmoidoscopy

Indications for Procedure: The patient is 75 years old. She has had an alteration in her bowel pattern and is being evaluated with a sigmoidoscopy.

Description of Procedure: She was given Fleet's enema preparation. She required no sedation. The CF100L video colonoscope was inserted and passed without difficulty to 50 cm. The mucosa were normal. No diverticulosis was observed. Some scybalous stool was present, but this was minimal. The patient tolerated the procedure well.

Assign appropriate CPT code(s) for the preceding procedures and indicate the index entries that were used to identify the codes. Assign only CPT codes (no E/M codes) and append any applicable modifiers.

Code(s):_____

Index entries:

_____

_____

Surgical Case #31

Operative Report

Diagnosis: Hodgkin's disease, nonsclerosing type

Operation: Placement of right subclavian Hickman catheter

Indications: The patient is a 35-year-old female with the diagnosis of Hodgkin's disease. Her indication for a Hickman catheter was chemotherapy infusion.

Procedure: The patient was taken to the operating room and placed in the supine position. The right chest and subclavian area, neck, and shoulder were prepped and draped in routine manner. A total of 48 cc of 1% Carbocaine without epinephrine was used for anesthesia. The subcutaneous area below the right clavicle was numbed with the Lidocaine down to the periosteum. The subclavian vein was stuck with the needle. Good blood flow was returned. The guide wire was passed. At this time, a 2-cm incision was made below the clavicle at the middle aspect. The Hickman catheter was then placed over the guide wire into the superior vena cava. This was documented with fluoroscopy. A second incision was made 3 cm below the first distance of 2 cm transverse. The area between the two incisions was then tunneled with a curved six. The distal aspect of the catheter was brought out through the second inferior incision. The teflon Hickman catheter was trimmed to the appropriate length with Teflon coating at the skin incision. The superior skin incision was closed with interrupted 3-0 nylon, as was the inferior skin incision. The patient tolerated the procedure well.

Assign appropriate CPT code(s) for the preceding procedures and indicate the index entries that were used to identify the codes. Assign only CPT codes (no E/M codes) and append any applicable modifiers.

Code(s):_____

Index entries:

_____

_____

Surgical Case #32

Operative Report

Preoperative Diagnosis: Ventral hernia

Postoperative Diagnosis: Ventral hernia

Operation Performed: Laparoscopic repair of ventral hernia

Anesthesia: General

Details of Procedure: The patient was taken to the operating room, placed in the supine position. The abdomen was prepped and draped in the usual sterile fashion. A Veress needle was then inserted in the left lateral abdominal wall. The abdomen was insufflated with CO_2 gas. A 10-mm Surgiport was then placed. The laparoscopic camera was then inserted. Additional 5-mm Surgiports were placed under direct vision, one in the left lower quadrant of the abdomen, the other in the left upper quadrant of the abdomen.

The 5-mm harmonic scalpel was used along with the dissecting forceps to take down the adhesions from within and around the hernia sac. There were a number of adhesions, primarily involving the omentum. These were all removed.

Two hernia defects were noted, one just above the umbilicus, perhaps 3 to 4 cm in diameter, and another toward the upper aspect of the midline incision, that had not been previously recognized.

It was elected to place an 18 × 24-cm segment of Gore-Tex dual mesh. #1 Prolene was sewn at each of the corners of this as well as in between, at the midpoint of each of the sides. Suitable locations were chosen for tying the anchoring sutures. The patch then was rolled around a grasper and inserted into the abdominal cavity through the 10-mm port. The patch was then unrolled and the orientation placed with the smooth side down against the bowel. An endo-close device was used to grasp each of the sutures and bring out through the previously placed incisions for the anchoring sutures. The patch was anchored at each of the six locations as noted above. Then, an auto suture protac was placed around the periphery of the patch. Additional staples were placed within the inner aspect of the patch using an Ethicon tacking stapler. The patch was noted to be quite taut and applied closely to the abdominal wall to prevent any movement of the patch. The abdomen was then desufflated and the ports withdrawn. Each of the skin incisions was closed with 4-0 clear PDS subcuticular suture and Steri-Strips. Tegaderm dressings were then applied. The patient tolerated the procedure well with no apparent difficulty. She was then taken to the postanesthesia recovery room for further postoperative care.

Assign appropriate CPT code(s) for the preceding procedures and indicate the index entries that were used to identify the codes. Assign only CPT codes (no E/M codes) and append any applicable modifiers.

Code(s):_____

Index entries:

_____

_____

Surgical Case #33

Operative Report

Preoperative Diagnosis: Right breast mammographic abnormality

Postoperative Diagnosis: Same

Indications: This is a 53-year-old woman who presented with a nonpalpable right breast mammographic abnormality. A stereotatic biopsy showed columnar cell hyperplasia without evidence of obvious malignancy; however, excision was recommended. Possible perioperative risks and complications and alternatives were discussed with her prior to surgery.

Details of Procedure: After informed consent was obtained from the patient, she was taken to the OR and placed on the table in the supine position. The right breast was noted to contain a localization wire. The films were reviewed. The breast was prepped with Betadine solution and draped sterilely. Sedation was administered by anesthesia. Local anesthesia was achieved with 1% lidocaine and 0.5% Marcaine with epinephrine. An incision was made over the course of the localization needle, and the underlying core of tissue surrounding the localization needle was excised using electrocautery. This was forwarded to radiology, which confirmed the presence of the previously marked mammographic abnormality within the specimen. It was then forwarded to pathology.

Wound was inspected for hemostasis, which was excellent. The deep tissues were approximated with interrupted 3-0 Vicryl, and a running 4-0 Monocryl subcuticular stitch was used to approximate the skin edges. Benzoin, Steri-Strips, and dry sterile dressing were applied. The patient was then awakened from anesthesia and returned to the recovery room in stable condition.

Assign appropriate CPT code(s) for the preceding procedures and indicate the index entries that were used to identify the codes. Assign only CPT codes (no E/M codes) and append any applicable modifiers.

Code(s):_____

Index entries:

_____

_____

Surgical Case #34

Operative Report

Preoperative Diagnosis: Chalazion, left lower lid

Postoperative Diagnosis: Same

Operation: Excision of mass, left lower lid

Procedure: Under adequate topical anesthesia and block anesthesia, the eye was prepared and draped in the usual manner. Chalazion speculum was applied. The left lower lid was everted and a vertical incision made. Excision of the mass was performed using curet, and a biopsy of the capsule of this 9-mm mass was made, as requested. Patient tolerated the procedure well and left the operating room in good condition after application of Cortisporin ointment and pressure patch.

Assign appropriate CPT code(s) for the preceding procedures and indicate the index entries that were used to identify the codes. Assign only CPT codes (no E/M codes) and append any applicable modifiers.

Code(s):_____

Index entries:

_____

_____

Surgical Case #35

Operative Report

Preoperative Diagnosis: Carpal tunnel compression, left, severe

Postoperative Diagnosis: Same

Operation: Release, left carpal tunnel

Procedure: After successful axillary block was placed, the patient's left arm was prepared and draped in the usual sterile manner. Tourniquet inflated. A curvilinear hypothenar incision was made and the palmaris retracted radially. The carpal tunnel and the transverse carpal ligament were then opened and completely freed in the proximal directions. It was noted to be severely tight in the palm with flattening and swelling of the median nerve. The carpal tunnel was opened distally in the hand and noted to be clear, out to the transverse palmar crease. The wound was then closed with 4-0 Dexon in subcuticular tissues. Sterile bulky dressing was applied, and the patient was awakened and taken to the recovery room in satisfactory condition.

Assign appropriate CPT code(s) for the preceding procedures and indicate the index entries that were used to identify the codes. Assign only CPT codes (no E/M codes) and append any applicable modifiers.

Code(s):_____

Index entries:

_____

_____

Surgical Case #36

Operative Report

Preoperative Diagnosis: Keratosis of glans penis

Postoperative Diagnosis: Same

Procedure: The penis was prepared and draped in the usual manner. Along the distal portion of the penis on the right side and adjoining the urinary meatus was a well-defined, firm area suggesting a keratosis. The entire lesion was excised and submitted for pathological examination. The pathologist confirmed the diagnosis of keratosis. The glans penis was then approximated with black silk. The patient returned to the recovery room in satisfactory condition.

Assign appropriate CPT code(s) for the preceding procedures and indicate the index entries that were used to identify the codes. Assign only CPT codes (no E/M codes) and append any applicable modifiers.

Code(s):_____

Index entries:

_____

_____

Surgical Case #37

Operative Report

Preoperative diagnosis: Herniated disc at L4–L5, L5–S1; good relief with previous two epidural blocks

Postoperative diagnosis: Same

Operation: Therapeutic epidural block

Procedure: The patient is kept on the left lateral side. The back is prepped with Betadine solution, and 1% Xylocaine is infiltrated at the L5–S1 interspace. Deep infiltration is carried out with a 22-gauge needle, and a 17-gauge Touhy needle is taken and an epidural is performed. After careful aspiration, which was negative for blood as well as for cerebral spinal fluid, about 80 mg of Depo-Medrol then were injected along with 5 cc of 0.25% Marcaine and 1 cc of 50 mcg of Fentanyl. The injection was done in a fractionated dose in a slow fashion. The patient was examined and evaluated following the block and found to have excellent relief of pain. The patient is advised to continue physical therapy and to come back in a month for further evaluation.

Assign appropriate CPT code(s) for the preceding procedures and indicate the index entries that were used to identify the codes. Assign only CPT codes (no E/M codes) and append any applicable modifiers.

Code(s):_____

Index entries:

_____

_____

Surgical Case #38

Operative Report

Procedure: Excision of left axillary lymph nodes

Indications for Procedure: This female patient had a lumpectomy for a breast lesion approximately two and a half years ago. She presents with palpable adenopathy in the left axilla.

Description of Procedure: The patient was brought into the operating room and placed on the OR table in the supine position. The left axilla was prepped and draped in the usual sterile fashion. After an adequate level of general anesthesia had been achieved, a knife with a #10 blade was used to make a curvilinear incision in the skin overlying the adenopathy.

This incision was carried down deep through the subcutaneous tissue using a Bovie knife. Babcock forceps were used to grasp the area of tissue surrounding the lymph node and was carefully dissected from the surrounding tissues using a Bovie knife and scissors. All vessels encountered were either Bovied or clipped.

The wound was irrigated and carefully examined for bleeders. The subcutaneous tissue was closed using a Vicryl suture placed in interrupted fashion, and the skin was reapproximated using staples. Drainage was achieved with a Jackson-Pratt drain brought out through a separate wound. Sterile dressings were applied, and the patient was taken to the Recovery Room in a stable postoperative condition.

Assign appropriate CPT code(s) for the preceding procedures and indicate the index entries that were used to identify the codes. Assign only CPT codes (no E/M codes) and append any applicable modifiers.

Code(s):_____

Index entries:

_____

_____

Surgical Case #39

Operative Report

Preoperative Diagnosis: Subepidermal nodular 1.5-cm lesion of the left side of the nose

Operation: Excision, lesion of nose

Procedure: Under local anesthesia, we excised the 1.5-cm lesion with 0.5-cm margins on all sides of the defect. The lesion was excised in fragments and submitted to pathology along with an ellipse of skin margins. Bleeding is controlled with electrocautery, and the wound is closed with four vertical mattress sutures of 5-0 nylon. Polysporin and dressing were applied.

Pathological Diagnosis: Well-organized basal cell carcinoma with no significant increase in activity or dysplasia of the cells

Assign appropriate CPT code(s) for the preceding procedures and indicate the index entries that were used to identify the codes. Assign only CPT codes (no E/M codes) and append any applicable modifiers.

Code(s):_____

Index entries:

_____

_____

Surgical Case #40

Emergency Department Physician Report

Chief Complaint:	Left eye, foreign body × 2 days
History of Present Illness:	The patient is a 29-year-old male who presents to the emergency room after having a piece of metal fly into his left eye yesterday. Since that time, he still continues to have the metal present. He denies any major disturbance in vision, although he states that his vision is slightly more blurry and irritated. He does complain of some pain.
Past Medical History:	Hypertension
Allergies:	None
Immunizations:	Unknown for tetanus
Social and Family History:	Noncontributory
Physical Exam of Eyes:	Reveals the left eye to have some periorbital erythema, but minimal swelling of the lids. PERRLA: No papilledema. EOMs intact. Vision intact. Inspection of the left eye shows a foreign body that resembles a piece of metal at 6 o'clock. At this time, Tetracaine was applied. The foreign body was successfully removed with the bevel of a 22-gauge needle. Two more drops of Tetracaine were applied, followed by Homatropine and Polysporin Ophthalmic ointment.
Assessment:	Foreign body of left eye, removed. The patient understood all instructions and agreed with the plan at which time he was discharged.

Assign appropriate CPT code(s) for the preceding procedures and indicate the index entries that were used to identify the codes. Assign only CPT codes (no E/M codes) and append any applicable modifiers.

Code(s):_____

Index entries:

_____

_____

Surgical Case #41

Operative Report

Preprocedure Diagnosis:	Left lower lobe lung nodule
Postprocedure Diagnosis:	Left lower lobe lung nodule
Operations Performed:	1. Left video-assisted thoracoscopy
	2. Wedge resection biopsy, left lower lobe times two
	3. Bronchoscopy with the right upper lobe, transbronchial biopsy times two

Indications for Procedure: The patient, who has been followed by both the Pulmonary Services as well as seen in the Thoracic Surgery Clinic, had had a long history of smoking. His chest CT had a nodule in the left lower lobe as well as an area in the right upper lobe that was consistent with some consolidation that had not increased in size. It was decided to perform a wedge biopsy of the left lower lobe lung nodule since this is a discrete mass, and bronchoscopy for the right upper lobe. Patient understood the previously mentioned procedures and approach. Informed consent was obtained.

Procedure: Patient was brought into the operating room, placed on the operating table in the supine position. After smooth induction of general anesthesia, endotracheal intubation, a Foley catheter was placed. The double-lumen endotracheal tube was placed. Patient was then turned into the left lateral decubitus position with the left side up and right side down. We prepped and draped with Hibiclens, alcohol, and Ioban. We then made a small incision in the posterior space with a scalpel, dissected down, bluntly entered into the chest cavity, placed a 5-mm port.

We then placed an additional port and moved the camera to the anterior inferior portion and placed another 5-mm trocar posterior inferior. We then used gross inspection of the chest. There were no adhesions and no pleural fluid to sweep out. No gross masses. Using a blunt grasper, we were able to palpate the left lower lobe posteriorly and feel the mass. We then used graspers retracted to the lung specimen up, used the EndoGIA staplers to perform wedge biopsies or initial wedge biopsy. We did not have the specimen. In this second wedge biopsy, we were able to get around from the green staple load and perform the biopsy and wedge out the mass lesion. This was then placed in a EndoCatch bag and removed. We were then able to palpate the mass, but the scalpel we opened had an appearance of an infectious etiology. Gram staining was sent and then it was sent for further dissection.

We then placed a #9 French pneumocath anteriorly under direct vision. There was no bleeding to speak of. We removed our trocars under direct vision. Lung was allowed to reinflate. Chest tube was placed to suction 10 cm to close the 10 × 12 site with 2-0 Vicryl and 4-0 Vicryl followed by Dermabond. Other trocar sites were closed with 4-0 Monocryl and Dermabond. Once this was completed, the patient was turned supine. We then performed a bronchoscopy. While in bronchoscopy, the trachea at the right appeared normal. On the right side, the bronchus intermedius appeared normal. We were able to cannulate the right upper lobe. We were able to then use the biopsy forceps to cannulate the apical segment of the right upper lobe. We sent several specimens with biopsy forceps for cytology as well as performed a biopsy with fluoroscopic guidance times two. We then removed the biopsy forceps.

We inspected the bronchus intermedius, the right medial lobe and right lower lobe orifices appeared normal. We then removed, pulled the scope back, advanced down the left main stem bronchus. All segments and lobes appeared

Surgical Case #41 (Continued)

normal. Through the bronchoscope, this point of procedure was terminated. Patient was extubated, transferred off the operating room table, awakened stable to the SICU. Dr. Howard was present for the entire procedure. There were no complications.

Assign appropriate CPT code(s) for the preceding procedures and indicate the index entries that were used to identify the codes. Assign only CPT codes (no E/M codes) and append any applicable modifiers.

Code(s):_____

Index entries:

_____

_____

Surgical Case #42

Operative Report

Preoperative Diagnosis: Arthritis of right acromioclavicular joint

Postoperative Diagnosis: Same

Operation: Mumford procedure, right shoulder

Procedure: The patient was brought to the operative room after general anesthesia. The patient was placed in the lounge chair position, the right shoulder was sterilely scrubbed and draped in the usual manner. Routine incision was taken down to the distal clavicle. The distal clavicle was identified subperiosteally. Retractors were put in place. At this time the clavicle was osteotomized using a saw and the distal end of the clavicle was removed. The wound was then irrigated. Marcaine with epinephrine was injected. The periosteum was closed with 0 Vicryl, subcu with 2-0 Vicryl, and the skin with staples. Dry sterile dressings were applied and the patient was sent to the recovery room in good condition.

Assign appropriate CPT code(s) for the preceding procedures and indicate the index entries that were used to identify the codes. Assign only CPT codes (no E/M codes) and append any applicable modifiers.

Code(s):_____

Index entries:

_____

_____

Surgical Case #43

Operative Report

Preoperative Diagnosis: Epidermal cyst

Postoperative Diagnosis: Awaiting permanent section by pathology

Operation: Excision of the area

Procedure: This 91-year-old female who resides in the Sunnybrook Nursing Home presented with a 1.25 × 1.25-cm enlarging tender granulomatous type lesion over the dorsum of the MCP joint of the left ring finger. Because of the patient's arthritis, she was left in the wheelchair while the procedure was done. The left hand was scrubbed for 10 minutes with sterile soap solution with Betadine, prepped with Betadine prep. The patient was draped with sterile towels and drapes exposing the area and then the area about the lesion was blocked with 1% Lidocaine without Epinephrine and then an ellipse was outlined with long axis vertical and the lesion was excised and then submitted to pathology. The total excised lesion including margins was 2.0 cm. It was closed with five sutures of 5-0 Prolene and dressed with Polysporin and a Band-Aid. The family was instructed that the Band-Aid could be changed and she was discharged to the home where I will follow her and remove the sutures in one to two weeks.

Pathological Diagnosis: Skin lesion, left ring finger: epidermal cyst, excised and actinic keratosis with extensive atypical basosquamous cell hyperplasia

Assign appropriate CPT code(s) for the preceding procedures and indicate the index entries that were used to identify the codes. Assign only CPT codes (no E/M codes) and append any applicable modifiers.

Code(s):_____

Index entries:

_____

_____

Emergency Department Case #44

Emergency Department Record

Chief Complaint: Injury to right fourth and fifth toes

History of Present Illness: Patient states that he was running for the phone when he stubbed his toes on a piece of furniture. Did this yesterday and has marked ecchymosis noted in the fourth and fifth toes of the right foot, slight swelling also. He states he has been able to ambulate and that his foot does not hurt, except for when he walks. Denies any numbness, tingling, or loss of sensation. He does also have an abrasion noted to the distal aspect of the fourth toe. He denies any further injury.

Past Medical History: Noncontributory

Allergies: Patient has no known medication allergies

Current Medications: None

Review of Systems: Negative

Physical Examination

Vital Signs: Blood pressure is 145/89. Temperature is 97.7°, pulse of 76, respirations 16.

General: Patient is alert, oriented, in no acute distress.

Extremities: Shows marked ecchymosis noted in the fourth and fifth toes and in the dorsal aspect of the foot adjacent to the fourth and fifth toes on the right foot. The patient is tender to palpation over the fourth and fifth digits proximal. Right foot is neurovascularly intact. Sensation is intact. Patient has an abrasion noted to the distal aspect of the right fourth digit. Range of motion is intact. Patient is able to ambulate with a slight limp due to pain. Remainder of physical exam is normal.

Emergency Department Course: An x-ray was taken of the patient's right foot with attention to the fourth and fifth toes. X-ray showed a fracture of the fourth and fifth proximal phalanx. X-ray was also reviewed by Dr. Smith, who agreed with this assessment. The patient's right fourth and fifth toes were digitally blocked with 2.5 cc of 2% lidocaine each. Abrasion on the fourth digit was prepped per protocol. Fractures were reduced in the fourth and fifth digits and buddy taped. Patient's right foot was again x-rayed. His postreduction film showed that the fractures were in better alignment. X-rays were also reviewed by Dr. Blevins, who agreed with this assessment. Patient was fitted for a postop shoe.

Impressions/Diagnosis: Patient has fractured, right fourth and fifth toes.

Plan:
1. Rest, ice, compress, and elevate the right foot.
2. Buddy tape × 2 weeks.
3. Follow-up with family medical doctor as needed.
4. Return if condition worsens. Patient refused any pain medication.

Disposition: Home

Assign appropriate CPT code(s) for the preceding procedures and indicate the index entries that were used to identify the codes. Assign only CPT codes (no E/M codes) and append any applicable modifiers.

Code(s):_____

Index entries:

_____

_____

Surgical Case #45

Operative Report

Preoperative Diagnosis: Lipoma of the right shoulder

Postoperative Diagnosis: Same

Procedure: Removal of lipoma

Description of Procedure: The patient was taken to the Operating Room and prepped and draped in the usual manner. A longitudinal incision was made centered over the palpable and visible mass, carried down through the skin. The subcutaneous layer was noted to be large lobulations and dissection was begun around the obvious palpable mass. This was dissected free and carried down through the deltoid muscle down to the level of the subscapularus tendon of the shoulder joint. Did not seem to have any major neurovascular attachments otherwise. Mass was dissected free through the muscle-slitting incision. The cephalic vein was retracted laterally. Bleeding was controlled with hemostats and bovie cautery. Estimated blood loss: 30 cc. The wound was then copiously irrigated after total removal was verified and the fascia was closed with 2-0 chromic gut, subcutaneous layer with 2-0 plain catgut and skin with 2-0 Dermalon. The patient tolerated the procedure well and left the OR in good condition after dressing was applied.

Assign appropriate CPT code(s) for the preceding procedures and indicate the index entries that were used to identify the codes. Assign only CPT codes (no E/M codes) and append any applicable modifiers.

Code(s):_____

Index entries:

_____

_____

Surgical Case #46

Operative Report

Preoperative Diagnosis: Ptosis, left upper eyelid

Postoperative Diagnosis: Same

Procedure: Frontalis ptosis, left upper eyelid

Anesthesia: Local

Description of Procedure: Topical tetracaine was applied to both eyes. The left upper lid and brow were infiltrated with Xylocaine with Epinephrine and Marcaine with Wydase. The patient was prepped and draped in the usual fashion for oculoplastic surgery. Incisions were made in the medial and lateral thirds of the lid, 3 mm above the lash line. Stat incisions were made at the medial and lateral thirds of the brow, approximately 5 mm above the brow and a single incision was made in the middle of the brow, approximately 1 cm higher than the previous two incisions. A 3-0 Prolene suture was passed from the lateral lid incision to the medial lid incision beneath the orbicularis, just above the tarsus. Suture was then passed beneath the brow and frontalis to emerge from the medial and lateral brow incisions respectively. Each end of the suture was then passed beneath the frontalis to emerge through the central brow incision. The suture was tied and tension was adjusted so that the lid level was just above the papillary border. The brow incisions were closed with interrupted sutures of 6-0 Prolene, the eye was dressed with Ocumycin ointment. The patient tolerated the procedure well and left the OR in good condition.

Assign appropriate CPT code(s) for the preceding procedures and indicate the index entries that were used to identify the codes. Assign only CPT codes (no E/M codes) and append any applicable modifiers.

Code(s):_____

Index entries:

_____

_____

Surgical Case #47

Operative Report

Preoperative Diagnosis: Displaced, rotated fractures of left index and long metacarpal shafts

Postoperative Diagnosis: Same

Procedure: Closed reduction and percutaneous pin fixation of displaced fractures of the left index and long metacarpal shafts

Description of Procedure: The patient is a 22-year-old, right-hand-dominant gentleman who sustained left index and long metacarpal shaft fractures while playing soccer. He was referred to my office and was found to have internal rotation and shortening deformities through the index and long metacarpal shaft fractures and subsequently is scheduled for closed, possibly open, reduction and percutaneous pin fixation or possible internal fixation of the above-mentioned fractures. The patient was placed in the supine position on the OR table and general anesthesia was admininstered. Left proximal arm tourniquet was placed and the left upper extremity was prepped and draped in the usual sterile fashion. The arm was exsanguinated with an Esmarch bandage and the tourniquet inflated to 250 mm of Mercury. Sterile finger traps and ropes were then applied to the left index and long fingers and 10 lb of weight were then applied over the end of the hand table. The fractures were then gently manipulated and multiple fluoroscopic views were obtained, which revealed satisfactory alignment. Attention was then turned to the index metacarpal shaft fracture, which was percutaneously pinned from its radial to ulnar aspect with excellent purchase being obtained on both sides. X-rays were then taken and revealed anatomic alignment. Attention was then turned to the long metacarpal shaft fracture, which was still slightly distracted and displaced. Additional manipulation was performed. A pin was initially inserted from radial to ulnar, which resulted in further distraction of the fracture. The pin was removed and another pin was inserted from ulnar to radial. This appeared to close the fracture gap and held the fracture in better alignment. A second pin was then placed just proximal and parallel to the original pin with resultant satisfactory alignment. There was still some slight gapping at the fracture site, but the rotation and angulation were corrected. The finger traps were removed and the fingers were flexed to the same degree. All fingertips appeared to point to the distal pole of the scaphoid without any evidence of angulation or rotation malalignment. The pins were trimmed and bent over at 90-degree angles. The pin sites were irrigated and Xeroform dressings were applied. Sterile gauze, lightly compressive hand dressing was then applied, reinforced with plaster splint with the hand placed in the intrinsic plus position and the PIP joint left free. The patient tolerated the procedure well and was sent to recovery in satisfactory condition.

Assign appropriate CPT code(s) for the preceding procedures and indicate the index entries that were used to identify the codes. Assign only CPT codes (no E/M codes) and append any applicable modifiers.

Code(s):_____

Index entries:

_____

_____

Surgical Case #48

Operative Report

Preoperative Diagnosis:	Symptomatic third-degree heart block
Postoperative Diagnosis:	Same
Operation:	Placement of permanent pacemaker with transvenous electrode
Anesthesia:	Local infiltration of Lidocaine 1%, total volume 13 cc
Complications:	None
Indications:	This 74-year-old gentleman was admitted with a diagnosis of third-degree heart block complicated by congestive cardiac failure. Patient is scheduled for placement of a permanent pacemaker today.
Procedure:	With the patient supine on the operating table with a shoulder roll placed beneath the thoracic spine, the chest was prepped and draped in a sterile fashion. In the right infraclavicular region, a subcutaneous pocket was created for containing the pulse generator. Using an introducer guide wire, a sheath technique bipolar targeted lead was introduced into the right subclavian vein. Under fluoroscopy control, this was directed into the right ventricle. Two initial locations were not satisfactory for pacing parameters. Finally, the pacemaker was positioned in satisfactory position with the following parameters: at the threshold 0.4 volts, current 1.5 milliamps and R wave 15. The pacing system analyzer was then turned to 10 volts output and the diaphragm observed for pulsations, which were not proven. The lead was then secured under the clavicle with a single suture of 2-0 Ethibond. It was then attached to a 5794 Medtronic low-profile VVI pacemaker programmed at 70 beats per minute. The pulse generator was then anchored in the subcutaneous pocket with a single 0 PDS suture. The subcutaneous tissue was then approximated with 2-0 PDS and the skin approximated with 4-0 Maxon. Sterile dressing was applied. A chest x-ray was obtained, which showed no pneumothorax and satisfactory position of the lead. The patient was then returned to the Coronary Care Unit in good condition.

Assign appropriate CPT code(s) for the preceding procedures and indicate the index entries that were used to identify the codes. Assign only CPT codes (no E/M codes) and append any applicable modifiers.

Code(s):_____

Index entries:

_____

_____

Surgical Case #49

Operative Report

Preoperative Diagnosis: Nasolacrimal duct obstruction, right eye

Postoperative Diagnosis: Same

Operation:
1. Probing right nasolacrimal duct
2. Balloon dilation, right nasolacrimal duct

Procedure: The patient was taken to the operating room and given general anesthesia by mask. The right upper punctum was then dilated and a #0 Bowman probe passed from the upper punctum into the lacrimal sac and down through the nasolacrimal duct with a small amount of resistance. A second probe was then passed under the right inferior turbinate and definite metal-on-metal contact established. The original probe was then withdrawn, and a #2 Lacricath was inserted from the upper punctum into the lacrimal sac and down through the nasolacrimal duct. Its position was confirmed in the nose. The balloon was inflated eight atmospheres for 90 seconds. It was then withdrawn 5 mm and again inflated eight atmospheres for 60 seconds. At this point, the Lacricath was withdrawn. A lacrimal cannula attached to a syringe containing normal saline dyed with Fluorescein was then inserted from the upper punctum into the lacrimal sac and fluid freely irrigated into the nose and was recovered with a suction catheter. A drop of a steroid antibiotic combination was then applied to the right eye and the patient awakened and returned to the recovery room in good condition.

Assign appropriate CPT code(s) for the preceding procedures and indicate the index entries that were used to identify the codes. Assign only CPT codes (no E/M codes) and append any applicable modifiers.

Code(s): _____

Index entries:

_____

_____

Emergency Department Case #50

Emergency Department Record

Chief Complaint: A laceration to the left lower leg

History of Present Illness: The patient is a 33-year-old male who presents to the ER today with a chief complaint of a laceration to his left lower leg. The patient states that he came to Cincinnati for a mountain bike competition, which he was in today. The patient stated that he was practicing before the competition when he accidentally cut the posterior aspect of his left leg on the pedal of his bike. The patient stated that the pedal was clean and that he had this accident on the pavement. There was no grass or dirt around at that time. The patient currently complains of pain to the area of the laceration. He is ambulatory with a limp. The patient stated that the accident happened approximately 1 hour prior to arrival at the emergency room. The patient denies any left calf pain. Denies any left knee pain. The patient did not have any head injury or any loss of consciousness. The patient's tetanus is up to date. The patient also denies any neck or back injury. The patient has no other complaints.

Review of Systems: See HPI; otherwise negative

Past Medical History: Unremarkable

Medications: None

Allergies: No known drug allergies

Emergency Department Case #50   (Continued)

Physical Examination:

Vital Signs:	Blood pressure is 128/68; temperature is 97.8; pulse 77; respirations 18
General:	The patient is a 33-year-old male who is in no acute distress. The patient is alert and oriented × 3.
Skin:	Pink, warm. Patient currently has a 5-cm gaping laceration to the posterior aspect of his left leg that is just inferior and medial to the left knee.
HEENT:	Within normal limits
Neck:	Supple, no cervical tenderness; no cervical adenopathy
Musculoskeletal:	The patient has full active range of motion of his left knee at this time. There is no edema, ecchymosis, or erythema noted to the left knee. However, the patient's posterior aspect of his left knee is indurated somewhat. The patient is nontender with palpation over the left gastrocnemius muscle. The patient's dorsalis pedis and posterior tibialis pulses are present and strong. Doppler was then used to pick up the patient's left popliteal pulse. This was present and strong, and when compared to the popliteal pulse of the right leg, it was the same strength. The patient is nontender with palpation of the left quadriceps as well as over the left hamstring muscles.
ED Course:	The patient was discussed with Dr. Ferguson. Dr. Ferguson also examined the patient. X-rays were then obtained of the patient's left tib/fib as well as the patient's left knee. X-rays were reviewed by both myself and Dr. Ferguson and were unremarkable. The patient was then given Keflex lg p.o. The patient was then given Lortab 5 mg p.o.
ED Procedure:	The patient's laceration was anesthetized using 15 cc of 1% lidocaine plain. The area was then cleansed using Betadine and normal saline solution. The wound was then explored for any evidence of foreign bodies. No foreign bodies were noted. Wound edges were then well approximated and brought together using three deep-layered sutures of 4-0 Vicryl and 7 mattress sutures of 4-0 nylon as well as one simple suture of 4-0 nylon. The area was then cleansed again using normal saline. Xeroform was applied as well as a 2 × 2 Kerlex wrap and Ace wrap. The patient was informed to remove the ace wrap prior to sleeping in the evening. The patient was also given a Lortab starter pack and informed to fill his antibiotic prescription. Patient was also informed to watch for any pain to his left calf. The patient understood this and stated that he would return if any pain occurred.
Impression/Diagnosis:	1. A 5-cm laceration left posterior leg, which was repaired
Plan:	1. Keep area clean and dry.
	2. Suture removal 10–12 days primary care physician.
	3. Wound care instructions: Watch for infection.
	4. Keflex 500 mg #20 no refills.
	5. Lortab 5 mg #10 no refills.
	6. Return with any worsening symptoms.

Assign appropriate CPT code(s) for the preceding procedures and indicate the index entries that were used to identify the codes. Assign only CPT codes (no E/M codes) and append any applicable modifiers.

Code(s):_____

Index entries:

_____

_____

Surgical Case #51

Operative Report

Preoperative Diagnosis:	Rule out bladder tumor
Postoperative Diagnosis:	Same
Procedures:	Cystoscopy, biopsy, and fulguration of bladder
Anesthesia:	Spinal
Indications:	This is a 68-year-old white female with a history of grade II superficial transitional cell carcinoma of the bladder. Cystoscopy showed a suspicious erythematous area on the right trigone. She presented today for cystoscopy, biopsy, and fulguration.
Findings:	The urethra was normal, the bladder was 1+ trabeculated, the mid and right trigone area were slightly erythematous and hypervascular, no papillary tumors were noted, no mucosal abnormalities were noted.
Description of Procedure:	The patient was placed on the table in supine position, satisfactory spinal anesthesia was obtained. She was placed in dorsolithotomy position and prepped and draped in the usual manner. #22 French cystoscopy sheath was passed per urethra in atraumatic fashion. The bladder was resected with a 70-degree lens with findings as noted above. Cup biopsy forceps were placed and 3 biopsies were taken of the suspicious areas of the trigone. These areas were fulgurated and the Bugby electrode, there was no active bleeding seen. The scope was removed, and the patient was returned to recovery in satisfactory condition.

Pathology Report

Bladder biopsy: chronic cystitis (cystica) with squamous metaplasia

Assign appropriate CPT code(s) for the preceding procedures and indicate the index entries that were used to identify the codes. Assign only CPT codes (no E/M codes) and append any applicable modifiers.

Code(s):_____

Index entries:

_____

_____

Surgical Case #52

Operative Report

Preoperative Diagnosis:	End-stage renal disease
Postoperative Diagnosis:	Same
Procedures Performed:	Tenckhoff catheter placement-permanent
	Acute hemodialysis catheter placement
Anesthesia:	IV sedation and 1% lidocaine with epinephrine local
Specimens:	None
Complications:	None

Indications for Procedure: This 74-year-old male patient had progressive renal disease secondary to diabetes and was suffering from increasing volume overload with inadequate renal function progressing to end-stage disease. Nephrology recommended peritoneal dialysis and acute hemodialysis for volume control.

Details of Procedure: With the patient supine and after sedation was administered, the left clavicular area was prepped and draped as a sterile field. 1% lidocaine was then infiltrated under the clavicle and a 7.4 French dual lumen acute hemodialysis catheter was placed. Access was gained with a needle and the guide wire passed and the dilator and catheter were placed without difficulty. The ports aspirated easily of venous blood and were flushed with heparinized saline solution. The catheter was secured with suture and dressing applied. A chest x-ray was obtained in the recovery room, which revealed good position of the catheter. The abdomen was then prepped and draped as a sterile field. 1% lidocaine was infiltrated in a left midabdominal area and a small transverse incision was made. The subcutaneous tissue and anterior rectus sheath were opened with cautery and then the posterior rectus sheath exposed after retracting the muscle. A small incision was made after infiltrating additional local. A separate stab incision was made in the left lateral abdomen and a Tenckhoff catheter tunneled in a curved fashion to exit at this site. A catheter guide was then placed over the catheter and this was used to insert the intra-abdominal portion into the pelvis. Two pursestring sutures of Vicryl were placed in the posterior rectus and peritoneum, and a good watertight seal was obtained. There was a moderate amount of ascites noted. The rectus was then closed with Vicryl and the subcutaneous tissue with Vicryl as well. The skin was closed with Monocryl. The catheter was connected to infusion of warm saline, and it flowed freely and good back flow was noted as well. A sterile dressing was applied. The patient tolerated the procedures well and was sent to recovery in good condition.

Assign appropriate CPT code(s) for the preceding procedures and indicate the index entries that were used to identify the codes. Assign only CPT codes (no E/M codes) and append any applicable modifiers.

Code(s):_____

Index entries:

_____

_____

Surgical Case #53

Endoscopy Report

Procedure:	Gastroenterology consultation/gastroscopy/esophageal dilatation
Indications:	This is a 72-year-old female who has had dysphagia for solids for some time. Barium swallow showed a smooth stricture at the LES. She is generally in good health otherwise except for hypertension. Because of her dysphagia, upper GI endoscopy is done today.
Details of Procedure:	She was premedicated with Versed. Conscious sedation was monitored in the usual fashion. The Olympus video endoscope was introduced into the esophagus. The distal esophagus has a tight stricture at the LES. The stomach, pyloric channel, duodenal bulb, and second part of the duodenum were normal. The scope was withdrawn, and she was serially dilated using Maloney dilators.

Assign appropriate CPT code(s) for the preceding procedures and indicate the index entries that were used to identify the codes. Assign only CPT codes (no E/M codes) and append any applicable modifiers.

Code(s):_____

Index entries:

_____

_____

Surgical Case #54

Operative Report

Preoperative Diagnosis:	Squamous cell carcinoma of the left forearm, 8 mm
Postoperative Diagnosis:	Same
Procedure:	Excision of the same with layered primary closure, 4 cm in length
Anesthetic:	Local
Brief Clinical History:	The patient had a biopsy-proven squamous cell carcinoma of the left forearm. After explanation of the risks, benefits, and alternatives, she agreed to re-excision and closure. She understood that there would be a scar as a result.
Details of Procedure:	The patient was taken to the outpatient operating area. An ellipse was taken around the primary lesion with 5 mm margins for excision around the lesion. The area was infiltrated with ½ % Xylocaine with 1:200,000 epinephrine and approximately 5 cc was used. The area was prepared with Betadine paint and draped in a sterile manner. The lesion was elliptically excised and closed in layers with 4-0PDS. The deep subcutaneous layer was closed separately and then a running subcuticular layer was performed. She tolerated the procedure well. She was given instructions for local care and will return in nine days for a checkup and suture removal.

Assign appropriate CPT code(s) for the preceding procedures and indicate the index entries that were used to identify the codes. Assign only CPT codes (no E/M codes) and append any applicable modifiers.

Code(s):_____

Index entries:

_____

_____

Surgical Case #55

Operative Report

Preoperative Diagnosis:	Right true vocal cord lesion
Postoperative Diagnosis:	Same
Operative Procedure:	Direct laryngoscopy with excision of right true vocal cord lesion
Findings:	Firm right true vocal cord lesion and some scarring on the right true vocal cord, otherwise normal laryngoscopy
Indication for the Procedure:	This is a 51-year-old gentleman who had a history of anterior commissure nodule that was biopsied back in 2001 and came back as benign. He was lost to follow-up, but came back with increasing hoarseness and was found on flexible laryngoscopy to have a mid-right-sided true vocal cord lesion. He was brought to the operating room today for laryngoscopy and removal of this lesion.
Details of the Procedure:	He was brought and placed in the supine position on the operating room table and mask anesthesia was induced. Once deeper anesthesia had been achieved, the table was turned towards the laryngoscopy instrumentation. Dedo laryngoscope was placed carefully into the mouth after the upper gums were protected using a wet gauze. The lingual surface of the epiglottis appeared normal as did the vallecula. The laryngeal surface of the epiglottis also appeared completely normal as did the arytenoids and false vocal cords bilaterally. The true vocal cords were bilaterally mobile. They were slightly edematous and there was an approximately 1.5 cm whitish nodule on the right vocal cord in the middle third of the cord. There was a small area of heaped mucosa near the anterior commissure that was slightly hard, but deemed normal and another one at the vocal process that again had normal mucosa, but was slightly firm like some scarring. Again, the left true vocal cord was completely normal except for slight edema. The posterior commissure area appeared normal. Again, the arytenoids were visualized and were thought to be completely normal. At this point, an LTA was sprayed and the patient was intubated. Completion of the direct laryngoscopy revealed a normal piriform sinus on the left normal postcricoid area and a normal right piriform sinus. At this point, the laryngoscope was replaced such that the right vocal cord was easily visualized and palpated. It was suspended at this time. At this point, the operating microscope was brought into place, through the #400 lens, the vocal cord was easily inspected and palpated. A right biting forceps was used to retract the mid-third of the right vocal cord and a leftward scissors was used to dissect the area where this lesion was noted on the vocal cord. This did include the medial aspect of the true cord on that side. Once this was excised in toto, it was sent off for permanent pathology. There was minimal bleeding at the site. The microscope and Dedo laryngoscope were taken out of the field, and the patient was returned to Anesthesia for reawakening, extubation, and transported to the Postanesthesia Care Unit in a stable condition. Dr. Fowler was present for this entire case.

Pathology Report

Specimen:	Right true vocal cord lesion
Gross description:	One specimen is received in formalin labeled with demographics and "right true vocal cord." It consists of a 0.2 × 0.1 × 0.1 cm white tissue fragment. The specimen is stained with eosin and entirely submitted in one cassette.
Microscopic Exam/ Diagnosis:	Squamous mucosa with focal moderate dysplasia

Assign appropriate CPT code(s) for the preceding procedures and indicate the index entries that were used to identify the codes. Assign only CPT codes (no E/M codes) and append any applicable modifiers.

Code(s):_____

Index entries:

_____

_____

Surgical Case #56

Operative Report

Preoperative Diagnosis: Previous history of polyps

Postoperative Diagnosis: Descending colon polyp

Operation: Colonoscopy total and polypectomy of descending colon polyp

Procedure: Patient was placed in the left lateral position. After adequate sedation the 168 cm videoscope was passed through the rectum, through the sigmoid colon, through descending colon, through transverse colon to the right colon. The position of the cecum was confirmed. The cecum and the right colon were found to be normal. The transverse colon was found to be normal. In the descending colon there was a small 3 mm size polyp. This was removed with use of cold knife forceps. The polyp was then given out for histopathology. The base of the polyp was electrocoagulated. The remainder of the colon was found to be normal except for diverticulosis involving sigmoid colon. Rectum was found to be normal except for hypertrophied anal polyp. The scope was removed. The patient tolerated the procedure well and was transferred to the recovery room in fair condition.

Assign appropriate CPT code(s) for the preceding procedures and indicate the index entries that were used to identify the codes. Assign only CPT codes (no E/M codes) and append any applicable modifiers.

Code(s):_____

Index entries:

_____

_____

Emergency Department Record Case #57

Operative Report (Emergency Room)

Preoperative Diagnosis:	Multiple lacerations to both ears
Preoperative Diagnosis:	Multiple lacerations to both ears, a laceration to the left ear and a series of four lacerations to the right ear
Anesthetic:	Local anesthetic was used, 1% Carbocaine plain
Indications:	The patient sustained the above-named lacerations when she was involved in a hay wagon accident.
Procedure:	The patient was treated in the Emergency Department. The right ear was dealt with first. The two smaller, more superficial lacerations, measuring 1.0 cm each were closed after the wound had been infiltrated with 1% Carbocaine and then cleaned copiously with Betadine, Saline, and Peroxide. They were closed with simple interrupted #6-0 Prolene sutures. The two other lacerations on the right ear, total of 3 cm in length, and two different lacerations were closed in the deep layer with #5-0 Vicryl suture after they had been infiltrated with 1% Carbocaine, prepped and draped in the appropriate fashion using Betadine, Peroxide, and Saline. The superficial layers were closed with interrupted #6-0 Prolene suture. After the right ear was completed the wounds were covered with Polysporin. The left ear was then dealt with after the 2.0 cm wound was infiltrated with 1% Carbocaine. After the wound was cleaned with Betadine, Saline, and Peroxide, the superficial layers were closed with interrupted #6-0 Prolene suture. The wounds were then covered with Polysporin.
Follow-Up:	The patient was instructed to follow up and take the sutures out in 6-7 days.

Assign appropriate CPT code(s) for the preceding procedures and indicate the index entries that were used to identify the codes. Assign only CPT codes (no E/M codes) and append any applicable modifiers.

Code(s):_____

Index entries:

_____

_____

Surgical Case #58

Operative Report

Preprocedure Diagnosis(es):
1. Backache, unspecified
2. Work-related back and leg pain

Procedure(s) Performed: Lumbar epidural steroid injection L5-S1 interspace

Indications for Procedure: The patient is a 41-year-old male with severe work-related back and leg pain, more left than right. The patient understands the reasons for the procedure and the risk associated with it. The patient is anxious and needed IV sedation and tolerated the pain associated with injection.

Details of Procedure: For the procedure, the patient was sedated with 2 mg of Versed and 1250 mg of Alfenta. The patient was monitored throughout the procedure and afterwards with pulse oximeter and Dinamap. The pulse oximetry ranged in the lower and upper 90 range. The patient tolerated the IV well; therefore, the procedure well.

For the procedure, the patient was placed prone on the fluoroscopy table with a pillow under his abdomen. We identified the sacral hiatus. Prepped the skin with alcohol and DuraPrep and applied drapes and anesthetized the skin with Xylocaine.

Next, we used fluoroscopy to guide the 17-gauge needle into the spinal canal through the sacral hiatus. This was advanced under AP and lateral fluoroscopic guidance with loss of resistance. We verified proper depth and placement with myelography injection.

The lumbar myelography injection was extradural in the lumbosacral area and consisted of 2 cc of Isovue 300. This showed we were in the spinal canal and highlighting the nerve roots at the lumbosacral region.

Next, we placed the catheter to the L5–S1 interspace. Through the catheter we injected steroid solution that contained 80 mg of Depo-Medrol, 3 cc of 0.75% Marcaine, and 4 cc of Omnipaque 300. This was injected under fluoroscopy, visualizing the nerve roots well throughout the lower lumbar area, more left than right. We cleared the catheter and needle of solution and removed them from the back. Permanent films were taken, and the patient was taken to the recovery room where he recovered in good condition.

Interpretation of Permanent Films: The permanent films afterwards verified the myelography and steroid solution were in the proper areas. On AP and lateral views, the solution highlighted the nerve roots at the lower lumbar area, but scar tissue is preventing the spread of medication throughout the entire region. Nerve roots do highlight in the lower lumbar spine. No evidence of dural puncture.

Assign appropriate CPT code(s) for the preceding procedures and indicate the index entries that were used to identify the codes. Assign only CPT codes (no E/M codes) and append any applicable modifiers.

Code(s):_____

Index entries:

_____

_____

Surgical Case #59

Operative Report

Preoperative Diagnosis: Bladder neck contracture, status post radical retropubic prostatectomy

Postoperative Diagnosis: Same

Procedure: Cystoscopy with dilation

Indications for Procedure: The patient is a 58-year-old male who underwent a radical prostatectomy in 2004. Postoperatively, he has had problems with bladder neck contractures requiring dilation. His last dilation was done in November 2004. He had been performing intermittent catheterization following this with good results of continence. Unfortunately, over the past several months, he had been unable to pass this catheter and appeared to be in urinary retention. He was scheduled for cystoscopy and dilation of bladder neck contracture accordingly. All alternative treatment options as well as risks and benefits and expected outcomes of the procedure were explained to the patient prior to the procedure and he understood these and wished to proceed.

Findings: Severe bladder neck contracture was noted. It was approximately #5 French in diameter.

Details of Procedure: After informed consent was obtained and the patient received 1 g of ampicillin and 100 mg of gentamicin IV, the patient was brought to the operating theater and placed in supine fashion. After adequate sedation, the patient was placed in the dorsal lithotomy position; his genitalia and perineum were prepped and draped in the usual sterile fashion. Using a # 22.5 French sheath, a scope was inserted into the patient's urethra and subsequently into the bladder. A long filiform was passed through the bladder neck contracture. Subsequent dilation from #8 French to #20 French was carried out. After approximately #16 French, it is very difficult to pass the dilator and therefore this was determined at the #20 French dilation. Another attempt at placing the filiform or followers was discontinued at approximately #14 French because of difficulty in passing the followers.

The filiform was then removed, and under direct visualization, an Amplatz super stiff guide wire was inserted into the bladder with the aid of a Pollack catheter to the #5 French open-ended catheter. The renal Amplatz dilators were then utilized to dilate the bladder neck contracture to #18 French. A #18 French Councill catheter was then inserted over the guide wire into the bladder. 10 cc was inflated into the balloon and the wire was removed. Irrigation confirmed that this was in the bladder. Patient was taken to the recovery room in satisfactory condition.

Assign appropriate CPT code(s) for the preceding procedures and indicate the index entries that were used to identify the codes. Assign only CPT codes (no E/M codes) and append any applicable modifiers.

Code(s):_____

Index entries:

_____

_____

Surgical Case #60

Operative Report

Preoperative Diagnosis:	Stab wound, left thigh
Postoperative Diagnosis:	Stab wound, left thigh with arterial bleeders secondary to branches off the deep femoral
Procedures Performed:	Exploration of left thigh stab wound with control of bleeding and repair of rectus femoris muscle
Indications for Procedure:	This 24-year-old gentleman was stabbed in the left anteromedial thigh earlier this morning. He presented to the emergency room, and the exam revealed a 1 cm stab wound about 20 cm below the inguinal ligament in the mid-thigh anteromedial. Posterior tibial pulses were equal bilaterally. There was no swelling in his foot or calf. He was explored in the emergency room, and it was obvious that there was a huge cavity within the rectus femoris muscle. Nothing further was done there and he was brought to the operating room.
Details of Procedure:	The patient was placed on the operating table in the supine position. General endotracheal anesthesia was induced, endotracheal tube was used. Left leg was prepped with Betadine and then draped. Enlarged the stab wound medial and laterally in oblique fashion, carried it down to the muscle, opened up the anterior fascia of the rectus femoris, got into a large cavity within it that went down almost to the femur. At the base of this there were two small pumping vessels that were electrocoagulated, which pretty much controlled the bleeding. There were then multiple small bleeders within the muscle belly itself that we coagulated. The wound was copiously irrigated, rechecked, and little bleeders Bovied and the bleeding was controlled. We evacuated all the hematoma that was present. Cleaned it out, irrigated it again, rechecked it, and no further bleeding. The anterior fascia was closed with interrupted 2-0 Vicryl, and subcutaneous tissue was irrigated and the skin closed with staples, 4 × 4 Kerlix and Ace wrap over that. The patient tolerated the procedure well. Estimated blood loss of the actual procedure was only about 50 cc. He was extubated and taken to the recovery room in stable condition.

Assign appropriate CPT code(s) for the preceding procedures and indicate the index entries that were used to identify the codes. Assign only CPT codes (no E/M codes) and append any applicable modifiers.

Code(s):_____

Index entries:

_____

_____

Appendix D

Answers to Chapter Review Exercises

Chapter 1: Introduction to Clinical Coding

Exercise 1.1 Introduction

1. The American Medical Association (AMA) updates the CPT codes, and the Centers for Medicare and Medicaid Services (CMS) updates the HCPCS National Codes (Level II).

2. Four

3. ICD-9-CM and HCPCS

4. a. Diagnosis: ICD-9-CM
      Procedure: HCPCS

   b. Diagnosis: ICD-9-CM
      Procedure: HCPCS

   c. UB-92 (CMS-1450)

5. ICD-9-CM

6. Procedure code 11440 is linked with diagnosis code #1 (216.3). Procedure code 82951 is linked with diagnosis code #3 (790.6).

   Note: Depending on the carrier, you may link more than one reference number in block 24E whereas some payers require just one. When reporting more than one code on a CMS-1500 claim, enter the code with the highest fee in line 1 of block 24 and the remaining in descending order of charges.

Chapter 2: Application of the CPT System

Exercise 2.1 Organization of CPT

1. Surgery
2. E/M services
3. Pathology and laboratory
4. Category II codes
5. Medicine
6. Radiology
7. Anesthesia
8. Category III codes
9. Maternal care and delivery
10. Case management services
11. Radiation oncology
12. Surgical pathology

Exercise 2.2 CPT Conventions

1. Repair blood vessel, direct; hand, finger
2. Two
3. Revised descriptor
4. Esophagoscopy, rigid or flexible, with insertion of plastic tube or stent
5. New descriptor
6. No
7. No
8. 13152, 13153
9. 40814
10. 37578, 31576

Exercise 2.3 Use of the Alphabetical Index

1. 23400   Green operation to scapulopexy
2. 10021   Aspiration, cyst, thyroid
3. 35556   Graft, *see* Bypass graft, Popliteal
4. 49555   Hernia repair, femoral, recurrent
5. 26991   Incision and drainage, bursa, hip
6. 01680   Anesthesia, shoulder
7. 31525   Laryngoscopy, direct
8. 72149   MRI to magnetic resonance imaging, spine, lumbar
9. 11055   Paring, skin lesion, benign hyperkeratotic, single lesion
10. 86701   HIV-1, antibody
11. 41105   Biopsy, tongue
12. 43239   Esophagogastro-duodenoscopy, *see* Endoscopy, gastrointestinal, upper, biopsy
13. 29881   Arthroscopy, surgical, knee
14. 95827   EEG, *see* Electro-encephalography, sleep
15. 65220   Removal, foreign body, cornea, without slip lamp
16. 58356   Endometrial Ablation; or Cryoablation, *see* Cryosurgery, *see* Destruction, endometrial

    Note: In CPT 2004, this code was 0009T. This is a good example of a Category III code being moved to Category I.
17. 4006F   Beta-blocker therapy, *see* Performance Measures
18. 0065T   Ocular Photoscreening
19. 76077   DXA, *see* Dual x-ray Absorptiometry, vertebral fracture
20. 25112   Ganglion, Cyst, Wrist Excision (25111–25112)

Exercise 2.4 CPT Coding Process

1. Colonoscopy and polypectomy
2. 45384–45385

3. How was the polyp removed (hot biopsy forceps, snare, and so on)?
4. "Was removed with hot biopsy forceps and retrieved"
5. 45384

Exercise 2.5 CPT Coding Process

1. Excision
2. Can be located under Excision, lesion, skin; or Lesion, skin, excision

    Selections: Benign   11400–11471
    Malignant 11600–11646
3. Pathological diagnosis indicates that the lesion was malignant (11600–11646).
4. Documentation is needed to code malignant lesion, size of lesion + margins (or size of excision) (2.0 cm + 0.5 cm + 0.5 cm = 3.0 cm excision site) and site (arm).
5. 11603

Exercise 2.6 CPT Coding Process

1. Hernia repair
2. Index entries: Hernia repair, umbilical; Hernia repair; Hernia, Repair, hernia, umbilical. Codes to review: 49580–49587
3. Age of patient; incarcerated or strangulated hernia
4. Review of documentation (38-year-old patient and no documentation for incarcerated/strangulated hernia). Using the abstracted documentation and process of elimination, the correct code would be 49585.
5. Wound closure would be an integral part of the procedure and would not be assigned a CPT code.

Exercise 2.7 Coding References

1. 45380
2. *CPT Assistant,* January 1996, page 7, instructs the coder to assign 45385. *CPT Assistant,* January 2004, states that if a small polyp is removed via cold knife biopsy, the appropriate code is 45380. This is a good example of the need to research the most current coding advice.

Exercise 2.8 Coding References

1. When a biopsy of a lesion is obtained and the remaining portion of the *same* lesion is then excised/fulgurated, only the code for the excision/fulguration should be used. When the biopsy is taken from a *different* lesion than the one excised, the biopsy code and an additional code for the removal of the separate lesion are reported. It would be appropriate to append modifier –59 to the code reported for the biopsy procedure.

2. Reference: In addition to the PRO letter, *CPT Assistant,* February 1999, page 11.

Exercise 2.9 Chapter 2 Review

1. Bullet

2. 11100 and 11101

3. Category III

4. 42320

5. 40843

6. Removal of <80% of vulvar area and there was removal of skin and deep subcutaneous tissue (See the note before CPT code 56405.)

7. Method of removal

8. No. Versed is a type of conscious sedation. The ⊙ symbol appears before code 43235; therefore, administration/monitoring of conscious sedation would be inherent in the procedure.

9. 76857, based on the definitions provided in the note before code 76830

10. 11730, 11732, 11732

Chapter 3: Modifiers

Exercise 3.1 Chapter 3 Review

1. 55

2. 77

3. 51

4. 62

5. 53

6. 64721–50   Carpal tunnel syndrome

7. 11730–FA   Avulsion, nails

8. 11043–73   Debridement, skin

9. 93922–52   Doppler scan, arterial studies, extremities

10. 19102–LT   Biopsy, breast

11. 28485–RT   Fracture, metatarsal, open

               (*Note:* –T9 is not applicable in this case because the procedure refers to the bones of the foot, not the toes.)

Chapter 4: Surgery

Exercise 4.1 Integumentary System

1. 11421   Excision, skin, lesion, benign; or

    11402   Lesion, skin, excision, benign

2. 17000   Lesion, skin, destruction, benign

    17003, 17003, 17003

3. 11642   Excision, skin, lesion, malignant; or Lesion, skin, excision, malignant

4. 11200   Skin, tags, removal

5. 11403   Lesion, skin, excision, benign

6. 11644   Lesion, skin, excision, malignant

7. 11641   Lesion, skin, excision, malignant

    11640

Exercise 4.2 Integumentary System

1. 11442   Excision, skin, lesion, benign; or Lesion, skin, excision, benign

Exercise 4.3 Integumentary System

1. 11308   Lesion, skin, shaving

Exercise 4.4 Integumentary System

1. 12002   Wound, repair; or Repair, wound, simple
2. 12032   Wound, repair; or Repair, wound, intermediate
3. 12041   Wound, repair; or Repair, wound, intermediate
    12002   Wound, repair; or Repair, wound, simple (sum of repairs)

Exercise 4.5 Integumentary System

1. 12001   Wound, repair; or Repair, wound, simple

Exercise 4.6 Integumentary System

1. 12032   Wound, repair; or Repair wound (simple and intermediate)
    12005

Exercise 4.7 Integumentary System

1. 13121   Wound, repair (complex)
    13122

Exercise 4.8 Integumentary System

1. 11603   Lesion, skin, excision, malignant
    12031   Wound, repair (intermediate)

Exercise 4.9 Integumentary System

1. 14021   Skin graft and flap, tissue transfer

Exercise 4.10 Integumentary System

1. 15120   Skin-thickness autograft
    11646   Excision, skin, lesion, malignant; or Lesion, skin, excision, malignant

Exercise 4.11 Integumentary System

1. 15100   Skin-thickness autograft
    15000
    15040   Harvesting, skin

Exercise 4.12 Integumentary System

1. 19000–LT   Breast, cyst, puncture aspiration

Exercise 4.13 Integumentary System

1. 19125–LT   Excision, breast, cyst; or Breast, excision, lesion by needle localization

    Note: The hospital also would assign 19290 for placement of the wire. The surgeon would not assign this code because the radiologist performed the procedure.

Exercise 4.14 Integumentary System

1. 19120–RT   Breast, excision, cyst; or Excision, breast, cyst

    Note: The entire nodule was excised, not just a piece of tissue, which is implied with the term *biopsy.*

Exercise 4.15 Integumentary System Review

1. 16020   Burn, dressings
2. 14020   Skin graft and Flap, tissue transfer

    Note: Excision of lesion is included and should not be assigned an additional code.
3. 12032   Wound, repair

    Note: Anatomic modifiers (LT, RT) are not appropriate.
4. 19102–LT   Breast, biopsy
    19295–LT   Breast, metallic localization clip placement

5. 11606   Lesion, skin, excision, malignant

6. 11770   Pilonidal cyst, excision (Single-layer closure indicates "simple.")

7. 11750–TA   Nails, removal

8. 15781   Dermabrasion

9. 17273   Skin, destruction, malignant lesion

10. 15931   Decubitus ulcer, *see* Debridement; Pressure Ulcer

Exercise 4.16 Musculoskeletal System

1. 25545–LT   Fracture, ulna, shaft, open treatment

2. 21800   Fracture, rib, closed treatment

    21800

3. 23605–RT   Fracture, humerus, closed with manipulation

4. 27532–RT   Fracture, tibia, closed treatment (initial cast application included with treatment code)

5. 27562–RT   Dislocation, patella, closed treatment

6. 27514–LT   Fracture, femur, distal

7. 24516–RT   Fracture, humerus, shaft, open

Exercise 4.17 Musculoskeletal System

1. 29515–RT   Splint, leg, short

    Note: E/M code 99283–25 is applicable in this case.

Exercise 4.18 Musculoskeletal System

1. 27788–LT   Fracture, fibula, closed treatment; or Fracture fibula, with manipulation

Exercise 4.19 Musculoskeletal System

1. 29875–LT   Arthroscopy, surgical, knee

2. 29827–RT   Arthroscopy, surgical, shoulder

3. 29846–LT   Arthroscopy, surgical, wrist

4. 29837–LT   Arthroscopy, surgical, elbow

Exercise 4.20 Musculoskeletal System

1. 29882–RT   Arthroscopy, surgical, knee

Exercise 4.21 Musculoskeletal System Review

1. 28475–LT   Fracture, metatarsal, closed

    28475–LT

2. 28285–T1   Hammertoe repair

3. 27766–RT   Fracture, ankle, medial

4. 20101   Wound, exploration

5. 23030   Hematoma, shoulder

6. 24343–RT   Ligament, repair, elbow

7. 28730–LT   Arthrodesis, tarsal joint

8. 29844–RT   Arthroscopy, surgical, wrist

9. 28108–T2   Excision, cyst, phalanges, toe

10. 27372–RT   Removal, foreign body, knee joint

Exercise 4.22 Respiratory System

1. 31255–50   Ethmoidectomy, endoscopic

2. 31238–LT   Endoscopy, nose; or Nose, endoscopy

3. 31233–50   Sinusoscopy, maxillary

Exercise 4.23 Respiratory System

1. 30520   Septoplasty

    31267–50   Endoscopy, nose, surgical

    30140–50   Turbinate, excision

Exercise 4.24 Respiratory System

1. 31540   Laryngoscopy, direct
2. 31577   Laryngoscopy, fiberoptic
3. 31510   Laryngoscopy, indirect
4. 31541   Laryngoscopy, direct

Exercise 4.25 Respiratory System

1. 31536   Laryngoscopy, direct

Exercise 4.26 Respiratory System

1. 31628   Bronchoscopy, biopsy
2. 31641   Bronchoscopy, removal, tumor
3. 31625   Bronchoscopy, biopsy

    31623   Bronchoscopy, brushings

Exercise 4.27 Respiratory System

1. 31623   Bronchoscopy, brushing

Exercise 4.28 Respiratory System Review

1. 32657   Thoracoscopy, surgical with wedge resection of lung
2. 30110   Polyp, nose, excision, simple
3. 31625   Bronchoscopy, biopsy
4. 30300   Removal, foreign bodies, nose
5. 31237   Endoscopy, surgical, nose
6. 30903–50   Epistaxis
7. 31540   Laryngoscopy, direct
8. 32420   Aspiration, lung puncture, *see* Pneumocentesis
9. 31576   Laryngoscopy, fiberoptic
10. 30130   Excision, inferior turbinate

Exercise 4.29 Cardiovascular System

1. 33207   Pacemaker, heart, insertion; or Insertion, pacemaker

Exercise 4.30 Cardiovascular System

1. 36590   Removal, venous access device

Exercise 4.31 Cardiovascular System

1. 36556   Insertion, venous access device, central

Exercise 4.32 Cardiovascular System Review

1. 33222   Pacemaker, revise pocket
2. 36833   Arteriovenous Fistula, Revision, hemodialysis fistula, with thrombectomy
3. 33824   Ductus Arteriosus, repair
4. 36215   Catheterization, brachiocephalic artery
5. 36582   Venous Access Device, replacement
6. 36870   Arteriovenous Fistula, thrombectomy, graft; or Thrombectomy, arteriovenous fistula, graft
7. 35493   Atherectomy, percutaneous, femoral
8. 33464   Valvuloplasty, tricuspid valve
9. 33246   Insertion, pacing cardio-defibrillator
10. 37720–50   Vein, stripping

Exercise 4.33 Digestive System

1. 43202   Endoscopy, esophagus, biopsy

    43217   Endoscopy, esophagus, removal, polyp

    Note: Modifier –59 would apply.

2. 45305   Proctosigmoidoscopy, biopsy

3. 43258   Endoscopy, gastrointestinal, upper, destruction of lesion

4. 45380   Endoscopy, colon, biopsy

5. 43264   Bile Duct, endoscopy, removal, calculi

Exercise 4.34 Digestive System

1. 43247   Endoscopy, gastrointestinal, upper, foreign body

Exercise 4.35 Digestive System

1. 45384   Colonoscopy, removal, polyp; or Endoscopy, colon, removal, polyp

Exercise 4.36 Digestive System

1. 45330   Sigmoidoscopy, exploration

Exercise 4.37 Digestive System

1. 49500   Hernia, repair, inguinal

2. 49561–RT   Hernia, repair, incisional, incarcerated

    49568   Implantation, mesh

3. 49651   Laparoscopy, hernia, recurrent

4. 49521   Hernia, repair, inguinal, incarcerated

5. 49585   Hernia, repair, umbilicus

Exercise 4.38 Digestive System

1. 49505–LT   Hernia, repair, inguinal

    Note: Mesh code is only coded with incisional and ventral hernia repairs.

Exercise 4.39 Digestive System Review

1. 46935   Hemorrhoids, destruction

2. 43644   Laparoscopy, gastric restrictive procedures

3. 0008T   Endoscopy, gastrointestinal, upper, suturing

4. 42200   Palatoplasty

5. 45383   Colonoscopy, destruction, lesion

6. 47564   Laparoscopy, cholecystectomy

7. 49521   Hernia Repair, inguinal, recurrent, incarcerated

8. 49322   Laparoscopy, aspiration

9. 46610   Anoscopy, removal, polyp

10. 42809   Removal, foreign body, pharynx

Exercise 4.40 Urinary System

1. 52332   Cystourethroscopy, insertion, indwelling ureteral stent

2. 52234   Cystourethroscopy, with fulguration, lesion/tumor

3. 52353   Cystourethroscopy, lithotripsy

4. 52282   Cystourethroscopy, insertion, urethral stent

Exercise 4.41 Urinary System

1. 52352   Cystourethroscopy, biopsy; or Cystourethroscopy, destruction, lesion

    52332–51–RT   Insertion, stent, ureteral

    Note: Because the stent was inserted at the conclusion of the procedure, one can presume it is an indwelling ureteral stent.

Exercise 4.42 Urinary System

1. 52234   Cystourethroscopy, with fulguration, lesion

Exercise 4.43 Urinary System Review

1. 51992 Sling Operation, stress incontinence
2. 53260 Excision, polyp, urethra
3. 52235 Cystourethroscopy, with fulguration, tumor
4. 51525 Cystotomy, excision, bladder diverticulum
5. 50200 Kidney, biopsy
6. 52351 Cystourethroscopy (range of codes)
7. 52290 Cystourethroscopy, with ureteral meatotomy (bilateral modifier not appropriate because code description specifies "unilateral" or "bilateral")
8. 51785 Electromyography, sphincter muscles, urethral, needle
9. 51701 Insertion, catheter, urethral
10. 50920 Fistula, ureter

Exercise 4.44 Male Genital System

1. 54057 Lesion, penis, destruction, laser surgery
2. 10060 Incision and drainage, abscess, skin
3. 55845 Prostatectomy, retropubic, radical
4. 54861 Epididymectomy, bilateral
5. 54150 Circumcision, with clamp, newborn

Exercise 4.45 Male Genital System

1. 55859 Prostate, brachytherapy, needle insertion

Exercise 4.46 Male Genital System

1. 54520–LT Orchiectomy, simple

Exercise 4.47 Male Genital System Review

1. 54840 Spermatocele, excision
2. 54415 Penile Prosthesis, removal, inflatable
3. 54690 Orchiectomy, laparoscopic
4. 54322 Hypospadias, one state, meatal advancement
5. 54820 Epididymis, exploration, biopsy
6. 55100 Scrotum, abscess, incision and drainage
7. 54240 Penis, plethysmography
8. 54060 Penis, lesion, destruction, surgical excision
9. 54640–50 Orchiopexy, inguinal approach
10. 55866 Laparscopy, prostatectomy

Exercise 4.48 Female Genital System

1. 58670 Laparoscopy, oviduct surgery
2. 58120 Dilation and curettage, corpus uteri
3. 59812 Abortion, incomplete
4. 49322 Laparoscopy, aspiration
5. 58545 Laparoscopy, removal, leiomyomata
6. 58262 Hysterectomy, vaginal, removal tubes/ovaries

Exercise 4.49 Female Genital System

1. 57461 LEEP Procedure

Exercise 4.50 Female Genital System

1. 58558 Hysteroscopy, surgical with biopsy

Exercise 4.51 Female Genital System Review

1. 57455   Colposcopy, biopsy (range of codes)
2. 56620   Vulvectomy, simple, partial (use definitions at beginning of section)
3. 58662   Laparoscopy, destruction, lesion
4. 58150   Hysterectomy, abdominal, total
5. 57023   Incision and Drainage, hematoma, vagina
6. 56605   Biopsy, vulva (external genitalia)
     57105   Biopsy, vagina
7. 58554   Hysterectomy, vaginal
8. 58561   Hysteroscopy, removal, leiomyomata
9. 58290   Hysterectomy, vaginal
10. 58356   Ablation, endometrium, ultrasound guidance

Exercise 4.52 Endocrine System Review

1. 60280   Thyroglossal Duct, cyst, excision
2. 60650   Laparoscopy, adrenal gland, excision

   Note: There are several misleading index entries for this example. Adrenalectomy, laparoscopic, leads to 50545. Same is true for Laparoscopy, adrenalectomy.

3. 60260–50   Thyroid Gland, excision, total, removal of all thyroid tissue
4. 10022   Thyroid gland, cyst, aspiration lists code 60001 (See note under CPT code for fine needle aspiration.)
5. 60500   Parathyroid Gland, excision

Exercise 4.53 Nervous System

1. 64445   Injection, nerve, anesthetic
2. 64702–F8   Neuroplasty, digital nerve
     69990   Operating microscope
3. 62281   Epidural injection
4. 64831–F5   Neurorrhaphy
     64832–F6

Exercise 4.54 Nervous System

1. 63075   Discectomies, *see* Diskectomy
     63076

Exercise 4.55 Nervous System Review

1. 64898–LT   Graft, nerve
     64902–59–RT   Graft, nerve
2. 64712   Neuroplasty, peripheral nerve
3. 64782   Excision, neuroma
4. 64840   Suture, nerve
5. 63272   Laminectomy (range of codes)
6. 62311   Epidural injection (range of codes)
7. 63688   Neurostimulators, removal, pulse generator
8. 63706   Myelomeningocele, repair
9. 64408   Nerves, injection, anesthetic
10. 61312   Craniotomy, surgery (range of codes)

Exercise 4.56 Eye and Ocular Adnexa

1. 66984–LT   Phacoemulsification, removal, extracapsular cataract

Exercise 4.57 Eye and Ocular Adnexa Review

1. 65222   Removal, foreign body, cornea with slit lamp
2. 67810–E1   Biopsy, eyelid
3. 68110   Lesion, conjunctiva
4. 67800–E3   Chalazion
5. 67311   Strabismus, repair, one horizontal muscle
6. 67700–E3   Eyelid, abscess, incision and drainage
7. 67906–E1   Blepharoptosis, repair, superior rectus technique, fascial sling
8. 67961   Eyelid, excisional
9. 67914   Ectropion, repair, suture
10. 67413–RT   Orbitotomy, with removal of foreign body

Exercise 4.58 Auditory System

1. 69436–50   Tympanostomy (–50 for bilateral)

Exercise 4.59 Auditory System Review

1. 69910   Labyrinthectomy with mastoidectomy
2. 69205–LT   Removal, foreign bodies, auditory canal
3. 69636   Tympanoplasty, with mastoidotomy, with ossicular chain reconstruction
4. 69005–LT   Abscess, ear, external, complicated (would expect to see documentation to explain why the procedure took an extensive amount of time)
5. 69401   Eustachian Tube, inflation, without catheterization

Exercise 4.60 Chapter 4 Review

1. 42305   Incision and drainage, abscess, parotid gland
2. 69436–50   Tympanostomy
3. 57455   Colposcopy, biopsy
4. 52234   Cystourethroscopy, excision of tumor; or fulguration
5. 19101–LT   Biopsy, breast
6. 12051   Repair, wound, skin and tissues
7. 26750–F5   Fracture, treatment, phalanx, finger, without manipulation
8. 31536   Laryngoscopy, direct
9. 36569   Venous access device, insertion
10. 45333   Sigmoidoscopy, removal of polyp
11. 49507–50   Hernia repair, inguinal
12. 29834–LT   Arthroscopy, elbow, surgical
13. 26010–FA   Finger, abscess
     26010–F1

Exercise 4.61 Chapter 4 Review

1. 61520–62   (physician #1) Cerebellopontine angle tumor to brain
    61520–62   (physician # 2) Tumor, excision
2. 59840   Abortion, induced by dilatation and curettage
3. 29821–RT   Arthroscopy, surgical, shoulder
4. 33208–55   Pacemaker, heart, insertion
5. 43268   ERCP to cholangio-pancreatography, endoscopic retrograde or bile duct or pancreatic duct
6. 58661–22   Laparoscopy, removal, fallopian tube

7. 68811–50 Nasolacrimal duct, with anesthesia

   Note: Exploration bilateral modifier applies because the code describes one duct.

8. 31267–50 Endoscopy, nose, surgery

9. 44151 Colectomy, total, with ileostomy

10. 27786–79 Fracture treatment, fibula, without manipulation

11. 15783 Dermabrasion

Chapter 5: Radiology

Exercise 5.1 Diagnostic Radiology

1. 74182 Magnetic resonance imaging, abdomen
2. 72131 CT Scan without contrast, spine
3. 72170 X-ray, pelvis
4. 74241 X-ray, gastrointestinal
5. 74430 Cystography

Exercise 5.2 Diagnostic Ultrasound

1. 76831 Hysterosonography, *see* Ultrasound; Sonohysterography
2. 76815 Ultrasound, pregnant uterus
3. 76645 Ultrasound, breasts

Exercise 5.3 Chapter 5 Review

1. 73090–26 X-ray, arm, lower
2. 72142–26 MRI to magnetic resonance imaging, spine, cervical, professional component
3. 74430 Cystography
4. 78460 Nuclear medicine, heart, myocardial perfusion
   78480
5. 76092 Mammogram, screening
6. 75994 Atherectomy, x-ray, renal artery

7. 70460–TC CT scan, with contrast, head
8. 76817 Ultrasound, pregnant uterus
9. 76942 Ultrasound, guidance, needle biopsy
10. 78306 Nuclear medicine, bone, imaging
11. 74270 Barium enema
12. 78205 Nuclear medicine, liver, imaging
13. 77404 Radiation therapy, delivery
14. 78707 Nuclear medicine, kidney, imaging
15. 71020 X-ray, chest
16. 77761 Radioelement, application
17. 72240 Myelography, spine, cervical
18. 76775 Ultrasound, retroperitoneal
19. 73540 X-ray, hip
20. 78262 Reflux study
21. 76775 Ultrasound, kidney Code 76775, limited, is for a single organ. (See *CPT Assistant,* May 1999.)
22. 73510-LT X-ray, Hip (unilateral, 2 views)
    72170 X-ray, pelvis (1–2 views)
23. 71010 X-ray, chest
24. 74241 X-ray, gastrointestinal
25. 70450 CT Scan, without contrast, head

Chapter 6: Pathology and Laboratory Services

Exercise 6.1 Chapter 6 Review

1. 88305   Pathology, surgical, prostate, TUR
2. 83880   Natriuretic
3. 80402   ACTH to adrenocorticotropic hormone, stimulation panel
4. 81003   Urinalysis, automated
5. 85055   Platelet assay
6. 88309   Pathology, surgical, breast mastectomy with regional lymph nodes
7. 86485   Candida skin test
8. 86689   Antibody, HTLV-1
9. 80061   Organ- or disease-oriented
   80051   panel, lipid panel, and electrolyte panel
10. 80198   Drug assay, theophylline
11. 82803   Blood gases—pO_2, pCO_2
12. 86706   Hepatitis antibody, B
13. 85730   Thromboplastin time, partial
    85610   Prothrombin time
14. 88027   Autopsy, gross and microscopic examination
15. 88331   Pathology, surgical, consultation, intraoperative

Chapter 7: Evaluation and Management Services

Exercise 7.1 Evaluation and Management (History)

1. HPI is brief (location, quality, and duration). Review of system(s) is problem specific. No PFSH documented. The history component of this visit would be expanded problem focused (brief HPI, problem-specific ROS, and expanded problem-focused PFSH including past, family and social history). The history component is equal to the lowest category documented.

2. HPI is brief (location, severity, and duration). Review of system(s) is extended (two to nine systems), and PFSH is pertinent (medications). The history is determined by the lowest level from all three categories; therefore, the history level would be expanded problem focused.

3. HPI is extended (location, severity, duration, and context). Review of systems is extended (two to nine systems). The PFSH is complete (two history areas documented). The history level is detailed; all three categories met this level.

Exercise 7.2 Evaluation and Management (Physical Exam)

1. Comprehensive exam: eight body systems were reviewed.

2. Expanded problem-focused exam: two systems reviewed (constitutional and integumentary)

3. Detailed exam. Note that the criteria for expanded problem focused and the detailed category are the same except in the level of specificity in the examination. Decisions on the level of specificity can be somewhat subjective.

Exercise 7.3 Evaluation and Management (Medical Decision Making)

1. Moderate complexity

Category	Documentation	Tabulation
Number of Diagnosis or Treatment Options	New problem; no additional workup planned	3 points = multiple (moderate complexity)
Amount and/or Complexity of Data Reviewed	Review and order clinical lab tests (1 point) Review and order test in radiology section of CPT (1 point)	2 points = limited (low complexity)
Level of Risk	Undiagnosed new problem with uncertain prognosis (presenting problem) Documentation of prescription drug management (mgmt. options)	Moderate complexity
Final Tabulation	Note that medical decision making is determined by the highest two of three	Moderate complexity

2. Low complexity

Category	Documentation	Tabulation
Number of Diagnosis or Treatment Options	Established problem; worsening	2 points = limited
Amount and/or Complexity of Data Reviewed	No data to be reviewed; no tests ordered	0 = minimal/low complexity
Risk Factors	Prescription drug management	Moderate complexity
Final Tabulation	One from each category—choose the middle	Low complexity

3. Straightforward

Category	Documentation	Tabulation
Number of Diagnosis or Treatment Options	Self-limited or minor	1 point = minimal
Amount and/or Complexity of Data Reviewed	No data	Minimal/low complexity
Risk Factors	Acute uncomplicated injury (presenting problem) and over-the-counter meds (management options)	Low complexity
Final Tabulation	Two out of three from straightforward category	Straightforward

Exercise 7.4 Evaluation and Management Case Study

Established Patient History

Elements of History	Documentation	Category
History of Present Illness	Location, duration, associated signs/ manifestations, severity	Extended
Review of Systems	Extended (2–9)	Detailed
PFSH	Complete (2 areas)	Complete
Result (equal to lowest category documented)	Extended is lowest category documented	Detailed history

Physical exam: A total of nine systems were reviewed for a comprehensive exam component.

Medical Decision Making

Category	Documentation	Tabulation
Number of Diagnosis or Treatment Options	New problem; no additional workup planned	3 points = multiple
Amount and/or Complexity of Data Reviewed	Chest x-ray	1 point = minimal/low complexity
Risk Factors	Prescription drug management	Moderate complexity
Final Tabulation	Highest two of three categories	Moderate complexity

1. Review the code descriptions for 99211–99215. Need two out of the three key components. The case study revealed a detailed history and comprehensive examination, and the medical decision making was of moderate complexity. The correct E/M code selection is 99214.

Exercise 7.5 Evaluation and Management

1. True
2. False
3. False
4. False
5. False
6. Extended—Four elements: yesterday (duration); getting ready to go to church (context); vomited bile (quality); deafness at the start (associated signs/symptoms)
7. Expanded problem focused—Systems reviewed: respiratory, integumentary, ENT (ears, throat), cardiovascular, gastrointestinal. Expanded problem focused (two to nine systems)
8. Pertinent—One area (past history)

Exercise 7.6 Chapter 7 Review

1. 99211
2. 99203
3. 99245
4. 99202
5. 99291
6. 99281
7. 99396
8. 99213
9. 99235
10. 99212
11. 99203

Chapter 8: Medicine

Exercise 8.1 Immunizations

1. 90471 Immunization administration
   90710 Vaccines, Measles, Mumps, Rubella and Varicella
2. 90471 Immunization administration
   90703 Vaccine, tetanus
3. 90471 Immunization administration
   90472
   90632 Vaccine, hepatitis A
   90658 Vaccine, influenza

Exercise 8.2 Injections and Infusions

1. 90471 Immunization administration
   90725 Vaccine, cholera
2. 90760 Infusion therapy, hydration
3. 90471 Immunization administration
   90748 Vaccines, hepatitis B and Hemophilus influenza B
4. 90782 Injection, intramuscular, therapeutic (Also, J3420 would be assigned for specific substance.)

Exercise 8.3 Psychiatry

1. 90885 Psychiatric diagnosis, evaluation of records
2. 90847 Psychotherapy, family
3. 90806 Psychiatric treatment, individual, insight oriented

Exercise 8.4 Dialysis

1. 90921 Dialysis, end-stage renal disease
2. 90945 Dialysis, peritoneal

Exercise 8.5 Ophthalmology

1. 92018 Gonioscopy (See note under code.)
2. 92004 Ophthalmology, Diagnostic, Eye Exam, New patient

Exercise 8.6 Cardiovascular Services

1. 93025 Cardiology, electro-cardiogram, Microvolt T-wave Alternans

2. 93510 Catheterization, cardiac, left

   93545 Injection, cardiac catheterization

   93556 Imaging, *see* Vascular Studies, cardiac catheterization

3. 92977 Thrombolysis, coronary vessels

4. 93015 Stress Tests, cardiovascular

5. 92995–LC Atherectomy, percutaneous, coronary

   92996–LD

   Note: Do not report angioplasty because it was performed on the same vessel.

6. 92982–LD Percutaneous Transluminal Angioplasty, coronary

   92984–RC

Exercise 8.7 Pulmonary Services

1. 94060 Pulmonary, spirometry

2. 94660 CPAP, *see* Continuous Postive Airway Pressure

3. 94450 Pulmonary, diagnostic, hypoxia response curve

Exercise 8.8 Allergy and Clinical Immunology

1. 95010 Allergy Test, skin, venoms

2. 95120 Allergen Immunotherapy

Exercise 8.9 Chemotherapy Services

1. 96413 Chemotherapy, intravenous
   96415 *Note:* J code for Cisplatin would also be assigned.

2. 96420 Chemotherapy, intra-arterial

Exercise 8.10 Physical Medicine and Rehabilitation

1. 97032 × 2 Physical Medicine, modalities, electric stimulation

2. 97113 × 2 Physical Medicine, aquatic therapy

3. 97006 Physical Medicine, athletic training

4. 97602 Wound debridement, non-selective

Exercise 8.11 Chapter 8 Review

1. 90937 Hemodialysis

2. 90707 Immunization, active, measles, mumps, rubella

   90471 Administration of immunization

3. 93010 EKG to electrocardiogram, evaluation

4. 96413 Chemotherapy, intravenous
   96415 x 2

5. 93600 Electrophysiology Procedure

6. 92556 Audiologic function tests, audiometry, speech

7. 90772 Injection, intramuscular,
   99070 therapeutic; supply, materials used during office visit

8. 90812 Psychotherapy, individual, interactive, office or outpatient

9. 92995 Atherectomy, percutaneous,
   92996 coronary; single vessel; additional vessel

10. 92014–25 Ophthalmology,
    92283 diagnostic, eye exam established patient; color vision exam

11. 92982 Percutaneous Transluminal Angioplasty, coronary

92973 Thrombectomy, percutaneous, coronary artery

92980 Coronary Artery, insertion, stent

12. 97520 × 3 Prosthesis training
13. 99050 Special services, after-hours medical services
14. 93925 Duplex scan, arterial studies, lower extremity
15. 95863 EMG to electromyography, needle, extremities
16. 96920 Psoriasis Treatment
17. 98926 Manipulation, osteopathic
18. 99502 Home Services, newborn care
19. 94640 Inhalation Treatment
20. 95807 Sleep Study

Chapter 9: Anesthesia

Exercise 9.1 Chapter 9 Review

1. 00406–P2 Anesthesia, breast
2. 01730–P1 Anesthesia, arm upper
99100
3. 00562–P4 Anesthesia, heart
4. 00540–P3 Anesthesia, lung
5. 00350–P1 Anesthesia, neck
6. 50240–P2 Nephrectomy, partial
7. 33945–P5 Heart transplant
99100
99140
8. 35301–P3 Thromboendarterectomy, carotid
99100
9. 47563–P1 Laparoscopy, cholecystectomy
10. 66984–P2 Cataract extraction, removal with prosthesis
99100

Chapter 10: HCPCS Level II

Exercise 10.1 Chapter 10 Review

1. E0196 Mattress, gel pressure
2. A4550 Surgical, tray
3. J3420 Vitamin, B$_{12}$
4. A4490 Surgical, stocking
5. J0560 Penicillin G benzathine and penicillin G procaine
6. 11975 Insertion, contraceptive capsules

A4260 Implant, contraceptive
7. 29540 Strapping, ankle
E0112 Crutches
8. 12011 Wound, repair

Note: CMS instructs coders not to assign a modifier: "Do not use a modifier to indicate an anatomical site location on body (modifier 50 or Level II modifiers) if the narrative definition of a code indicates multiple occurrences."

9. 11730–TA Avulsion, nails
11732–T1
10. 26055–F8 Trigger finger repair

Chapter 11: Reimbursement in the Ambulatory Setting

Exercise 11.1 Chapter 11 Review

1. Incorrect. Because all repairs were of the same type (simple) and same site classification, the lacerations may be added together. The correct CPT code is 12014. Note that the use of modifiers is not appropriate with these codes.
2. Incorrect. The CPT codebook provides codes 11200–11201 to report any type of removal of skin tags. The correct code is 11200.

3. Incorrect. A diagnostic colonoscopy is included in a surgical colonoscopy; only the code for the surgical colonoscopy is assigned (45385).

4. Incorrect. Code 52214 is in the urethra and bladder section and does not correctly identify the procedure. The correct code is 52354.

5. Incorrect. Code 58720 is identified as a separate procedure and thus should not be used with 58150.

6. Incorrect. Code 80076 is an incorrect code. The test to measure alanine amino transferase (ALT) (SGPT) was not performed. Total protein was not performed. The correct answer is 82040, 82247, 82248, 84075, 84450.

7. Incorrect. The D&C is included in the hysteroscopy code and does not warrant the additional code of 58120. NCCI lists 58558 as comprehensive code and 58120 as a component.

8. Correct.

9. Incorrect. The lesion was incorrectly coded as benign. CPT code 11642 is the correct code.

10. Incorrect. CPT code 31622 is a separate procedure code and should not be used with 31623. The only code needed is 31623.

Glossary

Abstracting: 1. The process of extracting information from a document to create a brief summary of a patient's illness, treatment, and outcome. 2. The process of extracting elements of data from a source document or database and entering them into an automated system

Acute care prospective payment system: The reimbursement system for inpatient hospital services provided to Medicare and Medicaid beneficiaries that is based on the use of diagnosis-related groups as a classification tool

Ambulatory care: Preventive or corrective healthcare services provided on a nonresident basis in a provider's office, clinic setting, or hospital outpatient setting

Ambulatory payment classification (APC) relative weight: A number reflecting the expected resource consumption of cases associated with each APC, relative to the average of all APCs, that is used in determining payment for hospital outpatient services provided to Medicare and Medicaid beneficiaries

Ambulatory payment classification (APC) system: The prospective payment system used since 2000 for reimbursement of hospitals for outpatient services provided to Medicare and Medicaid beneficiaries

Ambulatory surgery: An elective surgical procedure performed on a patient who is classified as an outpatient and who is usually released from the surgical facility on the day of surgery

Ambulatory surgery center or ambulatory surgical center (ASC): Under Medicare, an outpatient surgical facility that has its own national identifier; is a separate entity with respect to its licensure, accreditation, governance, professional supervision, administrative functions, clinical services, record keeping, and financial and accounting systems; has as its sole purpose the provision of services in connection with surgical procedures that do not require inpatient hospitalization; and meets the conditions and requirements set forth in the Medicare Conditions of Participation

Ambulatory surgical center (ASC) list: The list of surgical procedures that the Centers for Medicare and Medicaid Services considers safe and appropriate in an outpatient setting and for which Medicare pays a prospectively determined ASC facility fee

Ambulatory surgical center (ASC) services: Services that a Medicare-approved ambulatory surgical center provides in connection with procedures on the ASC list

American Health Information Management Association (AHIMA): The professional membership organization for managers of health record services and healthcare information systems as well as coding services; provides accreditation, certification, and educational services

American Hospital Association (AHA): The national trade organization that provides education, conducts research, and represents the hospital industry's interests in national legislative matters; membership includes individual healthcare organizations as well as individual healthcare professionals working in specialized areas of hospitals, such as risk management

Ancillary services: Tests and procedures ordered by a physician to provide information for use in patient diagnosis or treatment

Attending physician: The physician primarily responsible for the care and treatment of a patient

Balanced Budget Act (BBA) of 1997: Public Law 105-33 enacted by Congress on August 5, 1997, that mandated a number of additions, deletions, and revisions to the original Medicare and Medicaid legislation; the legislation that added penalties for healthcare fraud and abuse to the Medicare and Medicaid programs

Bundled: The grouping of CPT codes related to a procedure when submitting a claim

Carrier, Medicare: An organization under contract with the Centers for Medicare and Medicaid Services to serve as the financial agent that works with providers and the federal government to locally administer Medicare eligibility and payments

Category I codes: Procedures or services identified by a five-digit CPT code and organized within the six sections

Category II codes: Codes located in the CPT codebook that represent performance measurement tracking; use is optional

Category III codes: Temporary emerging technology codes located within the CPT codebook

Centers for Medicare and Medicaid Services (CMS): The division of the Department of Health and Human Services that is responsible for developing healthcare policy in the United States and for administering the Medicare program and the federal portion of the Medicaid program; called the Health Care Financing Administration (HCFA) prior to 2001

Certified coding associate (CCA): An AHIMA credential awarded to entry-level coders who have demonstrated skill in classifying medical data by passing a certification exam

Certified coding specialist (CCS): An AHIMA credential awarded to individuals who have demonstrated skill in classifying medical data from patient records, generally in the hospital setting, by passing a certification examination

Certified coding specialist—physician based (CCS–P) An AHIMA credential awarded to individuals who have demonstrated coding expertise in physician-based settings, such as group practices, by passing a certification examination

Charge code: The numerical identification of a service or supply that links the item to a particular department within the charge description master

Chargemaster: A financial management form that contains information about the organization's charges for the healthcare services it provides to patients; *see* **charge description master (CDM)**

Chief complaint: The principal problem a patient reports to a healthcare provider

Claim: Itemized statement of healthcare services and their costs provided by a hospital, physician's office, or other healthcare provider; submitted for reimbursement to the healthcare insurance plan by either the insured party or the provider

Claims processing: The process of accumulating claims for services, submitting claims for reimbursement, and ensuring that claims are satisfied

Classification system: 1. A system for grouping similar diseases and procedures and organizing related information for easy retrieval. 2. A system for assigning numeric or alphanumeric code numbers to represent specific diseases and/or procedures

Clean claim: A claim that has all the billing and coding information correct and can be paid by the payer the first time it is submitted

Clinic: An outpatient facility providing a limited range of healthcare services and assuming overall healthcare responsibility for patients

Clinical abstract: A computerized file that summarizes patient demographics and other information, including reason for admission, diagnoses, procedures, physician information, and any additional information deemed pertinent by the facility

Clinical coding: The process of assigning numeric or alphanumeric classifications to diagnostic and procedural statements

Clinical data: Data captured during the process of diagnosis and treatment

CMS-1500: A Medicare claim form used to bill third-party payers for provider services, for example, physician office visits

CMS-1450: A Medicare form used for standardized uniform billing

Code: In information systems, software instructions that direct computers to perform a specified action; in healthcare, an alphanumeric representation of the terms in a clinical classification or vocabulary

Code editor: Software that evaluates the clinical consistency and completeness of health record information and identifies potential errors that could affect accurate prospective payment group assignment

Code of Federal Regulations (CFR): The official collection of legislative and regulatory guidelines that are mandated by final rules published in the *Federal Register*

Coded data: Data that are translated into a standard nomenclature of classification so that they may be aggregated, analyzed, and compared

Coder: A person assigned solely to the function of coding

Coder/biller: A person in an ambulatory care or a physician office setting who is generally responsible for processing the superbill

Coding: The process of assigning numeric representations to clinical documentation

Coding Clinic: A publication issued quarterly by the American Hospital Association and approved by the Centers for Medicare and Medicaid Services to give coding advice and direction for ICD-9-CM

Coding specialist: The healthcare worker responsible for assigning numeric or alphanumeric codes to diagnostic or procedural statements

Community of Practice (CoP): A Web-based electronic network for communication among members of the American Health Information Management Association

Consolidation: The process by which the ambulatory patient group classification system determines whether separate payment is appropriate when a patient is assigned multiple significant procedure groups

Consultation: The response by one healthcare professional to another healthcare professional's request to provide recommendations and/or opinions regarding the care of a particular patient/resident

Conversion factor: A monetary multiplier that converts relative value units into payments

Correct Coding Initiative (CCI): A national initiative designed to improve the accuracy of Part B claims processed by Medicare carriers

CPT Assistant: The official publication of the American Medical Association that addresses CPT coding issues

CPT-5 Project: The AMA initiative to improve CPT to address the needs of hospitals, managed care organizations, and long-term care facilities

Current Procedural Terminology, Fourth Edition (**CPT**): A comprehensive, descriptive list of terms and numeric codes used for reporting diagnostic and therapeutic procedures and other medical services performed by physicians; published and updated annually by the American Medical Association

Denial: The circumstance when a bill has been accepted, but payment has been denied for any of several reasons (for example, sending the bill to the wrong insurance company, patient not having current coverage, inaccurate coding, lack of medical necessity, and so on)

Department of Health and Human Services (HHS or DHHS): The cabinet-level federal agency that oversees all the health- and human-services-related activities of the federal government and administers federal regulations

Diagnosis: A word or phrase used by a physician to identify a disease from which an individual patient suffers or a condition for which the patient needs, seeks, or receives medical care

Diagnosis chiefly responsible for services provided (outpatient): The diagnosis, condition, problem, or reason for an encounter/visit that is chiefly responsible for the services provided

Diagnostic codes: Numeric or alphanumeric characters used to classify and report diseases, conditions, and injuries

Diagnostic services: All diagnostic services of any type, including history, physical examination, laboratory, x-ray or radiography, and others that are performed or ordered pertinent to the patient's reasons for the encounter

Discharge diagnosis: Any one of the diagnoses recorded after all the data accumulated during the course of a patient's hospitalization or other circumscribed episode of medical care have been studied

Discharge status: The disposition of the patient at discharge (that is, left against medical advice, discharged to home, transferred to skilled nursing facility, or died)

Documentation: The recording of pertinent healthcare findings, interventions, and responses to treatment as a business record and form of communication among caregivers

Durable medical equipment (DME): Medical equipment designed for long-term use in the home, including eyeglasses, hearing aids, surgical appliances and supplies, orthotics and prostheses, and bulk and cylinder oxygen; *see* **home medical equipment (HME)**

Durable medical equipment regional carrier (DMERC): A fiscal intermediary designated to process claims for durable medical equipment

Edit: A condition that must be satisfied before a computer system can accept data

E/M coding: *See* **evaluation and management codes**

Emergency: A situation in which a patient requires immediate medical intervention as a result of severe, life-threatening, or potentially disabling conditions

Emergency patient: A patient who is admitted to the emergency services department of a hospital for the diagnosis and treatment of a condition that requires immediate medical, dental, or allied health services in order to sustain life or to prevent critical consequences

Encoder: Specialty software used to facilitate the assignment of diagnostic and procedural codes according to the rules of the coding system

Encounter: The direct personal contact between a patient and a physician or other person who is authorized by state licensure law and, if applicable, by medical staff bylaws to order or furnish healthcare services for the diagnosis or treatment of the patient

Episode of care: A period of relatively continuous medical care performed by healthcare professionals in relation to a particular clinical problem or situation

Established patient: A patient who has received professional services from the physician or another physician of the same specialty in the same practice group within the past three years

Evaluation and management (E/M) codes: CPT codes that describe patient encounters with healthcare professionals for assessment counseling and other routine healthcare services

Facilities, health: Buildings, including physical plant, equipment, and supplies, necessary in the provision of health services (for example, hospitals, nursing homes, and ambulatory care centers)

Federal Register: The daily publication of the U.S. Government Printing Office that reports all changes in regulations and federally mandated standards, including HCPCS and ICD-9-CM codes

Fee schedule: A list of healthcare services and procedures (usually CPT/HCPCS codes) and the charges associated with them developed by a third-party payer to represent the approved payment levels for a given insurance plan; also called table of allowances

Fee-for-service (FFS) reimbursement: A method of reimbursement through which providers retrospectively receive payment based on either billed charges for services provided or on annually updated fee schedules

Fiscal intermediary (FI):   An organization that contracts with the Centers for Medicare and Medicaid Services to serve as the financial agent between providers and the federal government in the local administration of Medicare Part B claims

Fraud: That which is done erroneously to purposely achieve gain from another

Fraud and abuse: The intentional and mistaken misrepresentation of reimbursement claims submitted to government-sponsored health programs

Freestanding facility: In Medicare terminology, an entity that furnishes healthcare services to beneficiaries and is not integrated with any other entity as a main provider, a department of a provider, or a provider-based entity

Geographic adjustment factor (GAF):   Adjustment to the national standardized Medicare fee schedule relative value components used to account for differences in the cost of practicing medicine in different geographic areas of the country

Geographic practice cost index (GPCI):   An index developed by the Centers for Medicare and Medicaid Services to measure the differences in resource costs among fee schedule areas compared to the national average in the three components of the relative value unit: physician work, practice expenses, and malpractice coverage

Global payment: A form of reimbursement used for radiological and other procedures that combines the professional and technical components of the procedures and disperses payments as lump sums to be distributed between the physician and the healthcare facility

Global surgery package: A CPT code denoting a normal surgical procedure with no complications that includes all the elements needed to perform the procedure

Group practice: An organization of physicians who share office space and administrative support services to achieve economies of scale, often a clinic or ambulatory care center

Grouping: A system for assigning patients to a classification scheme via a computer software program

Hard code: A code applied through a healthcare organization's chargemaster

Hard coding: The process of attaching a CPT/HCPCS code to a procedure located on the facility's chargemaster so that the code will automatically be included on the patient's bill

HCFA-1500:   Previous name for **CMS-1500**

HCFA-1450:   *See* **CMS 1450**

HCFA Common Procedure Coding System (HCPCS):   Previous name for the **Healthcare Common Procedure Coding System**

Health Care Financing Administration (HCFA):   Previous name for the **Centers for Medicare and Medicaid Services**

Health Insurance Portability and Accountability Act of 1996 (HIPAA):   The federal legislation enacted to provide continuity of health coverage, control fraud and abuse in healthcare, reduce healthcare costs, and guarantee the security and privacy of health information. The act limits exclusion for preexisting medical conditions, prohibits discrimination against employees and dependents based on health status, guarantees availability of health insurance to small employers, and guarantees renewability of insurance to all employees regardless of facility size

Health record: A paper- or computer-based tool for collecting and storing information about the healthcare services provided to a patient in a single healthcare facility; also called a patient record, medical record, resident record, or client record, depending on the healthcare setting

Healthcare Common Procedure Coding System (HCPCS): A classification system that identifies healthcare procedures, equipment, and supplies for claim submission purposes; the three levels are as follows: I, *Current Procedural Terminology* codes, developed by the AMA; II, codes for equipment, supplies, and services not covered by *Current Procedural Terminology* codes as well as modifiers that can be used with all levels of codes, developed by CMS; and III (eliminated December 31, 2003 to comply with HIPAA), local codes developed by regional Medicare Part B carriers and used to report physicians' services and supplies to Medicare for reimbursement

Healthcare provider: A provider of diagnostic, medical, and surgical care as well as the services or supplies related to the health of an individual and any other person or organization that issues reimbursement claims or is paid for healthcare in the normal course of business

HIPAA: *See* **Health Insurance Portability and Accountability Act of 1996**

History: The pertinent information about a patient, including chief complaint, past and present illnesses, family history, social history, and review of body systems

Home health prospective payment system (HH PPS): The reimbursement system developed by the Centers for Medicare and Medicaid Services to cover home health services provided to Medicare beneficiaries

Hospital: A healthcare entity that has an organized medical staff and permanent facilities that include inpatient beds and continuous medical/nursing services and that provides diagnostic and therapeutic services as well as overnight accommodations and nutritional services for patients

Hospital ambulatory care: All hospital-directed preventive, therapeutic, and rehabilitative services provided by physicians and their surrogates to patients who are not hospital inpatients

Hospital-based ambulatory care center: An organized hospital facility that provides nonemergency medical or dental services to patients who are not assigned to a bed as inpatients during the time services are rendered (an emergency department in which services are provided to nonemergency patients is not considered an ambulatory care center)

Hospital-based ambulatory surgery center: A department of an inpatient facility that provides same-day surgical services using the facility's equipment, staff, and support services

Hospital-based outpatient care: A subset of ambulatory care that utilizes a hospital's staff, equipment, and resources to render preventive and/or corrective healthcare services

Hospital outpatient: A hospital patient who receives services in one or more of a hospital's facilities when he or she is not currently an inpatient or a home care patient

Hospital outpatient care unit: An organized unit of a hospital that provides facilities and medical services exclusively or primarily to patients who are generally ambulatory and who do not currently require or are not currently receiving services as an inpatient of the hospital

Hospitalization insurance (Medicare Part A): A federal program that covers the costs associated with inpatient hospitalization as well as other healthcare services provided to Medicare beneficiaries

Individual provider: A health professional who delivers, or is professionally responsible for delivering, services to a patient, is exercising independent judgment in the care of the patient, and is not under the immediate supervision of another healthcare professional

International Classification of Diseases, Ninth Revision, Clinical Modification (ICD-9-CM): A classification system used in the United States to report morbidity and mortality information

International Classification of Diseases, Tenth Revision (ICD-10): The newest revision of the disease classification system developed and used by the World Health Organization to track morbidity and mortality information worldwide (not yet adopted by the United States)

Item description: An explanation of a service or supply listed in the chargemaster

Level of service: 1. The relative intensity of services given when a physician provides one-on-one services for a patient (such as minimal, brief, limited, or intermediate). 2. The relative intensity of services provided by a healthcare facility (for example, tertiary care)

Line item: A service- or item-specific detail of a reimbursement claim

Local medical review policies (LMRPs): Documents that define Medicare coverage of outpatient services via lists of diagnoses defined as medically reasonable and necessary for the services provided

Managed care: 1. Payment method in which the third-party payer has implemented some provisions to control the costs of healthcare while maintaining high-quality care. 2. Systematic merger of clinical, financial, and administrative processes to manage access, cost, and quality of healthcare

Managed fee-for-service reimbursement: A healthcare plan that implements utilization controls (prospective and retrospective review of healthcare services) for reimbursement under traditional fee-for-service insurance plans

Medicaid: An entitlement program that oversees medical assistance for individuals and families with low incomes and limited resources; jointly funded between state and federal governments

Medical care unit: An assemblage of inpatient beds (or newborn bassinets), related facilities, and assigned personnel that provide service to a defined and limited class of patients according to their particular medical care needs

Medical consultation: *See* **consultation**

Medical history: A record of the information provided by a patient to his or her physician to explain the patient's chief complaint, present and past illnesses, and personal and family medical problems; includes a description of the physician's review of systems

Medical nomenclature: A recognized system of preferred terminology for naming disease processes

Medical record: *See* **health record**

Medicare: A federally funded health program established in 1965 to assist with the medical care costs of Americans sixty-five years of age and older as well as other individuals entitled to Social Security benefits owing to their disabilities

Medicare Advantage (Part C):   Optional managed care plan for Medicare beneficiaries who are entitled to Part A, enrolled in Part B, and live in an area with a plan; types include health maintenance organization, point-of-service plan, preferred provider organization, and provider-sponsored organization; formerly **Medicare+Choice**

Medicare economic index (MEI):   An index used by the Medicare program to update physician fee levels in relation to annual changes in the general economy for inflation, productivity, and changes in specific health-sector expense factors including malpractice, personnel costs, rent, and other expenses

Medicare fee schedule (MFS):   A feature of the resource-based relative value system that includes a complete list of the payments Medicare makes to physicians and other providers

Medicare Part A: *See* **hospitalization insurance**

Medicare Part B: *See* **supplemental medical insurance**

Medicare Part C: *See* **Medicare Advantage**

Medicare+Choice: former name of **Medicare Advantage**

Medicare prospective payment system: *See* **acute care prospective payment system, home health prospective payment system, outpatient prospective payment system,** and **skilled nursing facility prospective payment system**

National Codes (HCPCS Level II codes):   Five-digit alphanumeric codes for procedures, services, and supplies that are not classified in CPT

National Correct Coding Initiative (NCCI):   A series of code edits on Medicare Part B claims

New patient: An individual who has not received professional services from the physician or any other physician of the same specialty in the same practice group within the past three years

Nomenclature: A recognized system of terms used in a science or art that follows preestablished naming conventions. A disease nomenclature is a listing of the proper name for each disease entity with its specific code number

Observation patient: A patient who presents with a medical condition with a significant degree of instability and disability and who needs to be monitored, evaluated, and assessed to determine whether he or she should be admitted for inpatient care or discharged for care in another setting

Omnibus Budget Reconciliation Act (OBRA) of 1989:   The federal legislation that mandated important changes in the payment rules for Medicare physicians; specifically, the legislation that requires nursing facilities to conduct regular patient assessments for Medicare and Medicaid beneficiaries

Operating room (OR) procedure: A predefined procedure that usually requires use of an operating room

Operation: *See* **surgical operation**

Operative report: A formal document that describes the events surrounding a surgical procedure or operation and identifies the principal participants in the surgery

Other diagnoses: All conditions (recorded to the highest documented level of specificity) that coexist at the time of admission, develop subsequently, or affect the treatment received and/or length of stay

Outpatient: A patient who receives ambulatory care services in a hospital-based clinic or department

Outpatient Code Editor (OCE):   A software program linked to the Correct Coding Initiative that applies a set of logical rules to determine whether various combinations of codes are correct and appropriately represent the services provided

Outpatient coder: An individual responsible for assigning ICD-9-CM and CPT/HCPCS codes to ambulatory surgery or emergency department cases

Outpatient prospective payment system (OPPS):   The Medicare prospective payment system used for hospital-based outpatient services and procedures that is predicated on the assignment of ambulatory payment classifications

Outpatient unit: A hospital-based ambulatory care facility organized into sections (clinics) whose number depends on the size and degree of departmentalization of the medical or clinic staff, available facilities, type of service needed in the community, and the needs of the patients for whom it accepts responsibility

Outpatient visit: A patient's visit to one or more units located in the ambulatory services area (clinic or physician's office) of an acute care hospital

Packaging: A payment under the Medicare outpatient prospective payment system that includes items such as anesthesia, supplies, certain drugs, and the use of recovery and observation rooms

Partial hospitalization: A term that refers to limited patient stays in the hospital setting, typically as part of a transitional program to a less intense level of service; for example, psychiatric and drug and alcohol treatment facilities that offer services to help patients reenter the community, return to work, and assume family responsibilities

Patient: A living or deceased individual who is receiving or has received healthcare services

Patient health record: *See* **health record**

Physical examination report: Documentation of a physician's assessment of a patient's body systems

Primary care physician (PCP):   1. Physician who provides, supervises, and coordinates the healthcare of a member of a managed care plan and who manages referrals to other healthcare providers and utilization of healthcare services both inside and outside the plan. 2. The physician who makes the initial diagnosis of a patient's medical condition; *see* **primary care provider**

Primary care provider (PCP):   Healthcare provider who provides, supervises, and coordinates the healthcare of a member of a managed care plan. PCPs can be family and general practitioners, internists, pediatricians, and obstetricians/gynecologists; other PCPs are nurse practitioners and physician assistants; *see* **primary care physician**

Primary diagnosis: *See* **principal diagnosis**

Principal diagnosis: The disease or condition that was present on admission, was the principal reason for admission, and received treatment or evaluation during the hospital stay or visit

Principal procedure: The procedure performed for the definitive treatment of a condition (as opposed to a procedure performed for diagnostic or exploratory purposes) or for care of a complication

Procedural codes: The numeric or alphanumeric characters used to classify and report the medical procedures and services performed for patients

Procedures and services (outpatient): All medical procedures and services of any type (including history, physical examination, laboratory, x-ray or radiograph, and others) that are performed pertinent to the patient's reasons for the encounter, all therapeutic services performed at the time of the encounter, and all preventive services and procedures performed at the time of the encounter

Professional component (PC): 1. The portion of a healthcare procedure performed by a physician. 2. A term generally used in reference to the elements of radiological procedures performed by a physician

Prospective payment system (PPS): A type of reimbursement system that is based on preset payment levels rather than actual charges billed after the service has been provided; specifically, one of several Medicare reimbursement systems based on predetermined payment rates or periods and linked to the anticipated intensity of services delivered as well as the beneficiary's condition; *see* **acute care prospective payment system, home health prospective payment system, outpatient prospective payment system,** and **skilled nursing facility payment system**

Provider: Physician, clinic, hospital, nursing home, or other healthcare entity (second party) that delivers healthcare services

Referral: A request by a provider for a patient under the provider's care to be evaluated and/or treated by another provider

Referred outpatient: An outpatient who is provided special diagnostic or therapeutic services by a hospital on an ambulatory basis, but whose medical care remains the responsibility of the referring physician

Reimbursement: Compensation or repayment for healthcare services

Rejection: The process of having a submitted bill not accepted by the payer, although corrections can be made and the claim resubmitted

Relative value unit (RVU): A measurement that represents the value of the work involved in providing a specific professional medical service in relation to the value of the work involved in providing other medical services

Resource-based relative value scale (RBRVS): A Medicare reimbursement system implemented in 1992 to compensate physicians according to a fee schedule predicated on weights assigned on the basis of the resources required to provide the services

Retrospective payment method: Type of fee-for-service reimbursement in which providers receive recompense after health services have been rendered

Revenue code: A three- or four-digit number in the chargemaster that totals all items and their charges for printing on the form used for Medicare billing

Significant procedure: A procedure that is surgical in nature or carries a procedural or an anesthetic risk or requires specialized training

Significant procedure ambulatory payment classification: A procedure that constitutes the reason for the visit, dominates the time and resources rendered during the visit, and is not subject to payment reduction/discounting

Skilled nursing facility prospective payment system (SNF PPS):   A per diem reimbursement system implemented in July 1998 for costs (routine, ancillary, and capital) associated with covered skilled nursing facility services furnished to Medicare Part A beneficiaries

Special care unit: A medical care unit in which there is appropriate equipment and a concentration of physicians, nurses, and others who have special skills and experience to provide optimal medical care for critically ill patients or continuous care of patients in special diagnostic categories

Superbill: The office form used for physician office billing that is initiated by the physician and states the diagnoses and other information for each patient encounter

Supplemental medical insurance (SMI) (Medicare Part B):   A voluntary medical insurance program that helps pay for physicians' services, medical services, and supplies not covered by Medicare Part A

Surgery: An umbrella term referring to the procedures of incision, excision, amputation, introduction, endoscopy, suture, and manipulation

Surgical operation: One or more surgical procedures performed at one time for one patient via a common approach or for a common purpose

Surgical procedure: Any single, separate, systematic process upon or within the body that can be complete in itself; is normally performed by a physician, dentist, or other licensed practitioner; can be performed either with or without instruments; and is performed to restore disunited or deficient parts, remove diseased or injured tissues, extract foreign matter, assist in obstetrical delivery, or aid in diagnosis

Tax Equity and Fiscal Responsibility Act of 1982 (TEFRA):   The federal legislation that modified Medicare's retrospective reimbursement system for inpatient hospital stays by requiring implementation of diagnosis-related groups and the acute care prospective payment system

Technical component (TC):   The portion of radiological and other procedures that is facility based or nonphysician based (for example, radiology films, equipment, overhead, endoscopic suites, and so on)

Third-party payer: An insurance company (for example, Blue Cross/Blue Shield) or healthcare program (for example, Medicare) that reimburses healthcare providers (second party) and/or patients (first party) for the delivery of medical services

UB-92:   *See* **Uniform Bill-92**

Unbundling: The practice of using multiple codes to bill for the various individual steps in a single procedure rather than using a single code that includes all the steps of the comprehensive procedure

Undercoding: A form of incomplete documentation that results when diagnoses or procedures that should be coded are missing

Uniform Bill-92 (UB-92): *See* **CMS-1450**

Unlisted procedure: A CPT procedure code assigned when the provider performs a procedure or service for which there is no CPT code

Upcoding: The practice of assigning diagnostic or procedural codes that represent higher payment rates than the codes that actually reflect the services provided to patients

Usual, customary, and reasonable (UCR): Method of evaluating providers' fees in which the third-party payer pays for fees that are "usual" in that provider's practice; "customary" in the community; and "reasonable" for the situation

Visit: A single encounter with a healthcare professional that includes all the services supplied during the encounter

World Health Organization (WHO): The United Nations specialized agency for health, established on April 7, 1948, with the objective, as set out in its constitution, of the attainment by all peoples of the highest possible levels of health; responsible for *The International Statistical Classification of Diseases & Related Health Problems* **(ICD-10)**

Index